Anaesthesia: Review 10

Contents of *Anaesthesia: Review 9*

ISBN 0 443 04564 X

Published April 1992

You can place your order by contacting your local medical bookseller or the Sales Promotion Department, Robert Stevenson House, 1–3 Baxter's Place, Leith Walk, Edinburgh EH1 3AF, UK
Tel: (031) 556 2424; Telex: 727511 LONGMN G; Fax: (031) 558 1278

Look out for *Anaesthesia Review 11* in June 1994

See final pages for Contents of *Anaesthesia Reviews 1–8*

Anaesthesia:
Review 10

Edited by

Leon Kaufman MD, FFARCS

Consulting Anaesthetist, University College Hospital, and St Mark's Hospital, London;
Honorary Senior Lecturer, Faculty of Clinical Sciences, University College, London, UK

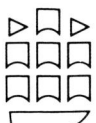

CHURCHILL LIVINGSTONE
EDINBURGH LONDON MADRID MELBOURNE NEW YORK AND TOKYO 1993

CHURCHILL LIVINGSTONE
Medical Division of Longman Group UK Limited

Distributed in the United States of America by Churchill
Livingston Inc., 650 Avenue of the Americas, New York,
N.Y. 10011, and by associated companies, branches and
representatives throughout the world.

© Longman Group UK Limited 1993

First published 1993

ISBN 0-443-04853-3
ISSN 0263-1512

British Library Cataloguing in Publication Data
A catalogue record for this book is available from the British Library.

Library of Congress Cataloguing in Publication Data is available

The
publisher's
policy is to use
**paper manufactured
from sustainable forests**

Produced by Longman Singapore Publishers Pte Ltd
Printed in Singapore

Contents

*Dedicated to the memory of my eldest brother,
a devoted general practitioner*

Preface

It is gratifying to record the support that this series has had from contributors and readers over the last decade. *Anaesthesia Review 10* like its predecessors attempts to bridge the gap between the literature appearing in the journals and in standard text books. There is a bias in *Review 10* towards physiology and this will appeal not only to anaesthetists in training but also to surgeons who now expect to be examined in critical care. Thus there are chapters on applied physiology in intensive care, oxygenation in the perioperative period, the endocrine response to surgery and factors affecting vascular tone. The modern management of burns and day case surgery are also of concern to anaesthetists and surgeons.

Anaesthetic apparatus is represented by an account of the measurement of gas flow and the development of the laryngeal mask airway. An interesting subject is that of information processing during sleep and anaesthesia. As in earlier volumes emphasis is placed on the application of medicine to anaesthesia and a whole chapter is devoted to advances in assessing cardiac function. The final chapter is an update of material previously presented.

The editor has enjoyed preparing this series and trusts that it has advanced the knowledge of the reader as much as it has enriched that of the editor. Constructive reviews of the series have been most welcome.

I am grateful to all the authors who have contributed to the series, particularly those who have contributed regularly. The assistance of my secretaries is not forgotten and I am grateful to Maria Pitts and Sylvia Wiggins for their continuous and persistent efforts. The publishers have been particularly helpful in accepting individual chapters after the start of the production process to avoid delay in publication. To mark the 10th volume in the series a list of contents of all previous volumes is included in this publication.

145 Harley Street   L. K.
London W1N 2DE
1993

Contributors

J. R. Brimacombe MB ChB FRCAnaes
Consultant Anaesthetist, Department of Anaesthesia and Intensive
Care, Cairns Base Hospital, Cairns, Queensland, Australia

J. Cooper BSc MB BS MRCP
Registrar in Cardiology, University College and Middlesex
Hospitals, London, UK

Joan P. Desborough MB ChB FFARCS
Senior Lecturer in Anaesthesia, St George's Hospital Medical School,
London, UK

George M. Hall MB BS PhD FIBiol FCAnaes
Professor of Anaesthesia, St George's Hospital Medical School,
London, UK

J. Gareth Jones MD FRCP FCAnaes
Professor of Anaesthesia, University of Cambridge, and Addenbrooke's
Hospital, Cambridge, UK

Leon Kaufman MD FFARCS
Consulting Anaesthetist, University College Hospital, and St Mark's
Hospital, London; Honorary Senior Lecturer, Faculty of Clinical Sciences,
University College, London, UK

Pushpinder S. Mangat MB ChB FCAnaes
Senior Registrar, Anaesthetic Department, Addenbrooke's Hospital,
Cambridge, UK

Rajesh Munglani MB BS DCH FRCAnaes
Research Fellow, Department of Anaesthesia, University of Cambridge,
and Addenbrooke's Hospital, Cambridge, UK

Nicholas Parkhouse DM(Oxon) MCh FRCS
Consultant Plastic Surgeon, and Director, Rainsford Burns Unit,
RAFT Department of Research into Plastic Surgery, Mount Vernon
Hospital, Northwood, Middlesex, UK

A. J. Pittard MB ChB
Registrar in Anaesthesia, Leeds General Infirmary, Leeds,
West Yorkshire, UK

N. Shorney MBBS FRCAnaes
Staff Anaesthetist, Cairns Base Hospital, Cairns, Queensland, Australia

Neil Soni FFARACS
Senior Lecturer, Anaesthesia and Intensive Care Unit, Charing Cross
and Westminster Hospital Medical School, London, UK

J. Malcolm Walker BSc MD FRCP
Consultant Cardiologist, University College and Middlesex Hospitals;
Clinical Director of the Hatter Cardiovascular Studies Unit, University
College Hospital; Honorary Senior Lecturer in Medicine University College
and Middlesex Schools of Medicine, London, UK

Nigel R. Webster BSc MB ChB PhD FFARCS
Consultant in Anaesthesia and Intensive Care; Senior Clinical
Lecturer, St James's University Hospital, Leeds, UK

David White MB BS FRCAnaes
Consultant Anaesthetist, Northwick Park Hospital and Clinical Research
Centre, Harrow, Middlesex, UK

David J. Wilkinson MB BS MRCS D(Obst)RCOG FFARCS
Consultant Anaesthetist, St Bartholomew's and Homerton Hospitals,
London, UK

1. Modern methods for assessing cardiac function

J. M. Walker   J. Cooper

Over the last 10 years there has been a rapid expansion in techniques available both for the diagnosis and treatment of cardiological disease. As with all new techniques, time is needed both to achieve the required skill for their optimum use and also to evaluate their effectiveness against other standard procedures. Inevitably some exciting developments will ultimately be disappointing whereas others with apparent limitations will prove to be valuable.

Prior to an anaesthetic, assessment is geared to determine the following points:

1. The likelihood of cardiac adverse events: their type, severity and potential preventive measures.

2. The risk of perioperative morbidity and mortality — needed to obtain informed consent and establish the suitability of operation.

3. Establish if prior correction of a cardiac abnormality will reduce risks.

The first part of this chapter outlines the methods of cardiovascular diagnosis and reviews the recent technical advances that have been made. The second part shows how they may help in the assessment of cardiac risk in patients undergoing anaesthesia, focusing attention on the four commonest conditions affecting cardiovascular risk: ischaemic heart disease, valvular heart disease, heart failure and paroxysmal arrhythmia.

ELECTROCARDIOGRAM (ECG)

The resting ECG is a simple, universally available investigation that may demonstrate changes of serious disease such as previous myocardial infarction or abnormal conduction. However, a normal resting ECG does not exclude serious cardiac pathology.

CHEST X-RAY

Both the degree of cardiac enlargement, which may give a rough estimate of the size of the cardiac chambers, and evidence of pulmonary oedema should alert the anaesthetist to possible heart disease. Like the resting ECG, a normal chest X-ray does not exclude serious cardiac disease.

1

Table 1.1 Minimum data set to establish cardiovascular risk

Condition	Echo	ETT	Holter	Other
Ischaemic heart disease				
Recent MI	+	if <6/52	ST mapping (?)	Only if emergency
MI 3/12	+	+	ST mapping (?)	
Suspected old MI	+	+	ST mapping (?)	
Valve disease				Antibiotic prophylaxis, anti-coagulant control in mitral stenosis, heart failure as in ventricular failure
Aortic stenosis	+	–	–	
Mitral stenosis	+	–	–	
Valvular regurgitation	+	?	?	
Ventricular failure				
Dilated heart	+	?	?	CVP, meticulous fluid management, postoperative ITU
Hypertrophied	+	?/ –	+	
Paroxysmal arrhythmia	N/A	?	+	ETT to establish propensity to stress-induced arrhythmia
Congenital heart disease	+	N/A	+	Arterial saturation, haematocrit, antibiotic prophylaxis

+ = Recommended; – = not recommended; ? = may be appropriate; N/A = not applicable.
Echo = Echocardiogram; ETT = Exercise tolerance test; Holter = 24 h ECG;
MI = Myocardial infarction; CVP = central venous pressure; ITU = Intensive treatment unit.

ECHOCARDIOGRAPHY

Without doubt, the single most important diagnostic investigation that has revolutionized cardiological diagnostic practice in the last 10 years is that of echocardiography. It allows a detailed analysis of both cardiac structures and flow of blood through the various chambers of heart and blood vessels. It is harmless to the patient and it is available in most general hospitals, unlike many other cardiac investigations which are restricted to cardiology centres. By describing cardiac anatomy and function preoperatively, anaesthesic risks and problems may to some degree be predicted.

The echocardiographic examination is made up of four different modalities: M-mode, two-dimensional (2D), Doppler and colourflow Doppler examination. Historically, this was the order that these modalities became available.

The principle behind echocardiography is that sound waves are transmitted to the heart and reflected back whenever a tissue interface is met; moving blood scatters the ultrasound. The time taken for the reflected beam to return gives the distance of the interface to the transducer. The transducer is placed on the chest and through a small acoustic window a series of reflected echoes are produced at different depths. This can be recorded against time to give a typical M-mode display. This image is useful to assess the timing of events accurately but has been largely superseded by the 2D image in assessing structural detail of the heart. Resolution is limited to objects greater than 2.5 mm in diameter. Structure and function of valves as well as chamber size, ventricular muscle thickness and contractile performance are easily and accurately assessed. Resolution does not allow examination of the coronary arterial tree.

Doppler echocardiography

The Doppler examination makes use of the change in frequency of ultrasound reflected from moving red cells. Direction and velocity of blood flow can be measured; as a general rule, all flow in the normal heart is <1 m/s. The velocity of blood flow increases either when there is obstruction to flow with a pressure gradient across the obstruction or when there is an increase in volume occurring across the same orifice. Using the modified Bernoulli equation, it is possible to calculate the pressure difference across a stenotic valve from: pressure (mmHg) $= 4 \times [\text{velocity (m/s)}]^2$.

The pressure and severity of regurgitant valves can be identified using Doppler echocardiography. Although more difficult to quantify accurately than jets across stenotic valves, semiquantifiable data can be achieved. The Doppler examination can be performed with a 2D imaging transducer and Doppler velocity measures taken from anatomically defined points within the heart. This is the pulsed-wave (PW) Doppler which allows good anatomical resolution, but accurate quantification of the velocities cannot be achieved. For this a continuous-wave (CW) Doppler is required, but here no simultaneous image is obtained and a high degree of operator skill is required to achieve reliable measurements.

More recently, colourflow Doppler has become available. This allows visualization of blood flow by colour coding for blood velocity and direction towards or away from the transducer. Colourflow is an expensive modality not easily given to quantification. Its great advantage is that it is able to identify shunts, high-velocity jets and abnormal flow directions superimposed on the anatomical 2D image of the heart. Very rapidly the operator will know if there is an abnormal flow pattern, which can be further assessed using PW and CW Doppler modalities. Colourflow Doppler has proven remarkably helpful in the assessment of congenital heart disease.

In practice, all four modalities in echocardiography are put together to provide a composite picture of heart function. The quality of the echocardiographic data obtained is now so high that many centres do not perform the invasive procedure of cardiac catheterization to confirm the severity of valvular heart disease prior to operation. This is particularly true of stenotic valvular lesions, the severity of which is accurately assessed using Doppler analysis; currently 90% of the surgery performed at the Mayo Clinic for stenotic lesions is performed without formal evaluation of valvular lesions by cardiac catheterization, although this is still required for assessment of intercurrent coronary artery disease.

The main limitation of transthoracic echocardiography is that it is not always possible to obtain satisfactory images. The acoustic window is large in children but gets smaller with age and is particularly small in patients with lung disease. This is primarily due to the interposition of the lung between the ultrasound probe and the heart, although imaging behind echogenic prosthetic heart valves is also a problem.

Transoesphageal echocardiography

To overcome the problems of imaging through the thorax, transoesophageal echocardiography may be performed. Images are obtained using an ultrasound transducer on a fibreoptic endoscope inserted into the oesophagus or gastric fundus. The images obtained show more clearly all structures of the heart, with the possible exception of the intraventricular septum. Aligning the probe for Doppler interrogation may be more difficult. The trade-off against this enhanced imaging is that the procedure is semi-invasive, requiring sedation, an endoscopy suite and increased numbers of staff.

Stress echocardiography

Echocardiography is normally performed with the heart at rest and thus abnormalities of cardiac function induced by ischaemia may not be seen. Recently however the technical problems involved in performing echocardiography with the heart under conditions of stress have to some extent been overcome. The patient undergoes echocardiography before, then immediately after exercise or after an infusion of a stressor agent such as dobutamine or dipyridamole. Using digital storage systems, it is possible to play back the images side by side, thus allowing comparison to detect subtle regional wall motion abnormalities caused by stress and indicative of ischaemia. Initially, it was thought that echocardiography would need to be performed during exercise but the regional wall motion abnormalities remain for several minutes after ischaemia has been induced. Therefore patients have time to lie down for the echocardiogram to be performed. If suitable images can be obtained, this technique may offer more detailed information than stress thallium radionuclide uptake investigations.

STRESS ELECTROCARDIOGRAPHY (THE EXERCISE TEST)

The normal 12-lead resting ECG often shows no abnormalities in patients who develop symptoms on exercise. The exercise test is therefore useful:

1. to ascertain whether symptoms are accompanied by any objective evidence of myocardial ischaemia, cardiac arrhythmia, hypertension or other events which would make an anaesthetic hazardous;

2. to reproduce the patient's symptoms so that they can be observed as they happen under standardized exercise conditions;

3. to assess the patient's functional capacity, i.e. the amount of work that can be performed before becoming limited by symptoms, and also how rapid is the recovery from exercise.

Modern exercise-testing regimes consist of an incremental load on either a treadmill or a cycle ergometer, in which the exercise load is started at an easily managed level, kept stable for 1.5–3 min at each load, and then serially increased with the aim of exhausting the subject within 15 min.

An ECG is continually monitored; ideally all 12 leads are recorded at frequent intervals to demonstrate ischaemia or arrhythmia and monitor the heart rate. The blood pressure is also recorded.

The exercise test is conclusively positive if the patient develops classical angina pain and if severe down-sloping (greater than 2 mm) ST segment depression is shown on the ECG.

A drop in blood pressure during exercise may be unaccompanied by ECG changes but is diagnostic of severe ischaemia. Minor degrees of ST depression are common, particularly in anxious individuals and especially young women, but are usually up-sloping. T-wave inversion is not necessarily ischaemic in origin. The sensitivity of the test may vary from 30% in simple step tests to between 75 and 96% in the more usual bicycle or treadmill protocols. Specificity is low in asymptomatic individuals and high in men with typical angina pain. Thus false-positive tests are common (10–25%) in healthy women with a low risk of having coronary disease.

AMBULATORY ECG ST SEGMENT MONITORING

An ambulatory ECG monitor is attached to the patient with two bipolar leads to record an inferior and lateral lead for a period of 24 h. The baseline is calibrated and ST segment depression is noted throughout the day (Raby et al 1989). It is apparent from such analysis that the majority of ST depression is not associated with chest pain and has therefore been named silent ischaemia (Mulcahy et al 1988). The importance of silent ischaemia is that the prognosis associated with it appears not to be affected by the presence or absence of concomitant pain (Schlant 1990).

RADIONUCLIDE IMAGING OF THE HEART

Myocardial perfusion imaging

Whilst various radiopharmaceuticals are available for perfusion imaging, the most commonly employed is the potassium analogue, thallium-201. This is injected into a vein and is taken up by myocytes in proportion to the perfusion and viability of the myocyte. The thallium-201 is detected using a gamma camera positioned at various angles over the patient, and used to determine the perfusion of the heart muscle. The initial perfusion test may be performed under conditions of stress by exercising the patient or by injecting the cardiac stimulant dobutamine. Dipyridamole or adenosine may also be used to provoke ischaemia. These are potent coronary vasodilators which create a steal phenomenon, accentuating differences in uptake between normal and abnormally perfused myocardium. Later images are obtained under resting conditions. Areas not initially perfused may therefore be reversible or irreversible, the former indicating myocardial ischaemia, the latter indicating myocardial damage. Areas of myocardium which would benefit from a revascularization procedure can thus be identified.

Multiple uptake gated acquisition (MUGA)

The patient's red blood cells are labelled with technetium-99m, using an in vitro or modified in vitro labelling technique. In order to increase resolution of the gamma camera image from the low level of emission, a large number of images are acquired over several cardiac cycles and the images from different phases of the cycle are averaged. The process is accomplished by gating, with reference to the ECG as a time marker, and dividing the cardiac cycle into a series of time intervals, for example, 30–50 ms. This allows the determination of peak systolic volume in relation to diastolic volume, which can be expressed as a percentage to give the ejection fraction. This is normally $\geqslant 50\%$. The resting MUGA scan can detect regional wall motion abnormalities, such as left ventricular aneurysms, whilst the calculated ejection fraction provides valuable prognostic information. For example, postinfarction there is a steep increase in 1-year cardiac mortality when the ejection fraction falls below 30% (Multicenter postinfarction research group 1983). In normal patients the ejection fraction increases by about 5% at peak exercise, whilst there is no such rise in those with significant coronary disease — indeed the prognosis is poor in those patients with <5% reduction in ejection fraction (Bonow et al 1984).

One major advantage of radionuclide investigations is that images can reliably be obtained in all patients in a regular heart rhythm. The major disadvantage is that it involves the injection of radioisotopes and is relatively expensive.

INVESTIGATING PATIENTS WITH HEART DISEASE

It is perhaps surprising that so few of the newer investigations used in the preoperative assessment have been shown adequately to predict outcome of patients undergoing anaesthesia, both in terms of morbidity and mortality. This may reflect the inadequacy of the studies that have looked into the use of these tests or that there are factors involved peri- or postoperatively that are far more significant. Although of limited prognostic importance, investigations which define more accurately the cardiac condition of a particular patient should allow an anaesthetic tailored to that individual and his or her cardiac status. It should also allow the more invasive and complex postoperative surveillance techniques to be concentrated on those individuals most likely to be at greatest risk of perioperative cardiac complications. In asymptomatic low-risk patients any number of sophisticated investigations will not improve an already excellent risk status.

Ischaemic heart disease (IHD)

Despite the obvious dangers of IHD being an underlying cause of arrhythmias or infarction, only myocardial infarction in the preceding 6 months and congestive cardiac failure have unequivocally been shown to be independent predictors of perioperative cardiac mortality (Reiz & Mangano 1989). Even recent myocardial infarction as an independent risk factor has been challenged by Rao et al (1983). Their results may reflect a particularly invasive approach to patient management with a detailed protocol entailing intra-arterial pressure, Swan–Ganz and central venous pressure monitoring in addition to prolonged care on the intensive care unit. This approach may be responsible for a reduction of perioperative mortality and illustrates the point that preoperative factors may be outweighed if appropriate peri- and postoperative precautions are taken. As perioperative mortality is reduced further, the size of studies required to detect an effect of various putative risk factors on morbidity and mortality will become larger, thus requiring complex multicentre randomized trials to be undertaken.

Stable angina has not been shown to be an independent risk factor for perioperative cardiac morbidity, and the prognosis of unstable angina has not been investigated (Reiz & Mangano 1989). However a possibility of selection bias in the type of patient referred for elective surgery cannot be excluded and management of symptomatic patients with ischaemic heart disease must be meticulous to avoid the expected complications of infarction, or sudden death.

ECG and exercise tolerance test

The resting ECG is an important determinant of perioperative cardiac mortality as it may demonstrate the changes of a recent myocardial infarction. Although preoperative exercise ECGs in conjunction with the resting ECG have been shown to identify those patients at higher risk of an adverse outcome from non-cardiac operations (Cutler et al 1981, McPhail et al 1988), this has not been confirmed by other investigators (Carliner et al 1985); exercise-testing in 200 patients over 40 undergoing major non-cardiac surgery failed to provide extra predictive power of cardiac complications over the routine preoperative ECG (Carliner et al 1985). However, the prognosis of patients with angina who are not undergoing surgery correlates closely with their exercise test tolerance during stress testing (Weiner et al 1984); Weiner et al studied 4083 medically treated patients with coronary artery disease. A high-risk subset was identified (12% of the population) with an annual mortality of ⩾5% when exercise workload was ⩽ Bruce stage 1 and the exercise ECG demonstrated ⩾1 mm ST segment depression. A low-risk subset (34% of the population) was identified with an annual mortality of <1%. These patients were able to exercise into ⩾ Bruce stage 3 and had a normal exercise ECG. It is likely therefore that patients at higher risk from anaesthesia may be identified using stress testing, and that the inability of Carliner et al (1985) to show the usefulness of the exercise test may reflect the inadequacy of their sample size.

Holter 24-h ST segment monitoring

In contrast to exercise ECGs, ambulatory ST segment monitoring has been shown to be an independent and highly significant predictor of postoperative adverse cardiac events in patients with peripheral vascular disease (Raby et al 1989). Of the 176 patients studied, 32 had episodes of ischaemic ST depression, of whom 12 had postoperative ischaemic events and 1 was fatal. Only 1 postoperative ischaemic event occurred in the 144 patients who did not have preoperative ischaemia (Raby et al 1989). The authors suggest that the predictive value of ST segment monitoring was insufficient to warrant further invasive assessment of the patients with ischaemia. However, it does suggest that a more cautious approach to the anaesthetic should be given to these patients. Furthermore, those patients in whom no ischaemia was demonstrated had an excellent postoperative prognosis (Raby et al 1989), obviating the need for complex invasive or other monitoring in these patients. Other investigators using a similar protocol have failed to reproduce these results (Mangano et al 1990). It may be concluded, therefore, that the role for preoperative ambulatory ECG monitoring remains uncertain. It provides a useful alternative to exercise testing and the required technology is increasingly available.

Nuclear medicine techniques

Dipyridamole-stressed thallium distribution has also been shown to be a strong independent risk factor for adverse cardiac events following operations for peripheral vascular disease (Boucher et al 1985). Of 54 patients studied, 16 patients had abnormal thallium redistribution and 8 of these had cardiac events. No such events occurred in the 32 patients whose thallium scan was normal or showed persistent defects, resulting from healed myocardial scar. Six other patients with reversible thallium defects underwent coronary angiography before vascular surgery. All had significant three-vessel coronary disease and 4 underwent coronary bypass surgery. All 6 had uncomplicated vascular surgery. Similar findings have been demonstrated by others (Cutler & Leppo 1987, Eagle et al 1989), although Eagle et al in a cohort of 254 patients undergoing preoperative thallium scanning found the presence of Q waves on the ECG gave similar power to predict postoperative cardiac events.

By combining clinical variables with thallium redistribution defects there was improved specificity and equivalent sensitivity to either clinical variables or thallium variables alone (Eagle et al 1989). They therefore suggested only performing routine preoperative thallium scanning in those with clinical variables suspicious of ischaemia, namely, advanced age, history of angina, Q wave on ECG, diabetes requiring treatment and history of ventricular ectopics requiring treatment. One group of investigators performed thallium scans preoperatively on 60 patients about to undergo vascular surgery and allowed it to be performed without the result being known (Mangano et al 1991b). Thallium scintigraphy was not found to be helpful in predicting adverse outcome in patients undergoing major non-cardiac surgery. The reason for the lack of effect may be due to intercentre variation in use of thallium imaging but as the only blinded trial on the effectiveness of thallium scanning, it casts a large shadow over the usefulness of this expensive investigation in assessing patients preoperatively.

Echocardiography

Stress (dipyridamole) echocardiography has recently been evaluated in a series of 109 patients undergoing peripheral vascular surgery. The results were remarkable in terms of their specificity and sensitivity for predicting postoperative cardiac events. Nine patients had positive scans; 7 of these had postoperative events. Only one event occurred among the 100 patients with negative studies (Tischler et al 1991).

Discussion

As these investigations have identified high-risk and low-risk populations, is there anything that can be done preoperatively to reduce the anaesthetic risk? At present there has been no trial taking patients with adverse prognostic indices and attempting to reduce their preoperative risk by introduction of medication or surgical revascularization. However, the coronary artery surgery study (CASS) registry experience suggests that coronary artery surgery may be effective in reducing mortality but not myocardial infarctions from major operations (Foster et al 1986); of 1201 patients who had significant coronary artery disease and underwent a major operation, the perioperative mortality was 0.9% in the 743 patients who had previous coronary artery bypass surgery and 2.4% in the 458 patients who did not receive coronary artery bypass surgery. Those initially selected for coronary artery bypass surgery had more severe disease and more severe symptoms at the time the decision to perform bypass grafting was made, making the difference even more striking. It may at face value seem advisable to take an aggressive stance to revascularization prior to non-cardiac surgery. However, the mortality from coronary bypass surgery in the best centres is in the region of 1% with significant morbidity (Cosgrove et al 1984), and has been found to be as high as 5.8% (Veterans study group 1984). Therefore unless a test can accurately pinpoint those patients at risk it is advisable to use the same criteria for coronary artery bypass grafting as in the patient who is not about to undergo surgery, that is, medical treatment for failure of angina, severe three-vessel or left main stem disease.

Perioperative factors. Whilst many studies have tried to identify preoperative factors that will help to predict adverse operative outcomes, others have looked at perioperative factors. In a prospective trial of 474 men with coronary artery disease or high risk from it, ambulatory ECG evidence of ischaemia postoperatively was the only variable found to be associated with adverse cardiac events (Mangano et al 1990). In this study postoperative ischaemia was common, occurring in approximately 40% of patients. The number of adverse cardiac events was only 18%. The test was highly sensitive (identifying those with cardiac events) but not specific (identifying those who did not have cardiac events). Interestingly, the operative period is not associated with an increased incidence of severity of ischaemia which is most severe during the postoperative period (Mangano et al 1991a). Whether the identification of this higher-risk group will allow differing postoperative management to be employed so that mortality is reduced is unknown, but worthy of further investigation.

Valvular heart disease

Sparse data are available on the risk of surgery in the patient with valvular heart disease. Early studies failed to identify an increased mortality of major operations in patients with mitral valve disease, although there was an approximately twofold increase in mortality in patients with aortic valve disease (Skinner & Pearce 1964). Similar findings were noted by Goldman et al (1977) who noted no increase in perioperative mortality in patients with mitral valve disease and a 13% (3/23) mortality in patients with important aortic stenosis. However, they did not find aortic regurgitation to be a significant risk factor.

In view of the increased mortality associated with aortic stenosis, the patient with a heart murmur should be evaluated preoperatively with care. If any doubt exists about the significance of the murmur an echocardiogram should be performed. The 2D transthoracic echocardiogram will normally demonstrate calcification or thickening of the valves in addition to demonstrating the degree of left ventricular hypertrophy that has developed as a result of the aortic stenosis. As a consequence of severe aortic stenosis the ventricle may eventually dilate and contract poorly. The Doppler echocardiogram will give an estimate of the gradient across the aortic valve. This figure should be taken in conjunction with the morphology of the valve and degree of left ventricular dysfunction to assess the severity of the stenosis, since severe aortic stenosis may be present in the presence of a low transaortic gradient if the left ventricular function is poor. As a general rule aortic gradients above 50 mmHg are regarded as significant and may lead to complications. Even if a valvular lesion is not haemodynamically significant the patient will still require appropriate antibiotic prophylaxis (see Table 1.2). In contrast, innocent flow murmurs unrelated to structural cardiac lesions will not.

Cardiac failure

Several studies have identified preoperative cardiac failure as a risk factor for cardiac events in the surgical population (Cooperman et al 1978, Goldman et al 1977, Rao et al 1983). The MUGA scan is one of the most reliable indicators of cardiac contractility and a decreased preoperative ejection fraction (less than 35%), determined by MUGA, has been found to correlate with early perioperative infarction (Pasternack et al 1985). As previously mentioned, the availability of radionuclide investigations is limited and an assessment of left ventricular function can readily be obtained from transthoracic echocardiography.

Echocardiography will also identify patients who have left ventricular hypertrophy either as a primary phenomenon (hypertrophic cardiomyopathy) or as a result of long-standing hypertension. Patients with left ventricular hypertrophy tend to exhibit abnormalities of myocardial relaxation and are particularly intolerant of large fluid loads, developing pulmonary oedema

Table 1.2 Antibiotic cover for patients with congenital heart disease or acquired valve disease receiving dental treatment or any operative procedure

1. Without anaesthetic or under local anaesthesia
   (a) Amoxycillin 3 g orally 1 h before procedure

For patients allergic to penicillin or who have had amoxycillin in the last month:
   (b) Erythromycin stearate 1.5 g orally 1 h before procedure plus a further 0.5 g 6 h later *or*
   (c) Clindamycin 600 mg orally 1 h before procedure

For children:
   Amoxycillin or erythromycin: half adult dose if under 10 years
                                quarter adult dose if under 5 years

2. Under General anaesthetic
   (a) Ampicillin 1 g intravenously with premedication plus 0.5 g orally 6 h later

For patients allergic to penicillin or who have had amoxycillin in the last month:
   (b) Vancomycin 1 g slowly intravenously over at least 1 h plus gentamicin 120 mg with premedication

For children:
   Vancomycin 20 mg/kg plus gentamicin 2 mg/kg intravenously

3. Special risk patients (prosthetic heart valves or previous history of infective endocarditis)
   Ampicillin 1 g plus gentamicin 120 mg intravenously with premedication, plus 0.5 g of amoxycillin orally at 6 h

   For penicillin allergy use 2(b)

readily. Furthermore, patients with hypertrophic cardiomyopathy are prone to ventricular arrhythmias and some may develop dynamic ventricular outflow tract obstruction if stimulants such as adrenaline or isoprenaline are administered. Despite these problems a retrospective study of 35 patients with hypertrophic obstructive cardiac myopathy undergoing general anaesthesia found no incidence of ventricular tachyarrythmias or perioperative death during 56 major surgical operations (Thompson et al 1985).

Arrhythmias and conduction defects

Arrhythmias are frequently a manifestation of an underlying cardiac disease, and it is the underlying disease rather than the arrhythmia that appears to be responsible for any adverse operative risk. For example, the frequency of ventricular premature beats correlates with left ventricular dysfunction and the severity of coronary artery disease (Schulze et al 1975, 1977), and thus frequent ventricular ectopic beats in patients with coronary artery disease are a risk factor for the development of cardiac complications perioperatively (Goldman et al 1977). This contrasts with ventricular ectopic beats in people with no underlying cardiac disease; this carries a normal prognosis (Kennedy et al 1985), and should not be considered as a risk factor for complications of non-cardiac surgery.

The management of patients with conduction defects follows the same lines as that of the non-surgical patient; that is, a pacemaker should be inserted in those patients with complete heart block. Several series have shown that bifascicular block is extremely unlikely to progress to complete heart block during the perioperative period, and thus unless there is a history of syncope or evidence of transient complete or Mobitz type II heart, the insertion of a pacemaker is unnecessary (Goldman & Braunwald 1992).

CONCLUSION

A carefully taken history and examination in conjunction with an ECG will often be all that is required in making a sensible anaesthetic assessment of the patient with cardiological disease. Whilst anaesthetists may have a large number of cardiological techniques available to establish diagnosis, their role at present in helping to determine anaesthetic risk is limited. By judicious use of the investigations the anaesthetist will be prepared for likely events in the perioperative period and be able to tailor the anaesthetic to the patient.

REFERENCES

Bonow R O, Kent K M, Rosing D R 1984 Exercise induced ischemia in mildly symptomatic patients with coronary artery disease and preserved left ventricular function: identification of subgroups at risk of death during medical therapy. N Engl J Med 311: 1339–1345
Boucher C A, Brewster D C, Darling R C et al 1985 Determination of cardiac risk by

dipyradamole-thallium imaging before peripheral vascular surgery. N Engl J Med 312: 389–394

Carliner N H, Fisher M L, Plotnick G H et al 1985 Routine preoperative exercise testing in patients undergoing major noncardiac surgery. Am J Cardiol 56: 51–58

Cooperman M, Pflug B, Martin E W et al 1978 Cardiovascular risk factors in patients with peripheral vascular disease. Surgery 84: 505–509

Cosgrove D M, Loop F D, Lytle B W 1984 Primary myocardial revascularization. J Thorac Cardiovasc Surg 88: 673–684

Cutler B S, Leppo J A 1987 Dipyradamole thallium 201 scintigraphy to detect coronary artery disease before abdominal aortic surgery. J Vasc Surg 5: 91–100

Cutler B S, Wheeler H B, Paraskos J A et al 1981 Applicability and interpretation of electrocardiographic stress testing in patients with peripheral vascular disease. Am J Surg 141: 501–506

Eagle K A, Coley C M, Newell J B et al 1989 Combining clinical and thallium data optimizes preoperative assessment of cardiac risk before major surgery. Ann Intern Med 110: 859–866

Foster E D, Davis K B, Carpenter J A et al 1986 Risk of noncardiac operation in patients with defined coronary disease: the coronary artery surgery study (CASS) registry experience. Ann Thorac Surg 41: 42–50

Goldman L, Braunwald E 1992 General anesthesia and noncardiac surgery in patients with heart disease. In: Braunwald E (ed) Heart disease. Saunders, Philadelphia

Goldman L, Caldera D L, Nussbaum S R et al 1977 Multifactorial index of cardiac risk in noncardiac surgical procedures. N Engl J Med 297: 845–850

Kennedy H L, Whitlock J A, Sprague M K et al 1985 Long-term follow-up of asymptomatic healthy subjects with frequent and complex ventricular ectopy. N Engl J Med 312: 193–197

McPhail N, Calvin J E, Shariatmadar A et al 1988 The use of preoperative exercise testing to predict cardiac complications after arterial reconstruction. J Vasc Surg 7: 60–68

Mangano D T, Browner W S, Hollenberg M et al 1990 Association of perioperative myocardial ischemia with cardiac morbidity and mortality in men undergoing noncardiac surgery. N Engl J Med 323: 1781–1788

Mangano D T, Hollenberg M, Fegert G et al 1991a Perioperative myocardial ischaemia in patients undergoing noncardiac surgery-1: Incidence and severity during the 4 day perioperative period. J Am Coll Cardiol 17: 843–850

Mangano D T, London M J, Tubau J F et al 1991b Dipyradamole thalium-201 scintigraphy as a preoperative screening test. A reexamination of its predictive potential. Circulation 84: 493–502

Mulcahy B, Keegan J, Crean P et al 1988 Silent myocardial ischaemia in chronic stable angina: a study of its frequency in 150 patients. Br Heart J 60: 417–419

Multicenter postinfarction research group 1983 Risk stratification and survival after myocardial infarction. N Engl Med J 309: 331–336

Pasternack P F, Imparato A M, Bear G et al 1985 The value of radionuclide angiography as a predictor of perioperative myocardial infarction in patients undergoing lower extremity revascularization procedures. Circulation 72: 13–17

Raby K E, Goldman L, Creagar M A et al 1989 Correlation between preoperative ischemia and major cardiac events after peripheral vascular surgery. N Engl J Med 321: 1296–1300

Rao T K, Jacobs K H, El-Etr A A 1983 Reinfarction following anesthesia in patients with myocardial infarction. Anesthesiology 59: 499–506

Reiz S, Mangano D T 1989 Anaesthesia and cardiac disease. In: Nimmo W S, Smith G (eds) Anaesthesia. Blackwell, Oxford

Schlant R C 1990 The prognosis of individuals with silent myocardial ischemia. Silent myocardial ischemia: a critical appraisal. Adv Cardiol 37: 187–201

Schulze R A, Rouleau J, Rigo P et al 1975 Ventricular arrhythmias in the late hospital phase of acute myocardial infarction: relation to left ventricular function detected by gated cardiac blood pool scanning. Circulation 52: 1006–1011

Schulze R A, Strauss H W, Pitt B 1977 Sudden death in the year following myocardial infarction: relation to ventricular premature contractions in the late hospital phase and left ventricular ejection fraction. Am J Med 62: 192–199

Skinner J F, Pearce M L 1964 Surgical risk in the cardiac patient. J Chronic Dis 17: 55–72

Thompson R A, Liberthson R R, Lowenstein E 1985 Perioperative anesthetic risk of non cardiac surgery in hypertrophic obstructive cardiomyopathy. JAMA 254: 2419–2421

Tischler M D, Lee T H, Hirsch A T et al 1991 Prediction of major cardiac events after peripheral vascular surgery using dipyradamole echocardiography. Am J Cardiol 68: 593–597

Veterans study group (The veterans administration coronary artery bypass surgery cooperative study group) 1984 Eleven-year survival in the Veterans Administration randomized trial of coronary bypass surgery for stable angina. N Engl J Med 311: 1333–1339

Weiner D A, Ryan T J, McCabe C H et al 1984 Prognostic importance of a clinical profile and exercise test in medically treated patients with coronary artery disease. J Am Coll Cardiol 3: 772–779

2. The respiratory system

L. Kaufman

PHYSIOLOGY

Clinical advances in pulmonary gas exchange have been reviewed by Wagner & Rodriguez-Roisin (1991). They found that limitation of alveolar capillary diffusion was an unlikely cause of hypoxaemia except during exercise at altitude. In asthma there is V_A/Q mismatch but no shunt and bronchodilators, although appearing to improve lung function as assessed by spirometry, have a deleterious effect on V_A/Q. Spirometry reflects the changes of bronchial tone of the large airways but gas exchange is more determined by the presence of mucus and oedema in the peripheral airways. Patients with high cardiac output such as in asthma and cirrhosis have less hypoxaemia than those with low cardiac output (e.g. pulmonary embolism).

In adult respiratory distress syndrome there are changes in V_A/Q but the major abnormality is underventilation of perfused areas (shunt). Positive end expiratory pressure (PEEP) not only reduces shunt but creates a high V_A/Q ratio. Vasoconstrictors improve gas exchange whereas vasodilators such as nitroprusside and diltiazem increase shunt. Although gas exchange is reduced, oxygen delivery may be increased by the increasing cardiac output.

In chronic lung diseases such as chronic obstructive pulmonary disease (COPD), shunt is minimal except during an acute exacerbation. Diffusion limitation is not implicated as a cause of hypoxaemia in COPD as in diffuse interstitial fibrosis. In primary pulmonary hypertension V_A/Q abnormalities are not significant but are marked in patients with pulmonary embolism. In hepatic cirrhosis PaO_2 can be maintained despite V_A/Q mismatch because of the high cardiac output but shunt can develop leading to severe hypoxia.

Respiratory failure is not only related to failure of gas exchange but also from failure of the ventilatory pump involving the central respiratory drive, disability of the respiratory muscles and defects in the chest wall. Ward & Macklem (1990) proposed an ingenious system of coupling in the respiratory system which forms a closed loop; there is evidence that failure or overloading of the respiratory muscles results in a negative feedback to motor neurons in the inspiratory centre, decreasing respiratory drive. Hyperinflation does not increase expiratory muscle recruitment during non-rapid eye movement (REM) sleep as it does during wakefulness (Begle & Skatrud 1990). During hyperventilation there is a reduction in skin blood flow with a corresponding

15

reduction in transcutaneous oxygen tension and therefore care should be taken with the interpretation of this measurement (Barker et al 1991).

The central nervous system and respiratory muscle coordination is also discussed by Cherniack (1990).

Diminished oxygen supply to tissues leads to an increase in cardiac output and red cell mass to maintain oxygen supply to the tissues. Carbon dioxide excretion is only impaired when lung disease is severe. The diaphragm contributes more to the increase in minute volume in response to hypoxaemia than to carbon dioxide (Bradley et al 1990).

The respiratory tract may be influenced not only by adrenergic and cholinergic nerves but also by non-adrenergic non-cholinergic (NANC) nerves. Although originally envisaged as a separate nervous system, it appears that the responses are mediated by the release of co-transmitters such as nitric oxide and vasoactive intestinal peptide (VIP) released from cholinergic nerves, and have inhibitory activity. Those with excitatory activity are mediated by the release of neuropeptide Y for adrenergic nerves, and bronchoconstrictor responses are associated with the release of tachykinins from unmyelinated sensory nerves. VIP is a potent relaxant of human bronchi and although calcitonin gene-related peptide is a potent vasodilator, it constricts human bronchi. Other peptides include bradykinin, which is a potent bronchoconstrictor especially in asthmatic patients; neuropeptide Y which appears to amplify the effects of noradrenaline; somatostatin which appears to have little effect on the airways and encephalin which appears to affect the release of neuropeptides. Although these peptides affect the respiratory tract and receptors have been discovered, their effect in disease has still to be evaluated (Barnes et al 1991a, 1991b). However Frostell et al (1991) found that inhalation of nitric oxide in animals reversed hypoxic pulmonary vasoconstriction and may have a place in the treatment of pulmonary hypertension. Nitric oxide (NO) is an endothelium-derived relaxing factor and should not be confused with nitrogen dioxide (NO_2) which is associated with air pollution leading to respiratory illness (Koo et al 1990). Cytochrome-P450, the production of oxygen radicals and oxidative phosphorylation, appears to be involved in hypoxic pulmonary vasoconstriction (Hampl & Herget 1991).

PERIOPERATIVE PULMONARY COMPLICATIONS

During anaesthesia atelectasis is a principal cause of abnormal gas transfer which occurs rapidly following induction of anaesthesia. The rapidity of the collapse as seen by computed tomography (CT) scan suggests that local compression is the cause and not the reduction of functional residual capacity. In a computer model, Westbrook & Sykes (1992) investigated the relationship between cardiac output and intrapulmonary shunt during anaesthesia and found that there were significant degrees of arterial desaturation as the cardiac output was reduced. They recommend plasma volume expansion when pulse oximeter readings show a decrease in oxygen saturation in the absence of other causes. Personal observations confirm these findings but it is possible that peripheral vasoconstriction may affect the readings.

Moller et al (1992) have also drawn attention to the incidence of hypoxaemia during operation and in the recovery area following elective surgical operations. The duration of hypoxaemia was much greater in the recovery area, as was noticed by Lanigan (1992), even following dental anaesthesia in children. This demonstrates the need for pulse oximetry in all recovery areas, and possibly even when the patient has returned to the ward. Rosenberg et al (1989) have demonstrated oxygen desaturation even on the third postoperative day, emphasizing the need for oxygen therapy not only in the recovery area.

Aldren et al (1991) studied 100 patients on the effects of laparotomy on postoperative hypoxaemia and pulmonary complications and found that there was a high incidence of hypoxaemia as assessed by pulse oximetry. Pulmonary complications were assessed clinically on respiratory symptoms and signs. On the first postoperative day 30 patients were hypoxaemic but 20 did not have pulmonary complications. There was a poor correlation between hypoxaemia and pulmonary complications on a day-to-day basis, but over a 5-day period the relationship between hypoxaemia and pulmonary complications was more obvious. The importance of this paper is to reaffirm that clinical assessment is not necessarily a guide to hypoxaemia and postoperative patients should be monitored routinely with a pulse oximeter and, by implication, oxygen therapy should not be restricted to the immediate postoperative period. The only predisposing factor to pulmonary complications in this study was age (85 years), although smoking, obesity and preoperative respiratory disorders are also generally accepted to be factors. Attempts to analyse the relationship between oxygen uptake and oxygen delivery in postoperative patients and those with septicaemia have not been fruitful in predicting the outcome of therapy (Vermeij et al 1991).

J G Jones (1991) described two phases of postoperative hypoxaemia — an early phase, and a late phase lasting up to a week which is associated with a reduction in functional residual capacity. The early phase is due to pulmonary collapse with intrapulmonary shunting and obstructive apnoea associated with postoperative sedation. In addition to oxygen monitoring and oxygen therapy, there may be a place for respiratory stimulants such as doxapram, especially after abdominal surgery (Jansen et al 1990). Almitrine bismesylate stimulates chemoreceptors and has been reported to be of value in COPD with hypoxaemia (Watanabe et al 1989) but as yet has not been assessed in anaesthesia.

Dilworth & Pounsford (1991) have demonstrated a decrease in the sensitivity of cough reflex to inhaled irritants in the immediate postoperative period following upper abdominal surgery. One factor was opiate analgesia; anaesthetic agents may also be involved while postoperative hypoxaemia may suppress the cough centre in the brainstem. Cough suppression is inadvisable as it leads to an increase in retention of bronchial secretions, and therapy designed to promote the effectiveness of cough has proved disappointing (Irwin & Curley 1991).

The irritability of the trachea during anaesthesia has been studied by Nishino et al (1990) in anaesthetized and paralysed patients. Tracheal irritation with water caused tracheal smooth muscle constriction which readily responded to intravenous atropine (0.03 mg/kg). There have been suggestions that hypercapnia might lead to bronchoconstriction and pulmonary collapse but this study showed that there was an individual variation in response. It was concluded that increased carbon dioxide cannot be considered an appropriate stimulus of the tracheal smooth muscle, despite its effect in animals.

DISEASE AND LUNG FUNCTION

Thyrotoxicosis

Dyspnoea is a common symptom in thyrotoxicosis. McElvaney et al (1990) found that the respiratory muscles which were weaker than those of controls improved with treatment, with corresponding rises in vital capacity, inspiratory capacity and total lung capacity. However on assessing breathlessness they found no difference in the intensity scores between patients and controls, or in patients before and after antithyroid therapy.

Myotonic dystrophy

Patients with myotonic dystrophy suffer from daytime somnolence which may not necessarily be related to carbon dioxide retention. There were frequent bouts of apnoea and hypopnoea with severe oxygen desaturation, especially during non-REM sleep. The apnoea could be either obstructive or central. Gilmartin et al (1991) concluded the abnormal respiratory function was not entirely due to respiratory muscle weakness. These findings reaffirm the view that sedation is particularly hazardous in these patients (Kaufman 1962).

Malignancy

Malignancy may be associated with syndromes resembling myasthenia which have been known to result in respiratory failure. Respiratory failure may also be due to malignant pleural effusions. Fernandez et al (1991) reported a patient who had respiratory failure from lung metastases from ovarian carcinoma. Respiratory failure was treated by prolonged mechanical ventilation which was discontinued following a successful course of chemotherapy.

Using high-dose chemotherapy and total body radiation in the management of patients receiving bone marrow transplant, the incidence of interstitial pneumonitis can be reduced to under 8% with a mortality of 1% (Jochelson et al 1990).

Sarcoid

In sarcoid there is a defect of diffusion and in some patients there is also fibrosis. High levels of fibronectin and hyaluronan (hyaluronic acid) and the presence of increased mast cells in bronchoalveolar lavage fluid reflect the degree of activity of the disease (Bjermer et al 1991).

Emphysematous bullae

Emphysematous bullae may cause pulmonary disability by compressing the lung tissue, by hyperinflation which increases the work of breathing and by increasing dead-space ventilation. Patients with a large bulla stand to benefit from surgical excision, but those with chronic bronchitis, hypercapnia and diffuse emphysema fared less well (Wade et al 1991).

Pulmonary embolism

Pulmonary embolism is believed to be the third most common cause of death in the USA and lung scan is widely used to diagnose the condition. Kelley et al (1991) evaluated the diagnostic techniques and agreed that a normal lung scan excludes the diagnosis of clinically important pulmonary embolism.

RESPIRATORY MUSCLE FATIGUE

This was considered in Review 9 (p 11) in which muscle fatigue was defined as a condition 'in which there is a reduction in force generating capacity of the muscle resulting from muscle activity underload which is reversible by rest'. Three types have been defined: central fatigue, transmission fatigue and contractile fatigue. Mador (1991) found that inspiratory muscle fatigue usually results in an increase in minute ventilation and respiratory rate, and a reduction in tidal volume. Paradoxical abdominal movement is often considered to be a sign of inspiratory muscle fatigue and this may be due to an increase in inspiratory load rather than to the fatigue itself. Fatigue may sometimes also result in a reduction rather than an increase in motor activity to the respiratory muscles. Although respiratory muscle fatigue can occur during exercise, training of the respiratory muscles by resistive breathing or hyperpnoea does not appear to improve exercise tolerance in patients with COPD (Fitting 1991). The extent of dyspnoea during sustained exercise is the product of intensity and duration. Halving the intensity and doubling the duration of activity markedly reduce the muscular efforts and dyspnoea (Kearon et al 1991).

SLEEP APNOEA SYNDROME (SAS)

SAS still continues to attract much interest, as reflected by the multiplicity of papers on the subject. SAS may be central, obstructive or mixed. In an analysis of over 1000 men Stradling & Crosby (1991) found that neck circumference, alcohol consumption and obesity were significant factors in predicting overnight episodes of hypoxia (see also Katz et al 1990). Posture has a significant effect on upper airway calibre but in patients with SAS, there is narrowing of the retropalatal airway and this may explain why patients prefer to sleep upright (Yildirim et al 1991).

The most common complaint in SAS patients is the inability to stay awake during the day and this appears to be not only related to disruption of sleep but also to nocturnal hypoxaemia (Bedard et al 1991). Nocturnal hypoxaemia apparently does not affect daytime somnolence (Colt et al 1991). Hypoxic drive apparently is a potent factor in determining ventilation following the period of apnoea; a mild increase in PCO_2 during apnoea affects ventilation partly by modulating the hypoxic response during sleep (Satoh et al 1991).

Williams et al (1991) have outlined the criteria for the diagnosis of obstructive sleep apnoea (OSA) based on clinical scoring and pulse oximetry. Clinically it was snoring, interrupted breathing during sleep, hypersomno-lence, obesity and essential hypertension. Hoffstein et al (1991a) agreed that there was a definite association between SAS and hypertension. Nocturnal pulse oximetry was useful in establishing the diagnosis and may obviate the need for nocturnal polysomnography. Oximetry alone is of value in detecting moderate or deep sleep apnoea syndrome (Cooper et al 1991) but abnormal flow–volume curves are of limited value for predicting sleep apnoea (Rauscher et al 1990).

OSA may occur in patients being treated for ventilatory insufficiency of COPD with a negative-pressure body ventilator. There was a significant fall in SaO_2 during sleep (Bach and Penek 1991).

Snoring is a feature of SAS and attempts have been made to assess the importance of pharyngeal volume. Green et al (1991) found that the volume of the pharynx in asymptomatic snorers was similar to that of non-snorers. On the other hand Gleadhill et al (1991) found that there were differences in upper airway collapsibility between normal patients who snore and those with SAS. Hoffstein et al (1991b) measured the changes in pharyngeal area in relation to lung volume and pharyngeal distensibility. Lung volume-associated changes in pharyngeal area were certainly related to the severity of sleep apnoea. Horner & Guz (1991) have discussed the anatomical and physiological factors which maintain the patency of the upper airway and these include upper airway geometry, negative intrapharyngeal pressure, activation of upper airway dilator muscles and sleep state.

Phenylephrine, an alpha-adrenergic agonist, increased pharyngeal cross-sectional area when applied locally to the nasal and pharyngeal mucosa. There was a decrease in pharyngeal resistance which is independent of the change in nasal resistance and may have a place in the management of SAS (Wasicko et al 1991). For details of nasal airway resistance see Eiser (1990).

Genioglossus muscle is a major pharyngeal dilator which is activated in response to upper airway negative pressure and it may well be that in SAS the response is reduced. In REM and non-REM sleep electromyogram activity of the genioglossus is reduced even in normal men (Wiegand et al 1990). Continuous nasal positive airway pressure ventilation is an effective treatment for SAS but there was no increase in pharyngeal volumes (Collop et al 1991). Delguste et al (1991) described a patient who developed upper airway obstruction during nasal intermittent positive pressure ventilation during sleep; they believed this was due to hypocapnia resulting in abrupt closure of the glottis with complete obstruction of the airway and cessation of respiratory movement.

In patients with SAS there was a shift to the right of the P_{50} with an increase in 2,3-diphosphoglycerate (2,3-DPG) and these may be protective mechanisms against the development of polycythaemia, pulmonary hypertension and cor pulmonale. Interestingly enough, following treatment the P_{50} and 2,3-DPG decreased and returned to normal (Maillard et al 1991).

The rate of desaturation is much less in central apnoea than in obstructive apnoea for the same duration and this may be because there is reduced oxygen consumption in the central type. Obstructive apnoea is often accompanied by intense muscular movement to overcome the obstruction (Fletcher et al 1991a). It might have been thought that erythropoietin would be raised following oxygen desaturation, but there is no relationship between nocturnal hypoxaemia and serum erythropoietin concentrations (Goldman et al 1991).

There are compensatory mechanisms to overcome the apnoea seen in SAS, such as hypercapnia. However there is also enhanced endogenous opioid activity in SAS which modulates the compensatory mechanisms, and this may lead to the development of chronic hypercapnia (Greenberg et al 1991).

SAS may be associated with a whole series of medical diseases including endocrine, upper respiratory, neurological and pulmonary disorders, e.g. acromegaly, hyperthyroidism, diabetes, micrognathia, poliomyelitis, obesity and chronic respiratory disorders. Significant intrathoracic airway obstruction was seen in patients with acromegaly and nocturnal hypoxaemia was common (Trotman-Dickenson et al 1991).

Another condition recently described is that of Prader–Willi syndrome which is characterized by hypotonia, obesity and short stature. These patients suffer from hypersomnia and underventilation even during the day, and die from cardiorespiratory failure (Kaplan et al 1991).

Malone et al (1991) found the obstructive type of SAS impaired left ventricular function in patients with cardiomyopathy and treatment with nasal continuous positive airway pressure (CPAP) led to significant improvement. The rate of desaturation is not influenced by the fall in cardiac output present before the apnoea or resulting from it (Fletcher et al 1991b). On the other hand, hypertension is common in this condition (Levinson and Millman 1991). Significant prolongation of QT interval can occur during a severe attack with abrupt shortening of the interval during the postapnoea hyperventilation period (Gillis et al 1991).

In the obstructive type there is increased diuresis during sleep and this is affected by an increase in the release of atrial natriuretic peptide (ANP).

The mean plasma levels of ANP correlated with the degree of hypoxaemia and the swings of oesophageal pressure during apnoea. Treatment with CPAP led to a decrease in the secretion of ANP (Krieger et al 1991). SAS is a contraindication to patient-controlled analgesia (PCA). VanDercar et al (1991) described an obese patient who subsequently was found to have the obstructive type of SAS and who developed respiratory failure following morphine administered by PCA.

UPPER AIRWAY

Gerhardt's syndrome is a condition in which there is overactivity of the adductor muscles of the larynx, and which had previously been ascribed to abductor paralysis. Injection of botulinum toxin abolished the stridor seen in this condition (Marion et al 1992). Gout may affect the larynx involving the cricoarytenoid muscle and Guttenplan et al (1991) described a patient who had a tophus on the vocal cord.

In laryngoscopy for patients with upper airway obstruction, high-frequency jet ventilation has been recommended but Desruennes et al (1991) reported on the possible dangers of hypoxaemia, barotrauma and also alveolar hypoventilation which may be due to limitation of gas entrainment or increased functional residual capacity.

ADULT RESPIRATORY DISTRESS SYNDROME (ARDS)

ARDS is characterized by interstitial lung oedema, reduced lung compliance, alveolar and small airway closure, a decrease in functional residual capacity and resistance hypoxaemia associated with shunt. The role of other factors has previously been discussed (Review 9). Campbell & Cone (1991) have outlined the management, mode of intervention and the use of PEEP. Pesenti et al (1991) have confirmed that there is increased respiratory resistance in ARDS and that PEEP increases this especially at levels of 10 cm H_2O or greater (Eissa et al 1991). In some patients the application of PEEP results in a volume displacement along the static inflation volume–pressure curve obtained during zero end-expiratory pressure without recruiting alveoli and with overdistention of the lung. In other patients there is alveolar recruitment with an upper shift of the volume–pressure curve (Ranieri et al 1991).

The management of ARDS is outlined by MacNaughton & Evans (1992); if lung damage is not severe, satisfactory oxygenation can be obtained by CPAP, but most patients will require mechanical ventilation with the use of PEEP. More recent techniques of ventilation include inverse-ratio ventilation and high-frequency jet ventilation. High peak airway pressures can lead to a reduction in cardiac output and barotrauma, but apparently if tidal volumes are reduced to 5 ml/kg with an inflation pressure of below 35 cm H_2O, satisfactory oxygenation can be obtained, despite hypercapnia which is well-tolerated. Extracorporeal membrane oxygenation has also been advocated. Cardiac output may be compromised and dobutamine is often required to maintain oxygen delivery to tissues. There is the danger of overloading the circulation and negative fluid balance is advocated. In addition, sepsis should be treated and enteral feeding which prevents absorption of septic material into the portal circulation should be encouraged. H_2-receptor blockers are often necessary as well as treatment of nosocomial pulmonary infection. A human monoclonal endotoxin antibody appears to reduce mortality when there is Gram-negative septicaemia.

ASTHMA

The morbidity and mortality from asthma appear to be increasing and attempts have been made to implicate beta$_2$-agonists which act as bronchodilators. Fenoterol in particular is said to be associated with increased mortality. Spitzer et al (1992) advised reassessment of patients who were on heavy doses of beta$_2$-agonists. Although catecholamines are bronchodilators Janssen & Tjiong (1991) noted that a patient with bronchial asthma improved after the removal of a phaeochromocytoma.

Serum creatine kinase activity increased in patients with brittle asthma treated with long-term subcutaneous terbutaline, and again it has been suggested that this was a sign of myocardial damage. However the cardiac isoenzymes were not raised and it is possible that the raised creatine phosphokinase may be due to drug-induced myositis (Sykes et al 1991). Lipworth & McDevitt (1992) also noted an increase in mortality with long-acting selective beta$_2$-agonists, but found the association was still unproven. However there is no doubt that the bronchodilator effect of salmeterol, which is a selective beta$_2$-adrenoceptor agonist, is more prolonged when compared with salbutamol (Spring et al 1992).

Inhalation of budesonide, a steroid, was found to be superior to terbutaline in newly detected mildly asthmatic patients (Haahtela et al 1991), but Maxwell (1990) noted that there were adverse effects of inhaling corticosteroids including oral candidiasis, adrenal suppression and osteoporosis. Nebulized atropine appears to be of little benefit in supplementing the bronchodilator effect of beta$_2$-agonists (Owens & George 1991). Attention is now focusing again on phosphodiesterase inhibitors, of which theophylline has been a drug in use for many years. With the discovery of phosphodiesterase isoenzymes, there is the possibility of using selective inhibitors for the treatment of asthma (Torphy & Undem 1991).

Acute asthma may result in hyperventilation leading to hypocapnia. Van den Elshout et al (1991) have found that a rise in end-tidal P_{CO_2} of 1 kPa caused a significant fall in respiratory resistance both in normal and asthmatic subjects. The corresponding fall in P_{CO_2} caused little effect in normal patients but a marked increase in respiratory resistance in asthmatic patients. Inhibition of NANC activity in the early morning may predispose to attacks of nocturnal asthma (MacKay et al 1991).

Although thiopentone is not viewed favourably as an anaesthetic agent for asthmatic patients, Grunberg et al (1991) found that continuous intravenous thiopentone with positive pressure ventilation improved the morbidity in patients suffering status asthmaticus.

CHRONIC OBSTRUCTIVE PULMONARY DISEASE

The management of COPD remains largely problematical in that treatment is palliative rather than curative. It is still quite difficult to correlate breathlessness with physical activity; the relationship between spirometric findings and walking distance for example is poor. P W Jones (1991) has discussed the quality of life in patients with COPD. COPD may be accompanied by increased mucus secretion, airway obstruction, hyperinflation of the lung, decreased compliance, V_A/Q mismatch, pulmonary hypertension, right ventricular failure and polycythaemia. Symptoms include cough, excess sputum, wheezing and breathlessness and these affect patients' physical, social, emotional, intellectual and economic activities.

Risk factors associated with acute exacerbations of respiratory failure with hypercapnia have been assessed by Jeffrey et al (1992). The adverse factors include age, acidosis, hypotension and uraemia. Arterial pH is the most important factor for survival and critical level appears to be 7.26 ($[H^+]$ greater than 55 nmol/l). The relationship between respiratory muscle weakness, pattern of breathing and carbon dioxide retention in COPD is also discussed by Rochester (1991). Apparently inspiratory muscle weakness and not fatigue is the major factor in COPD. This weakness leads to a reduction in tidal volume and an increase in the ratio of dead space to tidal volume, resulting in hypercapnia. Oxygen therapy is known to produce hypercarbia in COPD and Dunn et al (1991a) have confirmed that this also occurs in patients who are being ventilated with an increase in V_D/V_T. This effect does not appear to be due to an increase in the V_A/Q mismatch.

The calibre of the bronchi may be reduced by tachykinins but not by abnormal autonomic control as seen in asthma (De Jongste et al 1991). As airway resistance to air flow increases there is an increase in the workload required for breathing and hyperinflation makes it more difficult for the diaphragm to contract. Studies by Similowski et al (1991) confirmed that inspiratory muscle weakness and not fatigue is a feature in COPD.

Treatment

In acute exacerbations inhalation of anticholinergic and beta-adrenergic agents improve pulmonary function; Karpel (1991) reported improvement with ipratropium and metaproterenol. In stable chronic conditions, Callahan et al (1991) found that oral steroids improved baseline FEV_1 by more than 20%. The inspiratory muscles become less effective and hyperinflation probably is a major factor in causing chronic hypoventilation in COPD patients (Haluszka et al 1990).

Gigliotti et al (1991) have shown that negative pressure ventilation led to a decrease in inspiratory muscle electromyogram activity, implying that respiratory muscle fatigue is a factor despite evidence to the contrary. However Montserrat et al (1991) found that although negative pressure ventilation resulted in a fall in Pa_{CO_2} and an increase in maximum inspiratory pressure, the Pa_{O_2} was unchanged, suggesting that gas exchange had deteriorated.

ARTIFICIAL VENTILATION

Ludwigs et al (1991) have reviewed the results of 11 years' experience of mechanical ventilation in medical and neurological disorders and although it was life-saving in the initial stages of the disease, mortality was high with patients with cerebrovascular disorders and malignancy. Although neuromuscular blocking drugs and sedation are routinely used in patients being ventilated for respiratory failure, there is a lack of consensus on the desirability, the efficacy and the adverse effects. Expense is not inconsiderable (Hansen-Flaschen et al 1991).

The various modes of positive pressure ventilation have been reviewed by Sassoon (1991). The review includes description of the laboratory and clinical studies as well as limitation of the techniques. For example, inverse ratio ventilation (IRV) causes discomfort and an abnormal breathing pattern with the result that patients require to be sedated or paralysed. IRV apparently does not make a significant improvement on mortality from ARDS. Airway pressure release ventilation (APRV) is still in an experimental stage but it does improve alveolar ventilation and decreases peak airway pressure, although it has little effect on oxygenation. Pressure support ventilation (PSV) has gained widespread clinical use but still requires conventional ventilation if PSV is ineffectual. Other modes include proportional assist ventilation (PAV) which may have a place in weaning patients as welll as mandatory minute volume (MMV) which has only gained limited acceptance. Irrespective of the pattern of ventilation, the mean airway pressure is the major factor in determining the degree of effect on the cardiovascular system (Goertz et al 1991). Valentine et al (1991) compared pulmonary gas exchange in patients ventilated by synchronized intermittent mandatory ventilation (SIMV), PSV and APRV and found that there was little change in the cardiovascular system, and oxygenation was adequate. In patients with autonomic failure, there is a fall in Pa_{CO_2} and an increase in mean arterial pressure due to peripheral vasodilation (Ornot et al 1991).

Branthwaite (1991) has outlined the techniques and apparatus available for non-invasive domiciliary ventilation while Pennock et al (1991) used a ventilatory support system combining a ventilatory nasal mask and PSV. Van de Graaff et al (1991) studied the patient-triggered, pressure-assisted, flow-cycled mode of mechanical ventilation (PS), but even at high levels of ventilator support there was some patient–ventilator asynchrony. Insufflation of the airway by percutaneous tracheostomy reduces dead space and minute ventilation and this appears to be related to the flow rate (Hurewitz et al 1991).

Weaning from mechanical ventilation still presents problems. The control of breathing during weaning from mechanical ventilation has been studied by Dunn et al (1991b), who concluded that carbon dioxide recruitment threshold is a better reference point for the adequacy of coping with ventilatory load than the arterial carbon dioxide during mechanical ventilation. This was also discussed by Goldstone & Moxham (1991); they listed some of the physiological variables associated with failure to wean successfully. These include:

Tidal volume	<5 ml/kg
Vital capacity	<10 ml/kg
Minute ventilation (MV)	>10 1/min
Maximum voluntary ventilation	$<2 \times$ MV
Maximum inspiratory pressure	> -20 cm H_2O
Alveolar–arterial oxygen tension difference	>300 mmHg
Dead space/tidal volume	>0.6

Infection

Nosocomial pneumonia is not infrequently associated with patients on ventilators, and although it does not increase the mortality it prolongs the stay of patients in the intensive care unit (Rello et al 1991). However Torres (1991) questioned the accuracy of the diagnosis. Selective decontamination of the digestive tract appears to improve respiratory infection (Vandenbroucke-Grauls & Vandenbroucke 1991), but Gastinne et al (1992) found that this did not improve survival.

OXYGEN

Siggaard-Andersen et al (1990) have reviewed the importance of the development of multiwavelength oximeters; it is now possible to calculate the oxygen extraction tension, the concentration of extractable oxygen and the oxygen compensation factor which reflects the increase in cardiac output required to maintain the mixed venous po_2 of 5 kPa. Oxygen status has also been studied in the critically ill by Tulli et al (1990), who found that there was no relationship between the uncompensated mixed venous oxygen tension (po_2uv) and actual pvo_2 (mixed venous oxygen tension) — i.e. derived units and actual measurements may not coincide in the critically ill; see Willis 1990). Dantzker et al (1991) comment that the relationship between increased oxygen requirement and reduced oxygen transport may in fact just be a normal physiological response other than signs of impaired oxygen extraction. In other experiments oxygen delivery was decreased by anaemia, hypoxia and cardiac tamponade. Below the critical level of oxygen delivery, lactic acidosis and decreased oxygen supply occurred regardless of the mechanism of impairment (Cilley et al 1991).

In addition to the use of new technology, outlined interpretation of data may depend on the circumstances of the measurement. The oxygen tension difference between alveolar and arterial blood ($AaPO_2$) may not be a reliable index of normal gas exchange in the presence of alveolar hypoventilation (Gray & Blalock 1991). In ARDS oxygen consumption remains constant irrespective of the increases of oxygen delivery, and the increased concentrations of plasma lactate or sepsis do not predict dependence of oxygen consumption on oxygen delivery (Ronco et al 1991). Mixed venous oxygen saturation (SaO_2) is said to reflect on the changes in cardiac index (CI), but in fact it depends on its baseline levels. In critically ill patients, the SvO_2 is only a satisfactory indicator of therapeutic response in cardiac index when the SvO_2 is <55% and the CI <2 1/min per m^2 (Jain et al 1991). Metabolic alkalosis results in deterioration of the ventilation : perfusion ratio in patients with marked respiratory failure and an infusion of hydrochloric acid improved the arterial oxygen tension (Brimioulle & Kahn 1990).

PULMONARY OEDEMA

There are a variety of causes of pulmonary oedema ranging from cardiac, pulmonary, central and even drug-induced. The drug-induced causes include narcotics such as heroin, tocolytics such as ritodrine, cyclosporine, tricyclics and bleomycin (Reed & Glauser 1991). Other causes include high altitude which appears to respond to nifedipine (Bartsch et al 1991, Reeves & Schoene 1991).

Allison (1991) has outlined the physiological approach aimed at reducing hypoxaemia and pulmonary capillary pressure. This involves supplementary oxygen by CPAP or endotracheal intubation with ventilation as well as reducing preload which in turn reduces pulmonary capillary pressure. The measures include sitting posture, loop diuretics, morphine and possibly sublingual nitroglycerine. Bersten et al (1991) reported favourably on the use of CPAP in cardiogenic pulmonary oedema while Sznajder & Wood (1991) discussed the benefits of reducing pulmonary oedema in patients with acute hypoxaemic respiratory failure (see also Brandes & Finkelstein 1990; Murphy & Jones 1991).

SMOKE INHALATION

Inhalation of smoke includes not only carbon monoxide but also hydrogen cyanide. The effects of inhalational injury may not be apparent in patients suffering from severe burns; however Baud et al (1991) found that elevated plasma lactate concentration correlated well with blood cyanide and it was a useful indicator of cyanide toxicity (see also Kulig 1991).

THEOPHYLLINE

Theophylline is widely prescribed for asthmatics although it appears to be no more effective than terbutaline in treating severe asthma as assessed by nocturnal oxygenation and sleep quality (Brander et al 1990). Other studies suggested that theophylline also improves diaphragmatic contractility but this is only in high dosage (Janssens et al 1991).

Unfortunately theophylline is attended by a whole series of interactions; its clearance is decreased markedly by erythromycin, cimetidine, propranolol, verapramil, nifedipine and frusemide while isoprenaline, phenytoin, phenobarbitone, benzodiazepines and felodipine promote its clearance. Theophylline has a narrow therapeutic concentration range and therefore changes in clearance of approximately 25% can have a major clinical effect (Upton 1991a,b).

DIAPHRAGMATIC FLUTTER

This is a rare disorder associated with dyspnoea, chest or abdominal wall pain and epigastric pulsations, and is caused by involuntary contractions of the diaphragm. The diagnosis is made on electromyography and simple pulmonary tests. The condition readily responds to carbamazepine (Vantrappen et al 1992).

REFERENCES

Aldren C P, Barr L C, Leach R D 1991 Hypoxaemia and postoperative pulmonary complications. Br J Surg 78: 1307–1308
Allison R C 1991 Initial treatment of pulmonary edema: a physiological approach. Am J Med Sci 302: 385–391
Bach J R, Penek J 1991 Obstructive sleep apnea complicating negative-pressure ventilatory support in patients with chronic paralytic-/restrictive ventilatory dysfunction. Chest 99: 1386–1393
Barker S J, Hyatt J, Clarke C, Tremper K K 1991 Hyperventilation reduces transcutaneous oxygen tension and skin blood flow. Anesthesiology 75: 619–624
Barnes P J, Baraniuk J N, Belvisi M G 1991a Neuropeptides in the respiratory tract. Part 1. Am Rev Respir Dis 144: 1187–1198
Barnes P J, Baraniuk J N, Belvisi M G 1991b Neuropeptides in the respiratory tract. Am Rev Respir Dis 144: 1391–1399
Bartsch P, Maggiorini M, Ritter M et al 1991 Prevention of high-altitude pulmonary edema by nifedipine. N Engl J Med 325: 1284–1289
Baud F J, Barriot P, Toffis V et al 1991 Elevated blood cyanide concentrations in victims of smoke inhalation. N Engl J Med 325: 1761–1766
Bedard M-A, Montplaisir J, Richer F, Malo J 1991 Nocturnal hypoxemia as a determinant of vigilance impairment in sleep apnea syndrome. Chest 100: 367–370
Begle R L, Skatrud J B 1990 Hyperinflation and expiratory muscle recruitment during REM sleep in humans. Respir Physiol 82: 47–64

Bersten A D, Holt A W, Vedig A E et al 1991 Treatment of severe cardiogenic pulmonary edema with continuous positive airway pressure delivered by face mask. N Engl J Med 325: 1825–1830

Bjermer L, Eklund A, Blaschke E 1991 Bronchoalveolar lavage fibronectin in patients with sarcoidosis: correlation to hyaluronan and disease activity. Eur Respir J 4: 955–971

Bradley T D, Takasaki Y, Orr D, Popkin J 1990 Differential activation of respiratory muscles by CO_2 and hypoxia in man. Chest 97 (suppl): 52S

Brander P E, Sovijarvi A R A, Salmi T et al 1990 Nocturnal oxygen saturation and body movement in asthmatics treated with controlled-release preparations of theophylline or terbutaline. Eur J Clin Pharmacol 39: 117–121

Brandes M E, Finkelstein J 1990 The production of alveolar macrophage-derived growth-regulating protein in response to lung injury. Toxicol Lett 54: 3–22

Branthwaite M A 1991 Non-invasive and domiciliary ventilation: positive pressure techniques. Thorax 46: 208–212

Brimioulle S, Kahn R J 1990 Metabolic alkalosis and pulmonary gas exchange. Am Rev Respir Dis 141: 1185–1189

Callahan C M, Dittus R S, Katz B P 1991 Oral corticosteroid therapy for patients with stable chronic obstructive pulmonary disease. A meta-analysis. Ann Intern Med 114: 216–223

Campbell G S, Cone J B 1991 Adult respiratory distress syndrome. Am J Surg 161: 239–242

Cherniack N S 1990 The central nervous system and respiratory muscle coordination. Chest 97 (suppl): 52S–68S

Cilley R E, Scharenberg A M, Bongiorno P F et al 1991 Low oxygen delivery produced by anemia, hypoxia, and low cardiac output. J Surg Res 51: 425–433

Collop N A, Block J, Hellard D 1991 The effect of nightly nasal CPAP treatment on underlying obstructive sleep apnea and pharyngeal size. Chest 99: 855–860

Colt H G, Haas H, Rich G B 1991 Hypoxemia vs sleep fragmentation as cause of excessive daytime sleepiness in obstructive sleep apnea. Chest 100: 1542–1548

Cooper B G, Veale D, Griffiths C J, Gibson G J 1991 Value of nocturnal oxygen saturation as a screening test for sleep apnoea. Thorax 46: 586–588

Dantzker D R, Foresman B, Gutierrez G 1991 Oxygen supply and utilization relationships. A reevaluation. Am Rev Respir Dis 143: 675–679

De Jongste J C, Jongejan R C, Kerrebijn K F 1991 Control of airway caliber by autonomic nerves in asthma and in chronic obstructive pulmonary disease. Am Rev Respir Dis 143: 1421–1426

Delguste P, Aubert-Tulkens G, Rodenstein D O 1991 Upper airway obstruction during nasal intermittent positive-pressure hyperventilation in sleep. Lancet 338: 1295–1297

Desruennes E, Bourgain J-L, Mamelle G, Luboinski B 1991 Airway obstruction and high-frequency jet ventilation during laryngoscopy. Ann Otol Rhinol Laryngol 100: 922–927

Dilworth J P, Pounsford J C 1991 Cough following general anaesthesia and abdominal surgery. Respir Med 85 (suppl A): 13–16

Dunn W F, Nelson S B, Hubmayr R D 1991a Oxygen-induced hypercarbia in obstructive pulmonary disease. Am Rev Respir Dis 144: 526–530

Dunn W F, Nelson S, Hubmayr R D 1991b The control of breathing during weaning from mechanical ventilation. Chest 100: 754–761

Eiser N 1990 The hitch-hikers guide to nasal airway patency. Respir Med 84: 179–183

Eissa N T, Ranieri V M, Corbeil C et al 1991 Effects of positive end-expiratory pressure, lung volume, and inspiratory flow on interrupter resistance in patients with adult respiratory distress syndrome. Am Rev Respir Dis 144: 538–543

Fernandez K, O'Hanlan K A, Rodriguez-Rodriguez L 1991 Respiratory failure due to interstitial lung metastases of ovarian carcinoma reversed by chemotherapy. Chest 99: 1533–1534

Fitting J W 1991 Respiratory muscle fatigue limiting physical exercise? Eur Respir J 4: 103–108

Fletcher E C, Goodnight-White S, Munafo D et al 1991a Rate of oxyhemoglobin desaturation in obstructive versus nonobstructive apnea. Am Rev Respir Dis 143: 657–660

Fletcher E C, Goodnight-White S, Munafo D et al 1991b Effect of cardiac output reduction on rate of desaturation in obstructive apnea. Chest 99: 452–456

Frostell C, Fratacci M-D, Wain J C et al 1991 Inhaled nitric oxide. A selective pulmonary vasodilator reversing hypoxic pulmonary vasoconstriction. Circulation 83: 2038–2047

Gastinne H, Wolff M, Delatour F et al 1992 A controlled trial in intensive care units of selective decontamination of the digestive tract with nonabsorbable antibiotics. N Engl J Med 326: 594–599

Gigliotti F, Duranti R, Fabiani A et al 1991 Suppression of ventilatory muscle activity in healthy subjects and COPD patients with negative pressure ventilation. Chest 99: 1186–1192

Gillis A M, Stoohs R, Guilleminault C 1991 Changes in the QT interval during obstructive sleep apnea. Sleep 14: 346–350

Gilmartin J J, Cooper B G, Griffiths C J et al 1991 Breathing during sleep in patients with myotonic dystrophy and non-myotonic respiratory muscle weakness. Q J Med 285: 21–31

Gleadhill I C, Schwartz A R, Schubert N et al 1991 Upper airway collapsibility in snorers and in patients with obstructive hypopnea and apnea. Am Rev Respir Dis 143: 1300–1303

Goertz A, Heinrich H, Winter H, Deller A 1991 Hemodynamic effects of different ventilatory patterns. A prospective clinical trial. Chest 99 1166–1171

Goldman J M, Ireland R M, Berthon-Jones M et al 1991 Erythropoietin concentrations in obstructive sleep apnoea. Thorax 46: 25–27

Goldstone J, Moxham J 1991 Weaning from mechanical ventilation. Thorax 46: 56–62

Gray B A, Blalock J M 1991 Interpretation of the alveolar–arterial oxygen difference in patients with hypercapnia. Am Rev Respir Dis 143: 4–8

Green D E, Block A J, Collop N A, Hellard D W 1991 Pharyngeal volume in asymptomatic snorers compared with nonsnoring volunteers. Chest 99: 49–53

Greenberg H E, Rapoport D M, Rothenberg S A et al 1991 Endogenous opiates modulate the postapnea ventilatory response in the obstructive sleep apnea syndrome. Am Rev Respir Dis 143: 1282–1287

Grunberg G, Cohen J D, Keslin J, Gassner S 1991 Facilitation of mechanical ventilation in status asthmaticus with continuous intravenous thiopental. Chest 99: 1216–1219

Guttenplan M D, Hendrix R A, Townsend M J, Balsara G B 1991 Laryngeal manifestations of gout. Ann Otol Rhinol Laryngol 100: 899–902

Haahtela T, Jarvinen M, Kava T et al 1991 Comparison of a β_2-agonist, terbutaline, with an inhaled corticosteroid, budesonide, in newly detected asthma. N Engl J Med 325: 388–392

Haluszka J, Chartrand D A, Grassino A E, Milic-Emili J 1990 Intrinsic PEEP and arterial PCO_2 in stable patients with chronic obstructive pulmonary disease. Am Rev Respir Dis 141: 1194–1197

Hampl V, Herget J 1991 Possible mechanisms of oxygen sensing in the pulmonary circulation. Physiol Res 40: 463–470

Hansen-Flaschen J H, Brazinsky S, Basile C, Lanken P N 1991 Use of sedating drugs and neuromuscular blocking agents in patients requiring mechanical ventilation for respiratory failure. A national survey. JAMA 266: 2870–2875

Hoffstein V, Chan C K, Slutsky A S 1991a Sleep apnea and systemic hypertension: a causal association review. Am J Med 91: 190–196

Hoffstein V, Wright S, Zamel N, Bradley T D 1991b Pharyngeal function and snoring characteristics in apneic and nonapneic snorers. Am Rev Respir Dis 143: 1294–1299

Horner R L, Guz A 1991 Some factors affecting the maintenance of upper airway patency in man. Respir Med 85 (suppl A): 27–30

Hurewitz A N, Bergofsky E H, Vomero E 1991 Airway insufflation. Increasing flow rates progressively reduce dead space in respiratory failure. Am Rev Respir Dis 144: 1229–1233

Irwin R S, Curley F J 1991 The treatment of cough. A comprehensive review. Chest 99: 1477–1484

Jain A, Shroff S G, Janicki J S et al 1991 Relation between mixed venous oxygen saturation and cardiac index. Chest 99: 1403–1409

Jansen J E, Sorensen A L, Naesh O et al 1990 Effect of doxapram on post-operative pulmonary complications after upper abdominal surgery in high-risk patients. Lancet 335: 936–938

Janssen J A M J L, Tjiong H L 1991 Bronchial asthma improved after removal of a phaeochromocytoma. Eur Respir J 4: 1021–1022

Janssens S, Derom E, Reid M et al 1991 Effects of theophylline on canine diaphragmatic contractility and fatigue. Am Respir Dis 144: 1250–1255

Jeffrey A A, Warren P M, Flenley D C 1992 Acute hypercapnic respiratory failure in patients with chronic obstructive lung disease: risk factors and use of guidelines for management. Thorax 47: 34–40

Jochelson M, Tarbell N J, Freedman A S et al 1990 Acute and chronic pulmonary complications following autologous bone marrow transplantation in non-Hodgkin's lymphoma. Bone Marrow Transplant 6: 329-331

Jones J G 1991 Management of post-operative hypoxaemia: the role of respiratory stimulants. Ther Express 30: 1-3

Jones P W 1991 Quality of life measurement for patients with diseases of the airways. Thorax 46: 676-682

Kaplan J, Fredrickson P A, Richardson J W 1991 Sleep and breathing in patients with the Prader-Willi syndrome. Mayo Clin Proc 66: 1124-1126

Karpel J P 1991 Bronchodilator responses to anticholinergic and beta-adrenergic agents in acute and stable COPD. Chest 99: 871-876

Katz I, Stradling J, Slutsky A S et al 1990 Do patients with obstructive sleep apnea have thick necks? Am Rev Respir Dis 141: 1228-1231

Kaufman L 1962 Disordered respiration in dystrophia myotonica. MD thesis, Edinburgh University

Kearon M C, Summers E, Jones N L et al 1991 Effort and dyspnoea during work of varying intensity and duration. Eur Respir J 4: 917-925

Kelley M A, Carson J L, Palevsky H I, Schwartz J S 1991 Diagnosing pulmonary embolism: new facts and strategies. Ann Intern Med 114: 300-306

Koo L C, Ho J H-C, Ho C-Y et al 1990 Personal exposure to nitrogen dioxide and its association with respiratory illness in Hong Kong. Am Rev Respir Dis 141: 1119-1126

Krieger J, Follenius M, Sforza E et al 1991 Effects of treatment with nasal continuous positive airway pressure on atrial natriuretic peptide and arginine vasopressin release during sleep in patients with obstructive sleep apnoea. Clin Sci 80: 443-449

Kulig K 1991 Cyanide antidotes and fire toxicology. N Engl J Med 325: 1801-1802

Lanigan C J 1992 Oxygen desaturation after dental anaesthesia. Br J Anaesth 68: 142-145

Levinson P D, Millman R P 1991 Causes and consequences of blood pressure alterations in obstructive sleep apnea. Arch Intern Med 151: 455-462

Lipworth B J, McDevitt D G 1992 Inhaled β_2-adrenoceptor agonists in asthma: help or hindrance? Br J Clin Pharmacol 33: 129-138

Ludwigs U G, Baehrendtz S, Wanecek M, Matell G 1991 Mechanical ventilation in medical and neurological diseases: 11 years of experience. J Intern Med 229: 117-124

MacKay T W, Fitzpatrick M F, Douglas N J 1991 Non-adrenergic, non-cholinergic nervous system and overnight airway calibre in asthmatic and normal subjects. Lancet 338: 1289-1292

MacNaughton P D, Evans T W 1992 Management of adult respiratory distress syndrome. Lancet 339: 469-472

Mador J 1991 Respiratory muscle fatigue and breathing pattern. Chest 100: 1430-1435

Maillard D, Fleury B, Housset B et al 1991 Decreased oxyhemoglobin affinity in patients with sleep apnea syndrome. Am Rev Respir Dis 143: 486-489

Malone S, Liu P P, Holloway R et al 1991 Obstructive sleep apnoea in patients with dilated cardiomyopathy: effects of continuous positive airway pressure. Lancet 338: 1480-1484

Marion M-H, Klap P, Perrin A, Cohen M 1992 Stridor and focal laryngeal dystonia. Lancet 339: 457-458

Maxwell D L 1990 Adverse effects of inhaled corticosteroids. Biomed Pharmacother 44: 421-427

McElvaney G N, Wilcox P G, Fairbarn M S et al 1990 Respiratory muscle weakness and dyspnea in thyrotoxic patients. Am Rev Respir Dis 141: 1221-1227

Moller J T, Jensen P F, Johannessen N W, Espersen K 1992 Hypoxaemia is reduced by pulse oximetry monitoring in the operating theatre and in the recovery room. Br J Anaesth 68: 146-150

Montserrat J M, Martos J A, Alarcon A et al 1991 Effect of negative pressure ventilation on arterial blood gas pressures and inspiratory muscle strength during an exacerbation of chronic obstructive lung disease. Thorax 46: 6-8

Murphy P G, Jones J G 1991 Acute lung injury. The quantitative evaluation of acute lung injury. Intensive Care 1: 110-117

Nishino T, Sugimori K, Hiraga K, Honda Y 1990 Effects of tracheal irritation and hypercapnia on tracheal smooth muscle in humans. J Appl Physiol 69: 419-423

Ornot I, Bernard G R, Biaggioni I et al 1991 Direct vasodilator effect of hyperventilation-induced hypocarbia in autonomic failure patients. Am J Med Sci 301: 305-309

Owens M W, George R B 1991 Nebulized atropine sulfate in the treatment of acute asthma. Chest 99: 1084–1087

Pennock B E, Kaplan P D, Carlin B W et al 1991 Pressure support ventilation with a simplified ventilatory support system administered with a nasal mask in patients with respiratory failure. Chest 100: 1371–1376

Pesenti A, Pelosi P, Rossi N et al 1991 The effects of positive end-expiratory pressure on respiratory resistance in patients with the adult respiratory distress syndrome and in normal anesthetized subjects. Am Rev Respir Dis 144: 101–107

Ranieri V M, Eissa N T, Corbeil C et al 1991 Effects of positive end-expiratory pressure on alveolar recruitment and gas exchange in patients with the adult respiratory distress syndrome. Am Rev Respir Dis 144: 544–551

Rauscher H, Popp W, Zwick H 1990 Flow–volume curves in obstructive sleep apnea and snoring. Lung 168: 209–214

Reed C R, Glauser F L 1991 Drug-induced noncardiogenic pulmonary edema. Chest 100: 1120–1124

Reeves J T, Schoene R B 1991 When lungs on mountains leak. Studying pulmonary edema at high altitudes. N Engl J Med 325: 1306–1307

Rello J, Quintana E, Ausina V et al 1991 Incidence, etiology, and outcome of nosocomial pneumonia in mechanically ventilated patients. Chest 100: 439–444

Rochester D F 1991 Respiratory muscle weakness, pattern of breathing, and CO_2 retention in chronic obstructive pulmonary disease. Am Rev Respir Dis 143: 901–903

Ronco J J, Phang P T, Walley K R et al 1991 Oxygen consumption is independent of changes in oxygen delivery in severe adult respiratory distress syndrome. Am Rev Respir Dis 143: 1267–1273

Rosenberg J, Dirkes W E, Kehlet H 1989 Episodic arterial oxygen desaturation and heart rate variations following major abdominal surgery. Br J Anesth 63: 651–654

Sassoon C S H 1991 Positive pressure ventilation. Alternate modes. Chest 100: 1421–1429

Satoh M, Hida W, Chonan T et al 1991 Role of hypoxic drive in regulation of postapneic ventilation during sleep in patients with obstructive sleep apnea. Am Rev Respir Dis 143: 481–485

Siggaard-Andersen O, Gothgen I H, Wimberley P D, Fogh-Andersen N 1990 The oxygen status of the arterial blood revised; relevant oxygen parameters for monitoring the arterial oxygen availability. Scand J Clin Lab Invest 50 (suppl 203): 17–28

Similowski T, Yan S, Gauthier A P et al 1991 Contractile properties of the human diaphragm during chronic hyperinflation. N Engl J Med 325: 917–923

Spitzer W O, Suissa S, Ernst P et al 1992 The use of β-agonists and the risk of death and near death from asthma. N Engl J Med 326: 501–506

Spring J, Clague J, Ind P W 1992 A comparison of the effect of salmeterol and salbutamol in normal subjects. Br J Clin Pharmacol 33: 139–141

Stradling J R, Crosby J H 1991 Predictors and prevalence of obstructive sleep apnoea and snoring in 1001 middle aged men. Thorax 46: 85–90

Sykes A P, Lawson N, Finnegan J A, Ayres J G 1991 Creatine kinase activity in patients with brittle asthma treated with long term subcutaneous terbutaline. Thorax 46: 580–583

Sznajder J I, Wood L D H 1991 Beneficial effects of reducing pulmonary edema in patients with acute hypoxemic respiratory failure. Chest 100: 890–891

Torphy T J, Undem B J 1991 Phosphodiesterase inhibitors: new opportunities for the treatment of asthma. Thorax 46: 512–523

Torres A 1991 Accuracy of diagnostic tools for the management of nosocomial respiratory infections in mechanically ventilated patients. Eur Respir J 4: 1010–1019

Trotman-Dickenson B, Weetman A P, Hughes J M B 1991 Upper airflow obstruction and pulmonary function in acromegaly: relationship to disease activity. Q J Med 79: 527–538

Tulli G, Vignali G, Guadagnucci A, Mondello V 1990 The oxygen status of the arterial blood in the critically ill. Scand J Clin Lab Invest 50 (suppl 203): 107–118

Upton R A 1991a Pharmacokinetic interactions between theophylline and other medication (part I). Clin Pharmacokinet 20: 66–80

Upton R A 1991b Pharmacokinetic interactions between theophylline and other medication (part II). Clin Pharmacokinet 20: 135–150

Valentine D D, Hammond M D, Downs J B et al 1991 Distribution of ventilation and perfusion with different modes of mechanical ventilation. Am Rev Respir Dis 143: 1262–1266

Vandenbroucke-Grauls C M J E, Vandenbroucke J P 1991 Effect of selective decontamination of the digestive tract on respiratory tract infections and mortality in the intensive care unit. Lancet 338: 859–862

Van de Graaff W B, Gordey K, Donseif S E et al 1991 Pressure support. Changes in ventilatory pattern and components of the work of breathing. Chest 100: 1082–1089

Van den Elshout F J J, van Herwaarden C L A, Folgering H Th 1991 Effects of hypercapnia and hypocapnia on respiratory resistance in normal and asthmatic subjects. Thorax 46: 28–32

Van Dercar D H, Martinez A P, De Lisser E A 1991 Sleep apnea syndromes: a potential contraindication for patient controlled analgesia. Anesthesiology 74: 623–624

Vantrappen G, Decramer M, Harlet R 1992 High-frequency diaphragmatic flutter: symptoms and treatment by carbamazepine. Lancet 339: 265–267

Vermeij C G, Feenstra B W A, Adrichem W J, Bruining H A 1991 Independent oxygen uptake and oxygen delivery in septic and postoperative patients. Chest 99: 1438–1443

Wade J F III, Mortenson R, Irvin C G 1991 Physiologic evaluation of bullous emphysema. Chest 100: 1151–1154

Wagner P D, Rodriguez-Roisin R 1991 Clinical advances in pulmonary gas exchange. Am Rev Respir Dis 143: 883–888

Ward M, Macklem P T 1990 The act of breathing and how it fails. Chest 97: 36S–39S

Wasicko M J, Leiter J C, Erlichman J S et al 1991 Nasal and Pharyngeal resistance after topical mucosal vasoconstriction in normal humans. Am Rev Respir Dis 144: 1048–1052

Watanabe S, Kanner R E, Cutillo A G et al 1989 Long-term effect of almitrine bismesylate in patients with hypoxemic chronic obstructive pulmonary disease. Am Rev Respir Dis 140: 1269–1273

Westbrook J L, Sykes M K 1992 Peroperative arterial hypoxaemia. The interaction between intrapulmonary shunt and cardiac output. A computer model. Anaesthesia 47: 307–310

Wiegand D A, Latz B, Zwillich C W, Wiegand L 1990 Geniohyoid muscle activity in normal men during wakefulness and sleep. J Appl Physiol 69: 1262–1269

Williams A J, Yu G, Santiago S, Stein M 1991 Screening for sleep apnea using pulse oximetry and a clinical score. Chest 100: 631–635

Willis N 1990 Parameters derived from a computed in vivo oxygen dissociation curve as an aid to oxygen therapy. Scand J Clin Lab Invest 50 (suppl 203): 13–16

Yildirim N, Fitzpatrick M F, Whyte K F et al 1991 The effect of posture on upper airway dimensions in normal subjects and in patients with the sleep apnea/hypopnea syndrome. Am Rev Respir Dis 144: 845–847

3. Medicine relevant to anaesthesia

L. Kaufman

DIABETES

The management of diabetic patients still presents many problems but with recent advances prospects for even the brittle diabetics have shown a marked improvement (Gill & Alberti 1991). There have also been marked improvements in the management of maternal diabetes but hazards for the fetus still remain, including macrosomia (abnormal fetal growth), hypertrophic cardiomyopathy, hypoglycaemia, hypocalcaemia and hypomagnesaemia, polycythaemia and hyperbilirubinaemia. However the incidence of respiratory distress syndrome has decreased (Rosenn & Tsang 1991).

Insulin secretion

Insulin secretion is controlled by glucose, glucose metabolites, adenosine triphosphate and acetyl coenzyme A. Lipid synthesis is also an important factor stimulating glucose metabolism and insulin release (Laychock 1990). This may be due to a variety of causes including mutation of the insulin receptor genes, effects on the receptor kinase, stress, uraemia, cirrhosis, ketoacidosis, obesity as well as other hormones including glucocorticoid growth hormone etc. Bumetanide, a loop diuretic, apparently has a direct effect on pancreatic beta cells and reduces insulin release (Sandstrom 1990). Insulin resistance may also be inherited (Moller & Flier 1991).

Somatostatin

Somatostatin which is secreted by the D cells in the pancreas is believed to inhibit the secretion of insulin and glucagon as well as growth hormone. However Kollind et al (1990) found that it interferes with the clearance of insulin in insulin-dependent diabetic patients. Diem & Robertson (1991) suggested that prophylactic treatment with somatostatin analogue octreotide (SM 201–995) was beneficial as it could decrease the risk of ketoacidosis. However it does reduce the glomerular filtration rate and kidney size by affecting the serum insulin-like growth factor-1 (IGF-1; Serri et al 1991).

Non-insulin-dependent diabetes mellitus (NIDDM)

This is usually treated with oral diabetic agents such as sulphonylureas, although insulin may be required to control blood sugar as ischaemic strokes appear to be related to blood sugar concentration in patients with NIDDM (Galloway 1990).

Complications

Hypoglycaemia

Diabetic patients who were formerly on animal insulin have claimed that they are unaware of hypoglycaemia because of the lack of symptoms. Patrick et al (1991) found that the symptoms and hormonal responses to acute hypoglyacemia were indistinguishable. However Egger et al (1991a) cautioned on transferring patients to human insulin as there appears to be an increased incidence of hypoglycaemia. Egger et al (1991b) noted a lack of concentration, confusion and restlessness (also see Editorial 1991). Hypoglycaemia may also occur spontaneously in those who produce anti-insulin antibodies. Redmon et al (1992) reported such a case in a patient with multiple myeloma in which there was increased plasma insulin and low plasma C-peptide concentration (Polonsky 1992).

Hypertension may be associated with diabetes but Nilsson et al (1990) found hyperinsulinaemia in hypertensive patients who have been on antihypertensive therapy.

Hyperglycaemia is not uncommon in patients with phaeochromocytoma and following removal it is not unusual for the blood sugar level to fall. However, Levin & Heifetz (1990) have reported a patient with severe and protracted postoperative hypoglycaemia.

Ketoacidosis

During recovery from diabetic ketoacidosis, hyperchloraemic acidosis may develop and this is due to the fact that prior to treatment there is a marked loss in bicarbonate, and this is masked by the presence of ketone ions (Oh et al 1990). Riley et al (1989) advocated the use of bicarbonate despite the fact that it inhibits the Bohr effect and the replenishment of 2,3,-diphosphogluconate takes a few days.

Non-ketotic hyperosmolar coma

Non-ketotic hyperosmolar coma may also be found in diabetic patients. Daugirdas et al (1989) have been able to differentiate four hyperosmotic syndromes based on serum sodium levels which are high in dialysis patients exposed to high glucose levels, in diabetic non-ketotic patients, in those receiving parenteral nutrition and in excessive burns.

Neuropathy

Hyperglycaemia is thought to result in neuropathy, but there are other factors such as increased polyol pathway activity, alteration in endogenous nerve growth factor as well as hypoxia and ischaemia (Leading article 1991). In patients with autonomic neuropathy the mortality increased fivefold (O'Brien et al 1991).

Nephropathy

Diabetic nephropathy appears to respond to enalapril, an angiotensin converting enzyme inhibitor. Apparently it is not due to the antihypertensive action of the drug but appears to be a specific effect of the converting enzyme inhibitor (Bjorck et al 1992). However Mogensen (1992) reported that renal damage was a side-effect of angiotensin converting enzyme inhibitors.

Lung function

Despite previous reports Maccioni & Colebatch (1991) found that there was no deterioration in pulmonary function in diabetic patients, although Chertow et al (1991) found that pleural effusions were more likely to occur. It was assumed that the origin was cardiac as the patients had a low left ventricular ejection fraction.

In type 1 diabetes there may be limitation of joint mobility, possibly due to glycosylation of tissue proteins. This may lead to difficulty in intubation if there is restriction of movement of the larynx and cervical spine. There may also be limited mobility of the joints in the hands and an incomplete 'palm print' may suggest difficult intubation (Reissell et al 1990).

Surgery

Milaskiewicz & Hall (1992) have reviewed the developments in the management of diabetes at operation that have occurred in the last decade. Although at their hospital the mortality of diabetic patients was 1½ times that of non-diabetic patients, they felt that there was no evidence to show that the short period of hyperglycaemia was harmful, although it was accepted that hypoglycaemia certainly needed to be avoided. The regime recommended by Alberti & Thomas (1979) has not found universal acclaim (Dunnet et al 1988). It involved the administration of glucose, insulin and potassium in the same bag of intravenous fluid and the whole bag had to be changed when the dose of insulin needed to be altered. Other regimes have been described but these have become less important in view of the introduction of the infusion pump for intravenous insulin administration and the ease of performing repeated blood glucose estimations. The non-insulin-dependent diabetic patients may require insulin in the immediate postoperative period, although there is a possible danger of hypoglycaemia in patients treated with long-acting oral antidiuretic drugs.

CENTRAL NERVOUS SYSTEM

Fatigue

The assessment of fatigue and chronic fatigue syndrome presents many difficulties in view of the fact that even in normal subjects fatigue fluctuates during the day. Fatigue is associated with disorders of mood and there are diurnal variations in perceived mental and physical energy (Wessley 1992, Wood et al 1992). An endocrine cause has also been implicated with impaired activation of the hypothalamic–pituitary–adrenal axis (Demitrack et al 1991). Studies on sternomastoid muscle may be of value in respiratory muscle fatigue in severely ill and breathless patients (Mak et al 1991).

Neuromuscular disorders

Kelly & Luce (1991) have reviewed the diagnosis and management of neuromuscular diseases causing respiratory failure. These include lesions of the upper motor neuron (hemiplegia, extrapyramidal disorders); lower motor neuron disorders (poliomyelitis, amyotrophic lateral sclerosis, Werdnig–Hoffmann disease); lesions of the peripheral neurons (Guillain–Barré syndrome, acute porphyria, toxins, polyneuropathies); myoneural junction (myasthenia gravis, botulism, Eaton–Lambert syndrome, organo-phosphate poisoning) and lesions of the muscle (muscular dystrophies, polymyositis). Despite muscle weakness the central drive in many of these patients is increased and minute volume is not an adequate reflection of this (Baydur 1991). In amyotrophic lateral sclerosis, pulmonary function tests and arterial gas measurements did not correlate with the pattern of nocturnal breathing or survival time and the more sensitive test is the maximal inspiratory pressure. The main cause of nocturnal oxygen desaturation was hypoventilation (Gay et al 1991). The Guillain–Barré syndrome has replaced poliomyelitis as the commonest cause of acute generalized paralysis which may affect respiration, swallowing and autonomic function. Treatment may involve ventilation and therapy with plasma exchange and gammaglobulin (Ropper 1992; also see Winer 1992).

Autonomic dysfunction produced by spinal cord injury differs from that caused by peripheral autonomic neuropathy in that there are reduced plasma noradrenaline levels, but there is no significant alteration in clearance (Krum et al 1990).

Myotonic dystrophy

Although many of the abnormalities in this condition have been reported, an increase of calcification in the bone of the skull is also a feature of myotonic dystrophy. Rodriguez et al (1991) have also reported calcification in the basal ganglia associated with hyperparathyroidism. There are also changes in the cardiovascular muscles and in those of the gastrointestinal tract. The external and internal anal sphincters are also affected reflecting myopathic changes, muscular atrophy as well as neurological deficits (Eckardt & Nix 1991).

Cerebral ischaemia

In animals protracted hypotension and cardiovascular shock may be followed by improved recovery, whereas in humans even a short period of cerebral hypoperfusion is associated with poor outcome. In a damaged brain the autoregulation system fails and the blood flow depends entirely upon cerebroperfusion pressure. Thus a high pressure may result in cerebral oedema and a low pressure in cerebral ischaemia. Cerebral oedema may result from cerebral ischaemia once the cerebral circulation has been restored. Interruption of cerebral circulation often leads to disseminated haemorrhagic infarction and nerve cell destruction in selected areas such as the hippocampus. Brief ischaemia may lead to a state of hyperexcitation of the vulnerable cells followed by a complete disappearance of nerve cell activities (Baethmann & Kempski 1991). Tests of cerebral collateral reserve can be evaluated by carotid compression and cerebral carbon dioxide reactivity (Norris et al 1990).

The pathophysiology of acute ischaemic stroke has been summarized by Pulsinelli (1992). Regions nearest the collateral vessels are less severely affected than those in more distal areas. Ischaemia of 5 min but less than 1 hour kills some of the vulnerable neurons but when it lasts more than an hour, infarction begins in the central area of diminished cerebral blood flow. Ischaemic brain damage affects many transmitters involving adenosine triphosphate, glutamate and aspartate, and there is an exchange of ions across the cell membrane. Calcium activates phospholipases which hydrolyse membranes and there may be a place for calcium channel blockers such as nimodipine in treatment. There is depletion of brain noradrenaline which might influence the cerebral blood vessels in response to decreased cerebral blood flow (Kobayashi et al 1990). There appears to be no correlation between changes in cardiac output and changes in cerebral blood flow irrespective of blood pressure autoregulation. Mannitol increases intravascular volume but the effect of cerebral blood flow is probably due to a decrease in blood viscosity rather than cardiac output augmentation (Bouma & Muizelaar 1990). Davies et al (1991) found that the electrocardiogram was a poor indicator for myocardial function following subarachnoid haemorrhage and there was a better relationship between the echocardiogram and the severity of neurological disorder. In animal studies, Sutton et al (1990) found that venous oxygen content in the jugular bulb probably affects the adequacy of cerebral blood flow when there is intracranial hypertension.

Subarachnoid haemorrhage is associated with an early reduction in cerebral oxygen uptake, presumably due to the ischaemic damage at the time of aneurysm rupture (Jakobsen et al 1990). Fibrinogen and lipid levels are just as important risk factors for ischaemic stroke as they are for ischaemic heart disease (Qizilbash et al 1991). The value of anticoagulants in patients with atrial fibrillation and transient ischaemic attacks is still under trial (Rothrock and Hart 1991, Sandercock 1991). Animal experiments suggest that pretreatment with drugs such as almitrine will increase oxygen availability and it may be of value (Benzi et al 1990). Also in animals indomethacin appears to have an action on preventing the incidence of post-ischaemic blood–brain barrier leakage of albumin in the phase of hyperaemia following middle cerebral artery occlusion (Ting 1990).

Thirty per cent of patients following a stroke experience difficulty in swallowing and it is estimated that the frequency of aspiration varies between 40 and 70%. Patients likely to aspirate are those with abnormal gag reflex and/or who are unable to cough adequately (Horner et al 1990). Although barbiturates are now hardly used for night sedation, they still have a place in the management of neurological disorders such as epilepsy (Smith & Riskin 1991), while the use of methohexitone may demonstrate an epileptic focus. There is also evidence that they can decrease intracranial pressure, cerebral oedema, cerebral blood flow and cerebral metabolism, but their use following brain injury is still unproven.

Parkinson's disease

The pathophysiology of Parkinson's disease is reviewed by Agid (1991): dopaminergic neurons appear to be particularly affected but other transmitters are also involved. These include noradrenaline, serotonin, acetylcholine, susbtance P, somatostatin, encephalins and corticotrophin-releasing factor. In 15–20% of patients dementia also occurs. The rate of the loss of dopaminergic neurons is said to be 1% per year and factors involved are genetic, environmental and ageing. The presence of Lewy bodies is diagnostic. Some symptoms are resistant to treatment and these include imbalance and postural instability, constipation, bladder dysfunction, pain, speech and psychological difficulties (Clough 1991). Drug treatment ranges from anticholinergic agents including benzhexol and orphenadrine; dopaminergic receptor agonists including bromocriptine, lysuride and pergolide; dopamine precursors including L-dopa monoamine oxidase B (MAO B) inhibitors such as selegiline. MAO B is responsible for the metabolism of dopamine in the brain and has little effect on MAO A which is present in the gut. No special precautions are necessary in the administration of selegiline regarding interactions with pethidine or catecholamines (Stewart & MacPhee 1991).

Migraine

Serotonin (5-HT) is involved in the pathophysiology of migraine. Sumatriptan is a selective agonist of $5-HT_1$-like receptor and is effective in treatment (The Subcutaneous Sumatriptan International Study Group 1991).

Depression

The various types of depression and treatment are reviewed by Potter et al (1991). Depression which may include melancholia is associated with psychotic features. Attempts to correlate biochemical stress with treatment are still unsatisfactory. Many patients have abnormalities of the pituitary, adrenal, thyroid and growth hormone. There may be abnormalities in sleep pattern including prolongation of rapid eye movement sleep. Therapy has involved tricyclic antidepressant drugs and MAO inhibitors: some drugs affect the MAO A type, some B type and others both. Newly introduced drugs selectively inhibit 5-HT uptake — such as fluoxetine which has a long half-life — can cause anxiety and interact with tricyclic agents; benzodiazepines are not particularly valuable. Other drugs have fewer side-effects such as anticholinergic actions, insomnia or cardiac arrhythmias but they produce other hazards. Maprotiline, which has a long half-life, may cause seizures. Amoxapine blocks dopamine D_2-receptors and may produce extrapyramidal lesions. Alprazolam is addictive while bupropion results in insomnia, tremor and psychosis.

Neuroleptic malignant syndrome

This involves the extrapyramidal system and occurs following the administration of neuroleptic drugs. Symptoms include akathisia, dystonia, parkinsonism and dyskinesia. The syndrome is not only related to drugs but also to organic brain damage, dehydration, exhaustion, external heat load and excessive sympathetic stimulation. The incidence of drug-induced dyskinesia is about 30% following prolonged treatment with neuroleptic agents (Saltz et al 1991). Renwick et al (1992) described a case of neuroleptic malignant syndrome where the high temperature and the alteration in patient's consciousness were confused by the fact that the patient had an infection which was thought to be the cause of the temperature. Nierenberg et al (1991) emphasized the need for prompt diagnosis. Fever, muscular rigidity, altered consciousness and autonomic dysfunction are diagnostic in a patient receiving a neuroleptic agent. Treatment consisted of withdrawing the neuroleptic agent, intravenous dantrolene and bromocriptine or dantrolene and levodopa or carbidopa (Ebadi et al 1990).

Neuroleptic malignant syndrome should not be confused with malignant hyperthermia where genetic screening may reveal patients who are susceptible (Ellis 1992). Heat stroke may also be related to abnormality of the skeletal muscle which is not identical to that of malignant hyperthermia (Hopkins et al 1991) (p. 227).

ANTIEMETICS

The use of the 5-HT$_3$ receptor antagonist, ondansetron (Zofran), appears to be effective in reducing vomiting in patients receiving highly emetic chemotherapy for cancer (Dundee et al 1992). Side-effects include headache, constipation or diarrhoea, transient elevation of serum liver enzymes but no extrapyramidal reactions (Drug and Therapeutics Bulletin 1992). Ondansetron now has a product licence and is effective even if given orally prior to operation (Kenny et al 1992). It is also claimed that a single dose of 4 mg intravenously prior to induction is also efficacious.

MacDonald (1991) has drawn attention to the drug interactions of metoclopramide and domperidone but neither antagonized the effects of dopamine on the kidney. Metoclopramide causes a marked rise and domperidone a small fall in aldosterone concentration. Metoclopramide reduces blood pressure and leads to a loss of potassium. It also has effects on adenosine triphosphate and plasma cholinesterase. In patients with hepatic cirrhosis there is a reduced clearance (Albani et al 1991).

H$_2$-receptors

Cimetidine binds to cytochrome P450 and inhibits the activity of microsomal enzymes. It is said to potentiate the activity of warfarin, but this effect may have been overstated as warfarin is a racemic mixture and cimetidine affects the clearance of the less active R-enantiomer (Niopas et al 1991). There is a possibility that H$_2$-receptor blockers may cause central nervous system toxicity including hallucinations, disorientation, confusion and irritability (Cantu and Korek 1991).

Omeprazole, which is a specific inhibitor of H^+K^+ adenosine triphosphatase or the proton pump, blocks acid secretion to all stimuli and is more effective in this respect than H$_2$-receptor blockers. It binds to cytochrome P450 and inhibits the oxidation of drugs such as phenytoin (Howden 1991).

KIDNEY

Acute renal failure

Acute renal failure occurs when there is an increase in plasma creatinine concentration by 5.65 mmol/l (0.5 mg/dl) or more if the baseline level is less than 34 mmol/l (3 mg/dl). If the baseline level is above 34 mmol/l (3 mg/dl) the level should be increased by 11.3 mmol/l (1 mg/dl). The causes of acute renal failure are prerenal, acute tubular necrosis, glomerular disease, urinary obstruction, valves and tubulointerstitial disorders. Most of the cases are due to prerenal disorders or tubular necrosis. Renal failure is not uncommon following surgery for obstructive jaundice. Antihypertensive drugs decrease systemic blood pressure, resulting in a decrease in glomerular pressure and in this respect angiotensin converting enzyme inhibitors may be particularly involved as they cause pronounced vasodilation of the efferent arterioles, as a result of which there is a pronounced decrease in glomerular capillary pressure. Even a single dose of 6.25 mg of captopril can result in a fall in urinary output and an increase in serum creatinine. The prior administration of a diuretic may augment this effect (Rahn 1991).

Acute tubular necrosis may be caused by nephrotoxins such as aminoglycosides, haem pigments or profound haemorrhage. The epithelium of the proximal tubule becomes flattened and the limb of Henle and distal convoluted tubule become dilated. The three mechanisms that contribute to tubular necrosis leading to a decrease in glomerular filtration rate may be due to tubular obstruction by cellular debris, a back-leak of filtrate through the damaged tubule or changes in haemodynamics in the renal vessels. As there is diminished tubular sodium reabsorption there may be an increase in renin which causes vasoconstriction of the afferent arteriole. Diuretics appear to wash out the tubular obstruction but unfortunately diuretics are often given once there is established acute tubular necrosis. The place of atrial natriuretic hormone (ANH), which is a potent vasodilator, has still to be evaluated.

Amoroso & Brunner (1992), in a survey of the management of acute renal failure in the critically ill patient, found that continuous arteriovenous haemofiltration and haemodialysis were the most popular methods of treatment. There may be a place for the ANH analogue in the future for animal experiments have shown that it can improve glomerular and tubular function in acute renal failure induced by cisplatin (Pollock et al 1991). Diuretics and mannitol are said to prevent renal failure before renal damage occurs but are ineffectual if administered afterwards. Experimental studies suggest that ANH is able to improve glomerular filtration rate even when ischaemic renal injury has taken place (Lieberthal 1990). Pain et al (1991) advocate adequate preoperative hydration as well as preoperative administration of lactulose or sodium deoxycholate, which decreases the incidence of portal and systemic endotoxaemia.

Chronic renal failure (CRF)

El Nahas & Wight (1991) reviewed some aspects of CRF. They maintain the time has come to reassess the value of low-protein diets as well as the value of restricting phosphate. Hyperlipidaemia is common in CRF but whether reduction in lipid levels affects the progression of renal disease is still unproven. Even management of hypertension with angiotensin converting enzyme inhibitors, calcium antagonists, antiplatelet drugs and anticoagulants is still far from conclusive. Anti-inflammatory agents reduce proteinuria but they can cause renal damage, as prostaglandins which have a vasodilator action are necessary to maintain renal function and protstaglandin E_1 appears promising in this respect. The result of immunosuppressive drugs are inconclusive and the various therapies that have been advocated in the management of CRF have still to undergo carefully controlled clinical trials.

Not widely appreciated is the fact that patients with CRF have reduced lung carbon monoxide transfer which is further reduced in those patients having dialysis. Following transplantation there was no improvement and in fact residual volume was also decreased. The reasons are probably that there is pulmonary oedema which is not readily detected and which leads to pulmonary fibrosis (Bush & Gabriel 1991). An endogenous inhibitor of nitric oxide (asymmetrical dimethylarginine) is excreted in the urine but in end-stage chronic renal failure as it is not excreted it inhibits nitric oxide synthesis, resulting in hypertension and dysfunction of the immune system (Vallance et al 1992). Endothelin, a vasoconstrictor, also constricts the afferent arteriole leading to an increase in glomerular filtration rate and is involved in the tubular glomerular feedback control mechanism (Takabatake et al 1991). In CRF there is decreased urine excretion of ammonia resulting in acid–base imbalance. The rate of ammonia excretion is greater than expected in view of the diminution in renal size and Dass & Kurtz (1990) have suggested there are other sources for urinary nitrogen including the metabolism of glutamine.

Physiology

In the distal tubule and collecting duct antidiuretic hormone stimulates and adrenaline (beta-adrenergic action) inhibits potassium secretion. Adrenaline may also increase reabsorption of sodium either by direct effect or due to its cardiovascular action (Honrath et al 1990). There are now two types of adenosine receptors within some membranes, A_1 and A_2, which account for the cardiovascular actions of the drug. Stimulation of A_1-receptors produces negative chrono- and inotropic effects upon the heart while A_2 receptors are responsible for vasodilatation and lowering blood pressure. Levens et al (1991) found that the adenosine agonist acting on A_2-receptors has a direct effect on renal haemodynamics but does not affect urine volume, sodium excretion or renin release. It is also possible that adenosine acts as a mediator in the juxtaglomerular apparatus (JGA) (Osswald et al 1991) especially as local blood flow is important (Skott et al 1991). These results are due to advances in morphology of the JGA (Rosivall et al 1991). It has even been shown there are now two components involved in the autoregulation of renal blood flow, one of low frequency and one of high frequency, the latter being due to intrinsic vascular myogenic mechanisms (Holstein-Rathlou et al 1991, Marsh et al 1991). Acute hyperkalaemia can cause renal vasodilatation and stimulate renin release either by direct action on the JGA or by affecting the delivery of fluid and sodium to the macula densa (Lin et al 1991).

Diuretics

Acetazolamide reduces blood volume leading to isosmotic hypovolaemia with intracellular volume expansion, resulting in metabolic acidosis (Brechue et al 1990). It increases the excretion of bicarbonate, sodium, potassium acids and ammonia.

Another interesting observation is that the upright posture reduces by 50% the diuretic action and loss of sodium and chloride in response to frusemide. This is probably due to greater activation of kallikrein in the supine position and less activation of plasma noradrenaline which is antinatriuretic (Okaniwa et al 1990). For the detailed discussion of atrial pressure and natriuresis see Firth et al (1990). For assessment of the role of peptides in the regulation of the micturition reflex see Maggi (1991).

Transplantation

The transplanted kidney may also suffer tubular damage, in particular the excretion of potassium. The use of diuretics such as frusemide and metolazone may uncover subclinical defects in secretion (Gehr et al 1991).

Morphine

It has been assumed that the antidiuretic effect of morphine has been due to mu-activity. Rimoy et al (1991) have demonstrated that spiradoline, a kappa agonist, reduces diuresis and the urine has a reduced osmolality. The mechanism is still unclear but it does not involve the antagonism of antidiuretic hormone or affect the renal blood flow. The effect is antagonized by naloxone in high doses.

REFERENCES

Agid Y 1991 Parkinson's disease: pathophysiology. Lancet 337: 1321–1324
Albani E A, Tame M R, De Palma R, Bernardi M 1991 Kinetics of intravenous metoclopramide in patients with hepatic cirrhosis. Eur J Clin Pharmacol 40: 423–425
Alberti K G M M, Thomas D J B 1979 The management of diabetes during surgery. Br J Anaesth 51: 693–710
Amoroso P, Brunner M 1992 Acute renal failure. Survey of the management of acute renal failure in the critically ill in England and Wales. Intensive Care 10: 92–97
Baethmann A, Kempski O 1991 The brain in shock. Secondary disturbances of cerebral function. Chest 100 (suppl): 205S–208S
Baydur A 1991 Respiratory muscle strength and control of ventilation in patients with neuromuscular disease. Chest 99: 330–338
Benzi G, Pastoris O, Marzatico F, Dagani F 1990 Influence of aging and drug treatment on the bioenergetics of hypoxic brain. Neurochem Res 15: 659–665
Bjorck S, Mulec H, Johnsen S A et al 1992 Renal protective effect of enalapril in diabetic nephropathy. Br Med J 304: 339–343.
Bouma G J, Muizelaar P 1990 Relationship between cardiac output and cerebral blood flow in patients with intact and with impaired autoregulation. J Neurosurg 73: 368–374
Brechue W F, Stager J M, Lukaski H C 1990 Body water and electrolyte responses to acetazolamide in humans. J Appl Physiol 69: 1397–1401

Bush A, Gabriel R 1991 Pulmonary function in chronic renal failure: effects of dialysis and transplantation. Thorax 46: 424–428

Cantu T G, Korek J S 1991 Central nervous system reactions to histamine-2 receptor blockers. Ann Intern Med 114: 1027–1034

Chertow B S, Kadzielawa B, Burger A J 1991 Benign pleural effusions in long-standing diabetes mellitus. Chest 99: 1108–1111

Clough C G 1991 Parkinson's disease: managment. Lancet 337: 1324–1327

Dass P D, Kurtz I 1990 Renal ammonia and bicarbonate production in chronic renal failure. Miner Electrolyte Metabolism 16: 308–314

Daugirdas J T, Kronfol N O, Tzamaloukas A H, Ing T 1989 Hyperosmolar coma: cellular dehydration and the serum sodium concentration. Ann Intern Med 110: 855–857

Davis K R, Gelb A W, Maie P H et al 1991 Cardiac fuction in aneurysmal subarachnoid haemorrhage: a study or electrocardiographic and echocardiographic abnormalities.

Demitrack M A, Dale J K, Straus S E et al 1991 Evidence for impaired activation of the hypothalamic–pituitary–adrenal axis in patients with chronic fatigue syndrome. J Clin Endocrinol Metab 73: 1224–1234

Diem P, Robertson R P 1991 Preventive effects of octreotide (SMS 201–995) on diabetic ketogenesis during insulin withdrawal. Br J Clin Pharmacol 32: 563–567

Drug and Therapeutics Bulletin 1992 Ondansetron to prevent chemotherapy-induced vomiting. Drug Ther Bull 30: 21–24

Dundee J W, McMillan C M, Yang J, Wright P M C 1992 Is ondansetron a less effective antiemetic against moderately emetic as compared with highly emetic chemotherapy? Br J Clin Pharmacol 33: 200–201

Dunnet J M, Holman R R, Turner R C, Sear J W 1988 Diabetes mellitus and anaesthesia. A survey of the perioperative management of the patient with diabetes mellitus. Anaesthesia 43: 538–542

Ebadi M, Pfeiffer R F, Murri L C 1990 Pathogenesis and treatment of neuroleptic malignant syndrome. Gen Pharmacol 21: 367–386

Eckardt V F, Nix W 1991 The anal sphincter in patients with myotonic muscular dystrophy. Gastroenterology 100: 424–430

Editorial 1991 Hypoglycaemia and diabetes control. Lancet 338: 853–855

Egger M, Davey Smith G, Hans Imhoof, Teuscher A 1991a Risk of severe hypoglycaemia in insulin treated diabetic patients transferred to human insulin a case control study. Br Med J 303: 617–621

Egger M, Smith G D, Teuscher A U, Teuscher A 1991b Influence of human insulin on symptoms and awareness of hypoglycaemia: a randomised double blind crossover trial. Br Med J 303: 622–624

Ellis F 1992 Detecting susceptibility to malignant hyperthermia. Br Med J 304: 791–792

El Nahas A M, Wight J P 1991 The management of chronic renal failure: 10 unanswered questions. Q J Med 81: 799–809

Firth J D, Raine A E G, Ledingham J G G 1990 The mechanism of pressure natriuresis. J Hypertens 8: 97–103

Galloway J A 1990 Treatment of NIDDM with insulin agonists of substitutes. Diabetes Care 13: 1209–1239

Gay P, Westbrook P R, Daube J R et al 1991 Effects of alterations in pulmonary function and sleep variables on survival in patients with amyotrophic lateral sclerosis. Mayo Clin Proc 66: 686–694

Gehr T W B, Sica D A, Brater D C et al 1991 Metolazone pharmacokinetics and pharmacodynamics in renal transplantation. Int J Clin Pharmacol 29: 116–123

Gill G V, Alberti K G M M 1991 Outcome of brittle diabetes. Br Med J 303: 285–286

Holstein-Rathlou N-H, Wagner A J, Marsh D J 1991 Dynamics of renal blood flow autoregulation in rats. Kidney Int 39 (suppl 32): S98–S101

Honrath U, Wilson, D R, Sonnenberg H 1990 The effect of isoproterenol on fluid and electrolyte transport in the inner medullary collecting duct. Can J Physiol Pharmacol 69: 771–775

Hopkins P M, Ellis F R, Halsall P J 1991 Evidence for related myopathies in exertional heat stroke and malignant hyperthermia. Lancet 338: 1491–1492

Horner J, Massey W, Brazer S R 1990 Aspiration in bilateral stroke patients. Neurology 40: 1686–1688

Howden C W 1991 Clinical pharmacology of omeprazole. Clin Pharmacokinet 20: 38–49

Jakobsen M, Eevoldsen E, Bjerre P 1990 Cerebral blood flow and metabolism following subarachnoid haemorrhage: cerebral oxygen uptake and global blood flow during the acute period in patients with SAH. Acta Neurol Scand 82: 174–182

Kelly B J, Luce J M 1991 The diagnosis and management of neuromuscular diseases causing respiratory failure. Chest 99: 1485–1494

Kenny G N C, Oates J D L, Leeser J et al 1992 Efficacy of orally administered ondansetron in the prevention of postoperative nausea and vomiting: a dose ranging study. Br J Anaesth 68: 466–470

Kobayashi H, Hayashi M, Handa Y et al 1990 Role of adrenergic activity in ischemic brain edema. In: Long D et al (eds) Advances in neurology vol 52. Raven Press; New York, Raven pp 127–132

Kollind M, Moberg E, Lins P E, Adamson U 1990 Exogenous somatostatin raises plasma insulin levels in patients with insulin-dependent diabetes mellitus. Horm Metab Res 22: 581–583

Krum H, Brown D J, Rowe P R, Louis W J, Howes L G 1990 Steady state plasma [^{3}H]-noradrenaline kinetics in quadriplegic chronic spinal cord injury patients. J Autonomic Pharmacol 10: 221–226

Laychock S G 1990 Glucose metabolism, second messengers and insulin secretion. Life Sci 47: 2307–2316

Leading article 1991 Understanding diabetic neuropathy. Lancet 338: 1496–1497

Levens N, Beil M, Schulz R 1991 Intrarenal actions of the new adenosine agonist CGS 21680A, selective for the A_2 receptor. J Pharmacol Exp Ther 257: 1013–1019

Levin H, Heifetz M 1990 Phaeochromocytoma and severe protracted postoperative hypoglycaemia. Can J Anaesth 37: 477–478

Lieberthal W 1990 Effects of atrial natriuretic factor in ischemic renal injury. Studies in the isolated erythrocyte-perfused rat kidney. Clin Res 8: 157–165

Lin H, Young D B, Smith M J 1991 Stimulation of renin release by hyperkalemia in the nonfiltering kidney. Am J Physiol 260: 170–176

Maccioni F J, Colebatch H J J 1991 Lung volume and distensibility in insulin-dependent diabetes mellitus. Am Rev Respir Dis 143: 1253–1256

MacDonald T M 1991 Metoclopramide, domperidone and dopamine in man: actions and interactions. Eur J Clin Pharmacol 40: 225–230

Maggi C A 1990 The role of peptides in the regulation of the micturition reflex. An update. Gen Pharmacol 22: 1–14

Mak V H F, Chapman F, James C, Spiro S G 1991 Sternomastoid muscle twitch maximum relaxation rate: prolonged slowing with fatigue and post-tetanic acceleration. Clin Sci 81: 669–676

Marsh D J, Yip K-P, Källskog O, Holstein-Rathlou N-H 1991 Oscillations and more complex dynamics in tubuloglomerular feedback. Kidney Int 39 (suppl 32): S94–S97

Milaskiewicz R M, Hall G M 1992 Diabetes and anaesthesia: the past decade. Br J Anaesth 68: 198–206

Mogensen C E 1992 Angiotensin converting enzyme inhibitors and diabetic nephropathy. Br Med J 304: 327–328

Moller D E, Flier J S 1991 Insulin resistance — mechanisms, syndromes, and implications. N Engl J Med 325: 938–948

Nierenberg D, Disch M, Manheimer E et al 1991 Facilitating prompt diagnosis and treatment of the neuroleptic malignant syndrome. Clin Pharmacol Ther 50: 580–586

Nilsson P, Lindholm L, Schersten B 1990 Hyperinsulinaemia and other metabolic disturbances in well-controlled hypertensive men and women: an epidemiological study of the Dalby population. J Hypertens 8: 953–959

Niopas I, Toon S, Rowland M 1991 Further insight into the stereoselective interaction between warfarin and cimetidine in man. Br J Clin Pharmacol 32: 508–511

Norris J W, Krajewski A, Bronstein N M 1990 The clinical role of the cerebral collateral circulation in carotid occlusion. J Vascular Surg 12: 113–118

O'Brien I A, McFadden J P, Corrall R J M 1991 The influence of autonomic neuropathy on mortality in insulin-dependent diabetes. Q J Med 79: 495–502

Oh M S, Carroll H J, Uribarri J 1990 Mechanism of normochloremic and hyperchloremic acidosis in diabetic ketoacidosis. Nephron 54: 1–6

Okaniwa T, Exhizen H, Ishizaki T et al 1990 Pharmacodynamic characterization of posture-related diuretic and saluretic responses to furosemide in humans. J Pharmacol Exp Ther 255: 716–723

Osswald H, Muhlbauer B, Schenk F 1991 Adenosine mediates tubuloglomerular feedback response. An element of metabolic control of kidney function. Kidney Int 39 (suppl 32): S128–S131

Pain J A, Cahill C J, Johnson C D et al 1991 Prevention of postoperative renal dysfunction in patients with obstructive jaundice: a multicentre study of bile salts and lactulose. Br J Surg 78: 467–469

Patrick A W, Bodmer C W, Tieszen K L et al Human insulin and awareness of acute hypoglycaemic symptoms in insulin-dependent diabetes. Lancet 338: 528–532

Pollock D M, Holst M, Opgenorth T J 1991 Effect of the ANF analog A68828 in cisplatin-induced acute renal failure. J Pharmacol Exp Ther 257: 1179–1183

Polonsky K S 1992 A practical approach to fasting hypoglycemia. N Engl J Med 326: 1020–1021

Potter W Z, Rudorfer M V, Manji H 1991 The pharmacologic treatment of depression. N Engl J Med 325: 633–642

Pulsinelli W 1992 Pathophysiology of acute ischaemic stroke. Lancet 339: 533–536

Qizilbash N, Jones L, Warlow C, Mann J 1991 Fibrinogen and lipid concentrations as risk factors for transient ischaemic attacks and minor ischaemic strokes. Br J 303: 605–609

Rahn K H 1991 Acute disturbances of renal function. Chest 100: 197S–199S

Redmon B, Pyzdrowski K L, Elson M K et al 1992 Brief report: hypoglycemia due to a monoclonal insulin-binding antibody in multiple myeloma. N Engl J Med 326: 994–998

Reissell E, Orko R, Maunuksela E-L, Lindgren L 1990 Predictability of difficult laryngoscopy in patients with long-term diabetes mellitus. Anesthesia 45: 1024–1227

Renwick D S, Chandraker A, Bannister P 1992 Missed neuroleptic malignant syndrome. Br Med J 304: 831–832

Riley L J, Cooper M, Narins R G 1989 Alkali therapy of diabetic ketoacidosis: biochemical, phsyiologic, and clinical perspectives. Diabetes/Metab Rev 5: 627–636

Rimoy G H, Bhaskar N K, Wright D M, Rubin P C 1991 Mechanism of diuretic action of spiradoline (U-62066E) — kappa opioid receptor agonist in the human. Br J Clin Pharmacol 32: 611–615

Rodriguez J R, Castillo J, Leira R et al 1991 Bone anomalies in myotonic dystrophy. Acta Neurol Scand 83: 360–363

Rosenn B, Tsang R C 1991 The effects of maternal diabetes on the fetus and neonate. Ann Clin Lab Sci 21: 153–170

Ropper A H 1992 The Guillain–Barré syndrome. N Engl J Med 326: 1130–1136

Rosivall L, Razga Z, Ormos J 1991 Morphological characterization of human juxtaglomerular apparatus. Kidney Int 39 (suppl 32): S9–S12

Rothrock J F, Hart R G 1991 Antithrombotic therapy in cerebrovascular disease. Ann Intern Med 115: 885–895

Saltz B L, Woerner M G, Kane J M et al 1991 Prospective study of tardive dyskinesia incidence in the elderly. JAMA 266: 2402–2406

Sandercock P 1991 Recent developments in the diagnosis and management of patients with transient ischaemic attacks and minor ischaemic strokes. Q J Med 78: 101–112

Sandstrom P-E 1990 Bumetanide reduces insulin release by a direct effect on the pancreatic B-cells. Eur J Pharmacol 187: 377–383

Serri O, Beauregard H, Brazeau P et al 1991 Somatostatin analogue, octreotide, reduces increased glomerular filtration rate and kidney size in insulin-dependent diabetes. JAMA 265: 888–892

Skott O, Salomonsson M, Persson A E G, Jensen B L 1991 Mechanisms of renin release from juxtaglomerular cells. Kidney Int 39 (suppl 32): S16–S19

Smith M C, Riskin B J 1991 The clinical use of barbiturates in neurological disorders. Drugs 42: 365–378

Stewart D A, MacPhee G J A 1991 New drugs in Parkinson's disease. Hosp Update, November: 900–913

Sutton L, Mclaughlin A C, Dante S et al 1990 Cerebral venous oxygen content as a measure of brain energy metabolism with increased intracranial pressure and hyperventilation. J Neuros 73: 927–932

Takabatake T, Ise T, Ohta K, Kobayashi K-I 1991 Endothelin effects on renal function and tubuloglomerular feedback. Kidney Int 39 (suppl 32): S122–S124

The Subcutaneous Sumatriptan International Study Group 1991 Treatment of migraine attacks with sumatriptan. N Engl J Med 325: 316–321

Ting P 1990 Indomethacin attenuates early postischemic vasogenic edema and cerebral injury. In: Long D et al (eds) Advances in neurology vol 52. Raven Press, New York; pp 119–126

Vallance P, Leone A, Calver A et al 1992 Accumulation of an endogenous inhibitor of nitric oxide synthesis in chronic renal failure. Lancet 339: 572–575

Wessely S 1992 The measurement of fatigue and chronic fatigue syndrome. J R Soc Med 85: 189–190

Winer J 1992 Guillain–Barré syndrome revisited. Br Med J 304: 65–66

Wood C, Magnello M E, Sharpe M C 1992 Fluctuations in perceived energy and mood among patients with chronic fatigue syndrome. J R Soc Med 85: 195–198

4. Applied physiology in intensive care

N. Soni

Intensive care is a young specialty evolving as a practical response to supporting patients in respiratory failure and then progressing to encompass support of not only the respiratory system but most other organ systems. In that regard the development of intensive care has been an interesting association between providing immediate practical care in order to sustain life and the acquisition of knowledge and techniques to diagnose and treat the cause of the problem and to recognize and anticipate associated pathology. While pattern recognition is still an important aspect of intensive care, understanding the physiology and pathophysiology of both the illness and the treatments is increasingly the key to diagnosis and management.

It could be said that intensive care is an exercise in applied physiology and well beyond the scope of a chapter. It is the purpose of this chapter to look at some areas of intensive care practice where the understanding of the physiology behind the problem has enabled either more appropriate management of the patient to take place or at least allows an objective assessment of the value of various treatment modalities.

SODIUM METABOLISM

Abnormalities of extracellular sodium concentration are common in hospital and often a reason for intensive care referral. Empirical treatment of the numbers is a recipe for disaster and a physiological appraisal is essential. The problems are most easily addressed in terms of hypo- and hypernatraemia.

Hyponatraemia

For the purpose of this discussion artefactual causes of hyponatraemia, pseudohyponatraemia, such as hyperlipidaemia, will not be discussed as in these situations it is the measurement system not the distribution of sodium which provides the problem.

Hyponatraemia is a low concentration of sodium in the blood although as this is in equilibrium with the extracellular space it would be more appropriately described as the extracellular concentration. Under normal circumstances a fall in serum sodium is associated with a fall in osmolality and

this results in the suppression of antidiuretic hormone (ADH) and consequently a water diuresis, which will tend to correct the hyponatraemia (Fig.
4.1).

Failure of these mechanisms and persistence of hyponatraemia are usually
due to excess retention of water, excess administration of water or a
combination of the two, or alternatively salt loss. It can also occur from rapid
shifts of water out of cells into the extracellular space or alternatively sodium
into the intracellular space. Translated to the common presentations, the
causes of excessive water intake include polydipsia and iatrogenic water
administration. Water retention results from failure to excrete water through
the kidneys either due to renal failure or, less commonly, inappropriate ADH
production. These all result in increased intravascular volume (Table 4.1).

Volume deficit, especially arterial volume depletion, activates the renin
angiotensin system and ADH secretion via arterial baroreceptors in the
carotid sinus and the juxtaglomerular apparatus. The stimulus provided by
volume depletion will over-ride input both from capacitance vessel baroreceptors and from osmoreceptors. The net result will be retention of salt and
water. There will be low glomerular filtration, low tubular flow and the
production of concentrated low sodium urine. This is seen with congestive

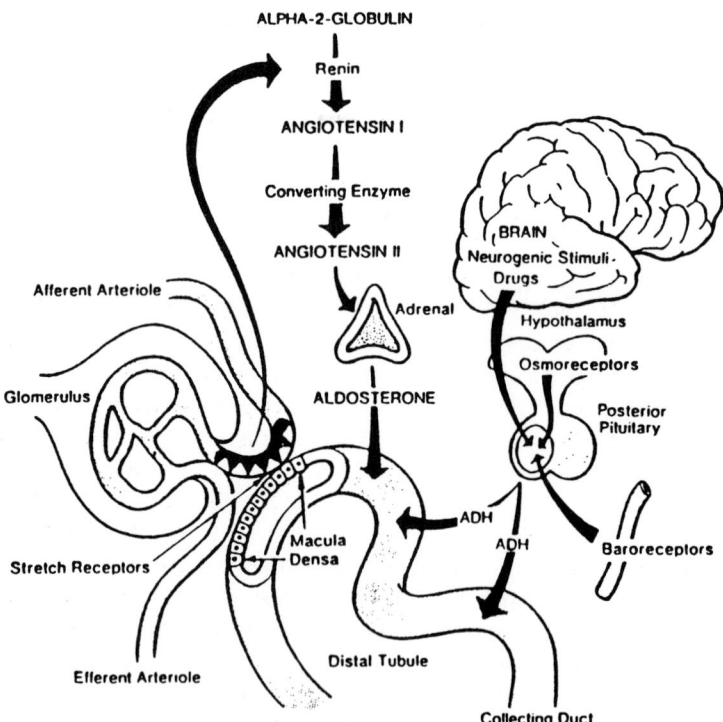

Fig. 4.1 Endocrine control of renal function. ADH = Antidiuretic hormone. Reproduced
with permission from Cousins & Skowronski (1990).

Table 4.1 Causes of hyponatraemia

Pseudohyponatraemia
   Hyperlipidaemia
   Hyperproteinaemia
Low arterial volume:
   Congestive cardiac failure
   Cirrhosis
   Nephrotic syndrome
   Sodium depletion
Normal arterial volume
   Polydipsia
   Iatrogenic water administration
   Renal failure
   Inappropriate antidiuretic hormone
Presence of solutes producing high serum osmolality, low sodium
   Mannitol
   Glucose

cardiac failure and cirrhosis. The patients have arterial volume depletion despite obvious oedema, which implies excessive salt and water retention, but still attempt to replete the intravascular volume and thereby the arterial volume by further salt and water retention.

Evaluation of patients with hyponatraemia may be difficult. The volume of urine being passed is crucial to accurate assessment. If the patient is clinically dehydrated, there will be little urine but it will be very concentrated. Excessive water intake will usually be matched by a large volume of dilute urine, appropriately low in salt. In clinically overhydrated patients a low volume of urine with high urine osmolality implies an element of renal failure, potent and appropriate ADH effect, or potent but inappropriate ADH effect. If there is an element of renal failure involved it will influence the clinical picture and should be biochemically easy to determine by the normal indicators of renal function. The main difficulty arises in determining whether impaired renal excretion is due to appropriate release of ADH to protect intravascular, or more precisely arterial, volume or inappropriate with no physiological basis. The result of both will be overhydration. Inappropriate ADH secretion is occurring when there is no physiological drive for water retention. This may be seen as hyponatraemia with hypo-osmolality, low urine output and normal or increased intravascular volume.

Interpretation of the underlying cause of the hyponatraemia will lead to the appropriate approach for management of the problem. If the extracellular fluid is depleted then the correct management is to replete the volume status of the patient, preferably with salt-containing solution. It is important to note that there will be a tendency to try to retain salt which will lead to water retention if inadequate salt is given in the replacement fluid. In overhydrated hyponatraemic patients with high urine output, a situation commonly seen in surgical wards, then the easiest and safest means of addressing the problem is to restrict the excess free water that they are being given and which they have to excrete. Restricting water intake usually leads to gradual correction of the problem over a matter of a few days. This is the commonest cause of hyponatraemia in hospitals where elderly small patients are regularly given large volumes of low salt solutions, classically 5% dextrose or dextrose/saline.

If a more aggressive approach to hyponatraemia is required then loop diuretics can be used to remove fluid, both salt and water, and then sodium-containing solutions can be given to replace the salt. In some circumstances it is deemed necessary to correct hyponatraemia rapidly. The essential consideration is whether the problems associated with hyponatraemia, cerebral oedema and fitting, outweigh the problems associated with rapid correction. Rapid treatment involves giving hypertonic saline to correct the sodium problem immediately. There are several potential problems, the first being that in a patient who has developed hyponatraemia slowly equilibration will have occurred with redistribution of electrolytes and solutes across the intra- and extracellular compartments. Rapid infusion of a hyperosmolar solution could cause water movement out of the cell and cellular dehydration with acute volume changes, especially in the central nervous system. The second problem is fluid overload as the hypertonic fluid will induce extracellular shift of water and a rapid expansion of the extracellular compartments. The third problem is that there appears to be an association between rapid changing of sodium concentrations and the development of central pontine myelinosis (Sterns et al 1986).

To add further difficulty to the decision as to whether rapid or slow correction is advisable, the literature on the subject is equivocal with some studies suggesting that rapid correction carries a lower morbidity than sustained hyponatraemia and others suggesting that slow correction is better. Nevertheless, a basic understanding of how the hyponatraemia has occurred in the first instance and a correct interpretation of the volume status of the patient should lead to appropriate management. The most difficult group are those with inappropriate ADH secretion and the key to management is identifying those with the genuine syndrome (Rose 1986, Oh & Carroll 1992).

Hypernatraemia

Hypernatraemia is a high concentration of sodium in the extracellular compartment. It occurs for a variety of reasons, including a net gain of sodium, a loss of water or intracellular shift of either salt or water. Common examples of water loss occurring in intensive treatment units are the polyuric phase of renal failure, secondary water losses to an osmotic diuresis from drugs given intentionally — mannitol or radiological contrast media — or glycosuria occurring incidentally in the critically ill patient. The net result is a mandatory loss of water and a gradual increase in sodium concentration. This leads to a shift of water from the cells into the extracellular space and consequently a loss of cell volume. This may not be of great significance except in the brain where a reduction in cell volume will eventually result in a reduction in brain volume and this, if it occurs very rapidly, can result in potential damage with tearing of vessels. In general circumstances the hypernatraemia occurs relatively slowly and there is time for cell volume regulation to occur. Electrolytes, including sodium, move intracellularly, associated with the intracellular accumulation of various organic solutes, largely amino acids such as taurine. This mechanism produces an osmotic component intracellularly which helps to correct the osmotic gradient, thereby protecting the volume of the cell from acute changes. This mechanism becomes pertinent and potentially damaging if aggressive medical management involves rapid correction of the hypernatraemia by infusing large volumes of 'free' water which will result in rapid increase in cell size.

Diagnosis is relatively straightforward. Water depletion alone results in a low volume of high-osmolality urine as water is avidly retained. The most common problem seen in intensive care is water loss from an osmotic diuresis. This may be induced, as with mannitol, or acquired through the accumulation or excretion of an osmotically active solute such as urea or glucose. There will be a large volume of urine with osmolality tending to be in the intermediate range, created largely by the solute inducing the diuresis. Diabetes insipidus also results in large volumes of urine associated with water loss (Blevins & Wand 1992). The osmolality is almost invariably low. The mechanism of diabetes insipidus is relevant. Central, neurological diabetes insipidus causes failure of ADH secretion which may not be complete and which may therefore respond to fluid deprivation with a gradual increase in urine osmolality. The thirst mechanism is often intact and is triggered by rising osmolality, leading to increased water intake, and the kidneys remain sensitive to ADH so that exogenous ADH will be effective. Conversely in nephrogenic diabetes insipidus the kidneys are insensitive to ADH levels so that there is no mechanism for alteration of the urine concentration (Table 4.2).

Management of the problems relating of hypernatraemia really requires interpretation of the mechanism underlying its development. Water deprivation responds to water. If there is an osmotic diuresis then identification and clearance or reduction in the quantity of the solute will enable water replacement to be effective. Diabetes insipidus will respond to ADH if it is neurogenic but not if nephrogenic.

Table 4.2   Diagnosis of hypernatraemia

	Urine osmolality	
>700 mosm/L	700 mosm/L to Posm	< Posm
Insufficient water intake	Partial DI	Complete DI
	Renal failure	Congenital Nephrotic DI
	Loop diuretics	
Osmoreceptor	Acquired nephrotic DI	Severe acquired nephrotic DI
	Osmotic diuresis	

DI = Diabetes insipidus; Posm = Plasma osmolality.
Modified from Oh & Carroll (1992).

Correction of hyponatraemia should occur in the same manner in which the hyponatraemia presented. So that if it has presented rapidly then rapid correction is probably appropriate. Under most circumstances it occurs relatively slowly, in which case slow correction is advisable. In these patients equilibration will have occurred between the intra- and extracellular space and if large volumes of fluid are then given there will be large water shifts intracellularly. The brain may be vulnerable to these fluid shifts. Management in these patients should follow interpretation of the physiological mechanism by which fluid has being lost, correction of the cause where possible and then correction of the hypernatraemia at an appropriate pace.

RENAL FAILURE

Acute renal failure in the intensive care unit is a relatively common problem but while there are many varieties of renal failure, acute tubular necrosis is the most common (Table 4.3). This is usually in association with either an ischaemic or nephrotoxic insult or a combination of the two. Indeed in many circumstances in intensive treatment units it may be a relatively mild ischaemic insult which becomes significant because of the presence of nephrotoxic substances, a traditional example being the aminoglycosides.

The vulnerability of the kidney to ischaemia is often overlooked. While 20% of cardiac output goes through the kidneys only 6% of this passes through the medulla which consequently has an excessively high oxygen extraction but a low oxygen tension. The thick ascending tubule, metabolically very active, is in the medulla and is therefore very vulnerable to ischaemia.

The development of ischaemic renal failure can be looked at as passing through various phases depending on the speed of onset and magnitude of the ischaemic insult. The first phase involves the insult triggering physiological mechanisms which are designed to protect the body against a reduction in intravascular and extracellular volumes. There is a reduction in renal perfusion and within the kidney there are attempts to conserve salt and water in order to maintain the integrity of the intravascular volume. The ischaemic insult is manifest as a combination of reduced oxygen delivery, lower blood flow, associated with increased metabolic activity, and hence oxygen demand, as the tubules strive to retain salt and water. As blood pressure falls and renal perfusion is reduced ADH and aldosterone are released to inhibit salt and water loss. There is diversion of blood flow with reduced cortical perfusion and hence glomerular filtration. As filtration decreases the resorption necessary within the ascending tubule is reduced. The oxygen requirements of the ascending tubule are reduced, protecting it from ischaemic damage. Therefore the consequence of these attempts to conserve salt and water will be initially an increase in metabolic activity as sodium is actively resorbed; this will be replaced by a fall in activity as glomerular filtration and thereby the quantity of filtrate presented to the tubules decreases and hence oxygen

Table 4.3   Causes of acute renal failure

Postischaemic acute renal failure
Nephrotoxic acute renal failure
Prerenal azotaemia
Vascular occlusion
   Thromboembolic disease
   Dissecting aortic aneurysms
   Renal artery stenosis
Renal vein thrombosis
   Dehydration (infants)
   Hypercoagulable states
   Neoplasms
Urinary obstruction (postrenal azotaemia)
   Intrarenal abnormalities
   Ureteral obstruction
   Diseases of bladder or urethra
Cortical necrosis
   Gram-negative sepsis
   Abruptio placentae
   Placenta praevia
   Renal allograft rejection
Papillary necrosis
   Diabetes mellitus
   Sickle cell disease
   Analgesic nephropathy
Thrombotic microangiopathy
   Thrombotic thrombocytopenic purpura
   Haemolytic–uraemic syndrome
   Postpartum renal failure
   Scleroderma
   Malignant hypertension
Glomerulonephritis
Acute interstitial nephritis
   Hypersensitivity reactions
   Immunological disorders
   Infections

requirements fall. here will be a reduction in urine volume and low urinary sodium but the osmolality of the urine will be high as there is still a mandatory requirement to excrete waste products such as urea. It is important to note that while creatinine and urea are both passed through the glomerulus only urea is resorbed to any extent. The rate of resorption is determined in part by tubular fluid flow so that as the urine flow through the tubules falls the amount of urea being resorbed increases. Consequently as urine flow falls a disparity will arise between the apparent urea and creatinine clearances. This can be accentuated by other changes occurring elsewhere in the body, as for example a urea load from blood in the gastrointestinal tract.

This scenario implies a gradual development of a prerenal problem but often in critical illness changes in intravascular volume or renal perfusion occur rapidly. If there is major haemodynamic alteration, as might occur in a shocked patient with a very significant or total reduction in renal blood flow, then ischaemic injury to the cells within the tubules will occur. Inevitably a fall in glomerular filtration will reduce the metabolic work of the tubules but the major insult will be a global loss of oxygen supply. Low blood flow also results in erythrocyte sludging in the medullary vessels accentuating endothelial cell oedema, which contributes further to impaired flow and ischaemia. The ischaemic cells within the tubules will fail to achieve their normal metabolic functions and will be unable to concentrate urine. This functional deterioration is followed later by cell death and tubule blockage with debris. This produces back-pressure inhibiting glomerular filtration. Analysis of the urine will show reduced urea and creatinine concentrations and blood concentrations of these substances will rise. The damaged cells have impaired or no function and the tubules will pass an ultrafiltrate and urine osmolality will fall.

In the early phases of acute tubular necrosis there are methods of differentiating prerenal failure from tubule damage which are logically derived from the interpretation of these pathophysiological events. An example of this would be the use of fractional excretion of sodium which will reflect tubule function.

$$FE_{Na} = \frac{U_{Na} \cdot P_{Cr}}{U_{Cr} \cdot P_{Na}} \times 100$$

where FE_{Na} is fractional excretion of sodium, usually less than 1 in prerenal failure and in the order of >3 in renal failure, U_{Na} is urinary count of sodium and P_{Cr} is plasma count of chromium.

The fractional excretion of sodium would be high in patients with functional damage who are unable actively to conserve sodium, and low in those who are producing a physiological response to hypovolaemia.

There can be functional damage without oliguria, a condition described as non-oliguric renal failure. In this circumstance the tubular cells are ineffective and the urine volume is sustained although the concentration ability is grossly impaired. This generally implies a lower degree of damage than if there is oliguric renal failure as there must be both glomerular filtration and tubular patency if the patient is non-oliguric. It may also be a feature of the recovery phase as tubular patency and filtration precede full cellular function. The recovering kidney is not homogeneous and the range of damage occurring across the tubules within the kidneys is extremely variable. This can be demonstrated as the patient enters the diuretic phase with more recruitment of tubules which become firstly patent and then develop their normal metabolic function and concentrating ability (Fig. 4.2).

The management of renal failure leads directly from the physiological appraisal of how the renal damage occurs. The concept of a hypoxic injury caused by a fall in oxygen supply in the face of ongoing metabolic demand provides two potential therapeutic approaches. The first is avoidance of a reduction in oxygen supply by maintenance of renal perfusion, or if the insult has already occurred, to re-establish or ensure adequate perfusion and thereby

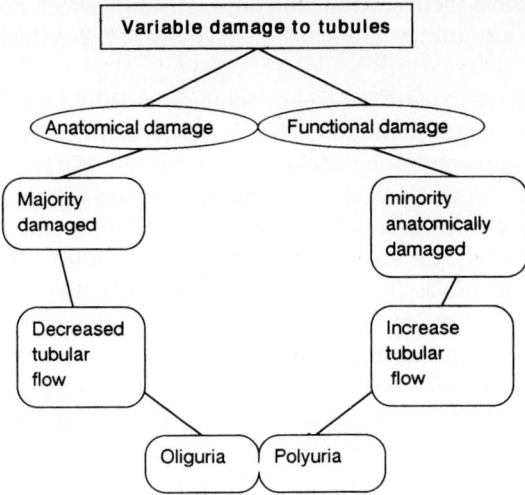

Fig. 4.2 Oliguric and polyuric renal failure.

avoid potentiating the injury. The second is the early use of agents to reduce metabolic activity and reduce the oxygen requirement — cytoprotection (Finn 1990).

Renal perfusion is dependent on an adequate intravascular and extracellular volume in association with optimal cardiovascular function. In many circumstances, early in the evolution of tubular necrosis, this alone will result in reversal of the trends towards ischaemic damage. Indeed optimization of the cardiovascular system in terms of extracellular fluid replacement and management of pressure and perfusion is mandatory whether in the evolutionary or established stages of acute tubular necrosis.

Pharmacological means of improving renal perfusion may also be useful. Renal dopamine, 0.5–3.0 μg/kg per min, activates dopamine receptors, enhancing perfusion although the efficacy of this in the presence of intense sympathetic activity is debatable. In one study, albeit of the mesenteric circulation, the combination of thoracic epidural and dopamine produced enhanced mesenteric flow and a fall in regional lactate production while dopamine alone did not (Lundberg et al 1990).

The apparent effects of dopamine may be blocked by prostaglandin inhibitors, implying other elements to its action. Dopamine certainly increases glomerular filtration rate, renal blood flow and sodium excretion in some patients with acute renal insufficiency and in some at risk of renal insufficiency (Parker et al 1981). In the latter group renal insufficiency was dramatically reduced in liver transplant patients treated with dopamine (Polson et al 1987). Despite these reports the effects of dopamine are still controversial, and there is little to support the use of the term 'renal dopamine' (Duke & Bersten 1992).

Other vasoactive agents include the prostaglandins which not only enhance blood flow but also inhibit the metabolic activity of the tubular cells (Finn et al 1987).

The mainstay of trying to influence acute renal failure has been the use of diuretic agents of various kinds. The rationale behind the use of osmotic diuretics such as mannitol include an increase in the extracellular fluid, both improving renal blood flow and reducing the impact of prerenal effects, the flushing effect of the diuretic sweeping away debris and toxins and the osmotic action reducing endothelial cell oedema. Other postulated mechanisms include its role as an oxygen scavenger. While there is some evidence to suggest mannitol might be beneficial in the initial stages leading to renal failure or if given as pretreatment (Hanley 1981), there is little or no evidence to suggest that mannitol is of benefit once there is organic damage.

Other diuretics such as frusemide have also been widely used to try and prevent or ameliorate renal failure. Frusemide has been clearly shown to increase renal blood flow, an effect reversed by prostaglandin inhibitors, and it also blocks metabolically active pumps in the ascending tubules, thereby sparing oxygen consumption. In isolated kidneys frusemide has been shown to protect these tubules, presumably due to its inhibitory action on metabolism (Brezis et al 1984). It is probable that beneficial effects of diuretics are a combination of increased blood flow, increased tubular flow and possibly an effect on metabolism. Data suggest pretreatment with either frusemide or mannitol limits ischaemic damage but there are no data convincingly showing amelioration of existing damage (Brown et al 1981). One negative aspect of the use of diuretics is that assessment of renal function by volume or content following their use is confusing and potentially misleading.

Cytoprotection is the newer area of approach to the treatment of acute renal failure and addresses the question of cellular damage being either in evolution or established. Methods are then sought of trying to minimize, reduce or reverse the cellular damage that will occur or has occurred. Calcium channel blocking agents, prostacyclins, and xanthine oxidase inhibitors have all been used, as have free radical scavengers (Schrier et al 1987, Wagner & Neumayer 1987). New agents that have shown benefit, at least in animals, include atrial natriuretic peptide and pentoxifyllin, although the mechanism of action of either of these is unclear.

Diagnosis of renal failure in the critically ill should be based on an evaluation and interpretation of the events which have provided the ischaemic or hypoxic insult. Management should then seek to correct not only these causative but also the ongoing physiological disturbances.

VENTILATION

Ventilatory failure is defined as a pathological reduction of the alveolar ventilation below the level required for the maintenance of normal arterial blood gas tensions (Nunn 1987). There are a large number of causes for ventilatory failure which can be categorized by site or by underlying pathophysiology or a combination of the two. In very general terms there may be problems with the mechanical aspects of ventilation, the ventilatory pump, or with the gas exchange mechanism. It is the intention in this section to consider not the vast subject of the pathophysiology of respiratory failure but the physiology of the mechanical management of the problem.

Ventilation in all its forms can be used to deal with the following problems. It can replace the ventilatory pump and move gas in and out of the lungs. It can be used to influence the impact of a reduced functional residual capacity (FRC), which is a common pathway of ventilatory failure, and it can be used to reduce the work of breathing. The first use is self-explanatory although the implications of ventilation are still relevant but the impact on FRC and the work of breathing are worthy of further discussion.

FRC represents the end-expiratory volume and in circumstances where it is reduced lung function is impaired for a combination of reasons. There is a decrease in the compliance of the lung and thorax unit, which increases the work of breathing, a reduced vital capacity and an alteration in ventilation–perfusion mismatch as both ventilation and perfusion are altered in different parts of the lung. The relative importance of these problems depends on which parts of lung volume are impaired.

With failing respiratory drive or neuromuscular problems all lung volumes are reduced. This is also the case with atelectasis or lobar pneumonia but in these latter situations there is also a large volume of the lung which is non-ventilated although still perfused, resulting in a major V/Q abnormality.

Injuries which prevent lung expansion, postoperative patients with pain or those with interstitial oedema result in a significant reduction in vital capacity with low tidal volumes and inefficient breathing, causing increased work.

Conditions with both a reduction in effective surfactant and an increase in interstitial oedema result in a reduction of residual volume and a change in compliance. There are large areas of perfused, underventilated lung in association with an increased ventilatory workload. This is seen in the range of conditions termed adult respiratory distress syndrome (ARDS).

In all of these situations the FRC is significantly reduced and intervention is aimed at attempting to increase the FRC, thereby improving the volume of lung actively involved in gas exchange, or alternatively to guarantee better ventilation of unaffected areas of the lung in the hope of compensating for the affected areas. The latter is important as there are some conditions such as lobar pneumonia where it is unlikely that ventilation will result in aeration of the diseased area and yet may result in better gas exchange taken as an overall view (Shapiro 1981).

The other aspect of ventilatory support is that of reducing work with the intrinsic oxygen cost. In critically ill patients, especially those with lung pathology, the work of breathing may have a substantial oxygen cost and ventilation may reduce this considerably (Marinii 1990).

Ventilation is a term loosely covering a large variety of modalities. While all address the issues of improvement of oxygenation, removal of carbon dioxide and reduction in workload, the emphasis on each varies, as do the physiological implications of each modality.

The influence of changed inspired gas concentrations will not be discussed but the influence of an increase in the FRC, a change in mean intrathoracic pressure and the consequent alterations in the cardiovascular system are pertinent.

Functional residual capacity

An increase in FRC has several effects which depend on whether the patient is breathing spontaneously, being ventilated or a combination of the two. In the former this can be achieved either by the use of end expiratory resistance, positive end expiratory pressure (PEEP), or by the use of high flow in association with an effective end expiratory resistance. Either will result in an increase in FRC and a change in the compliance of the lung–chest wall unit. In Figure 4.3 a reduction in FRC (FRC$_1$) results in a shift to the right of the compliance curve. To achieve the same tidal volume (V$_T$) a larger pressure change (P$_2$) is required. Addition of PEEP moves the FRC back to its original

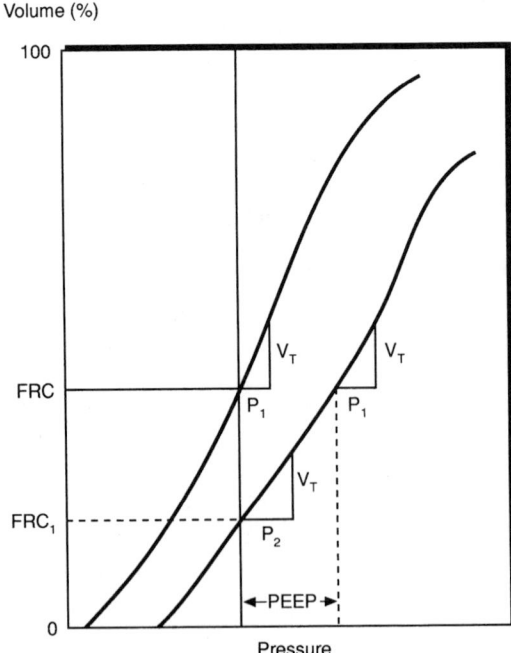

Fig. 4.3 Influence of functional residual capacity (FRC) on the compliance of the lung–chest wall.

position and gives the original pressure change (P_1) required. Breathing is more efficient and work is therefore reduced. If continuous positive airways pressure (CPAP) is applied then positive pressure in the system throughout inspiration will further reduce the work of inspiration (Fig 4.3).

As FRC increases it is hoped that the increased volume of alveoli will include many of those alveolic previously non- or underventilated and hence improve the $V : Q$ ratio within the lung. This is not guaranteed as the alveoli already open will be more compliant than the smaller previously occluded alveoli and it may result in further diversion of inspired gas to distended or overdistended alveoli. In the supine patient there is evidence to suggest that the posterior aspects of the lungs are underventilated and relatively non-compliant whilst it is also these gravitationally dependent areas which are well-perfused. This is potentially more deleterious. When positive pressure ventilation is used there is potential for a decrease in ventilation of these dependent areas, which may result in worsening of the $V : Q$ abnormality.

Cardiovascular system

A rise in the mean intrathoracic pressure by whatever means has an influence on the cardiovascular system. There is a reduction in venous return as the extrathoracic–intrathoracic gradient is reduced, which will tend to reduce right ventricular preload. Furthermore pulmonary vascular resistance can be influenced. At low FRC the interstitial pressure can result in reduced capillary diameter and increased resistance. As FRC is increased this allows expansion of the capillaries but then at higher volumes excessive intra-alveolar pressure causes distention of alveoli which compress pulmonary capillaries, again raising resistance. The rise in pulmonary vascular resistance may adversely add to the reduced venous return and contribute to a fall in cardiac output. It may also influence the quantity and quality of capillary perfusion and thereby the $V : Q$ ratio. The capacitance of the capillary bed is reduced as intrathoracic pressure rises above normal, forcing fluid out from the pulmonary vasculature by enhancing venous return to the left atrium. Paradoxically the gradient between inside the chest and outside is the gradient that the left ventricle has to overcome to push blood out systemically so that in some circumstances the rise in end-expiratory pressure reduces the gradient and may augment cardiac output. It can be seen that a series of relatively unpredictable but interdependent advantages and disadvantages are relevant when end-expiratory pressures are applied. As ventilation is often used primarily to improve oxygenation of the patient, success must be determined not by blood oxygenation alone but by the resultant oxygen delivery to the tissues. There is a balance between the positive effects of intrathoracic pressure on blood oxygenation and the negative effects on haemodynamics and oxygen delivery and it is this balance which must be correctly interpreted (Pinsky 1990).

A further haemodynamic consequence of positive intrathoracic pressure is the effect on renal function. There is a reduction in renal perfusion, in particular cortical flow, and a fall in glomerular filtration rate. These are probably due to the rise in venous pressures but changes in intravascular volume, cardiac output and ADH release mediated by baroreceptors probably all play a role (Annat et al 1983).

Specific types of ventilation

Positive pressure ventilation is now feasible in many forms. The physiology of ventilation described above can be applied to any of these forms and there is little point in providing a list. There are several modes which illustrate some of these points.

CPAP increases the FRC and the work of inspiration is reduced by the positive pressure in the system. A raised intrathoracic pressure has the expected haemodynamic effects, although as the patient breathes spontaneously the intrathoracic pressures are less than with positive pressure ventilation. A variation on this theme is airway pressure release ventilation (APRV), where CPAP is applied but periodically the system is opened to atmosphere and the pressure falls (Downs & Stock 1987). The peak airway pressures are no higher than the CPAP and the mean airway pressures will be lower than CPAP. There will be an effective increase in FRC as with CPAP but this may be in part jeopardized by the periods of low pressure. Haemodynamic effects should be similar to CPAP.

Inverse ratio ventilation is pressure-controlled ventilation in which inspiratory time exceeds expiratory time. The prolonged application of pressure is more effective in recruiting alveoli as longer application of positive pressure will allow opening of the less compliant alveoli. The decelerating flow modifies the pressure waveform to lower peak pressure effectively but mean pressure is inevitably higher. In conditions with a reduced FRC and non-ventilated alveoli, this should aid recruitment but the raised mean intrathoracic pressure would be expected to have haemodynamic consequences (Sassoon 1991). The clinical benefits of this method are not yet convincing.

Inspiratory pressure support allows triggered breaths from a ventilator to be supplemented by pressure-limited flow from a ventilator. This augments a weak inspiratory effort, the level of augmentation being determined by the pressure limit. This is in effect positive pressure ventilation and has similar costs and benefits. The main advantages are that it will effectively allow a small amount of work to produce adequate ventilation, thereby mechanically enhancing breathing efficiency, and is often well-tolerated by patients. It is a useful weaning tool.

Negative pressure ventilation is now an uncommonly used mode of ventilation in which negative pressure is generated in a cuirass or tank outside the thorax to augment the normal pattern of breathing. There is a decrease in mean intrathoracic pressure which influences both venous return and ventricular afterload. There is enhanced venous return but the reduced intrathoracic pressure requires the left ventricle to generate larger transmural pressures to eject blood, although this is not usually a problem. In circumstances of an impaired ventilatory pump this method is of benefit and will not embarrass existing $V : Q$. In conditions of reduced lung compliance and thereby a reduced FRC, it is likely to be ineffective in recruiting alveoli. This is conjectural rather than factual as in neonates with respiratory distress syndrome the use of negative pressure ventilation has been very successful and reports have indicated improved oxygenation with this method. This may reflect the synergistic benefits of exogenous ventilatory pump support, minimal cardiovascular compromise and improved oxygen delivery (Stern et al 1970).

From these examples it can be seen that the interpretation of the potential benefits and disadvantages of any modality of ventilation should be predictable from a consideration of the physiological effects. The balance of these effects in any individual is far more difficult but not impossible to predict.

OXYGEN DEMAND AND SUPPLY

One of the most important and yet fundamental changes in intensive care practice in the last decade has been the introduction and popularization of the concept of oxygen supply and demand. In a wide range of pathophysiological conditions the final common pathway is the delivery of oxygen to the tissues. Indeed when this fails at lung, cardiovascular, cellular or mitochondrial level the end-point for the tissues is potentially the same. Instead of complex clinical descriptions of conditions such as shock, oxygen transport theory can be used to describe the problems in a physiological context which then lends itself both to classification and to corrective rather than symptomatic management.

Tissue oxygenation is dependent on three main factors: oxygen uptake in the lung, oxygen binding in the blood and oxygen delivery to the tissues by the cardiovascular system.

Oxygen passes from the lungs to the blood and is then distributed through the body as far as the capillaries where it diffuses to the cells. The central transport mechanisms are cardiac output and oxygen carriage determined by haemoglobin concentration, Sao_2 and oxygen affinity (P_{50}) and peripherally local capillary perfusion and the distance and obstacles between capillary and cell. Under normal circumstances the delivery of oxygen satisfies the tissue demands and as these increase so does the delivery. Small increases in demand can be met by either an increase in supply, via cardiac output, or by an increase in the extraction ratio but larger increases in demand will rapidly exhaust the compensatory increase in extraction ratio and necessitate an increase in delivery (Fig. 4.4). In exercise, when the delivery is exceeded by demand, aerobic energy production is supplemented by anaerobic metabolism. This occurs at the point named the anaerobic threshold, defined as the oxygen consumption above which a sustained lactic acidosis occurs (Wasser-

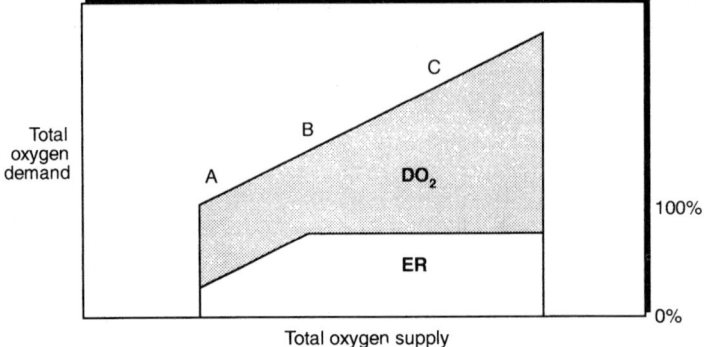

Fig. 4.4   Increase in tissue oxygen delivery is a combination of changing extraction from blood and the amount of oxygen delivered by the blood. The areas ER and DO_2 refer to the amount extraction (ER) and blood volume (DO_2) contribute to total oxygen supply. At point A the oxygen demand is met by the oxygen delivered and a low ER. As demand increases the amount extracted can increase as ER increases without changing the volume of blood delivered (B). When the extraction ratio is maximal and can increase no further, the increased demand is met by increasing the volume of blood delivered (C).

man 1986). In pathophysiological circumstances, when oxygen consumption increases, delivery may be unable to meet these demands and a comparable situation may exist.

Peripheral mechanisms may contribute to the shortfall in delivery to the cells themselves. In sepsis there often appears to be a functional block of extraction from blood to cell.

Oxygen is transported with the majority bound to haemoglobin (1.39 g/ml) with a tiny amount dissolved in the blood (0.00314 Pa_{O_2} ml/dl). The amount of oxygen delivered to the body is then a function of the cardiac output. If a pulmonary artery catheter is in situ, allowing measurement of cardiac output, and the mixed venous oxygen saturation is known, the amount of oxygen delivered to the tissues and the quantity returning unused can be calculated quite easily (inverse Fick method). The difference is the amount of oxygen consumed (Table 4.4). Alternatively total body oxygen consumption can be measured by the breath by breath analysis of the respiratory gases. These methods enable the total body oxygen delivery and consumption to be quantified, but not regional delivery.

Probably the most important aspect of oxygen transport is the consequences of inadequate supply. These are failed adenosine triphosphate production from anaerobic metabolism with increased lactate production, recruitment, in brain, heart and muscle of stored phosphocreatine to supplement the adenosine triphosphate supply, allowing some cell function to continue and the ongoing use of existing and new adenosine triphosphate. As this is broken down hydrogen ions are liberated (Busa & Nuccitelli 1984). The net result is increased lactate and hydrogen ion production — lactic acidosis. Plasma lactate levels are therefore used by many as a marker of anaerobic metabolism,

Table 4.4 The calculation of oxygen transport variables

1 DO_2	=	$CI \times CaO_2 \times 10$	(ml/min per m^2)
	=	$CI \times [Hb] \times SaO_2 \times 1.31 \times 10$	
2 Unused O_2	=	$CI \times CvO_2 \times 10$	(ml/min per m^2)
	=	$CI \times [Hb] \times SvO_2 \times 1.31 \times 10$	
3 VO_2	=	$CI \times (CaO_2 - CvO_2) \times 10$	(ml/min per m^2)
Where:			
DO_2	=	Total oxygen delivery/m^2	(ml/min per m^2)
VO_2	=	Total oxygen consumption/m^2	(ml/min per m^2)
CI	=	Cardiac index	
	=	Cardiac output/body surface area	(l/min per m^2)
CaO_2	=	Arterial oxygen content	(ml/dl)
CvO_2	=	Mixed venous oxygen content	(ml/dl)
SaO_2	=	Arterial oxyhaemoglobin saturation	(%)
SvO_2	=	Mixed venous oxyhaemoglobin saturation	(%)
[Hb]	=	Haemoglobin concentration	(g/dl)

but the interpretation of lactate levels is complex. Red blood cells lack mitochondria and produce lactate which accounts for about 25% of basal concentrations. The other 75% is produced by brain, myocardium, skin and muscle.

There is a high daily turnover of lactate as various tissues utilize or clear lactate. Some lactate is used for gluconeogenesis but most is oxidized for energy production. Muscle, liver, kidney and heart all utilize lactate readily. Catecholamines increase lactate production as an energy substrate, as does respiratory alkalosis. The latter induces an increased rate of glycolysis and a tendency to hyperlactaemia. Lactate clearance is heavily influenced by organ perfusion and alterations in the perfusion of liver, kidney and skeletal muscle also influence lactate levels (Brooks 1986).

Under normal circumstances oxygen supply tends to match the sum of demands imposed by the tissues, thereby avoiding anaerobic metabolism (Denison 1981). As demands increase, as during exercise, so does supply and if they reduce, as in sleep, the supply will also reduce and as with most physiological systems, there is a large margin of safety. However, when delivery is reduced artificially in dogs, Cain demonstrated that initially there was no change in oxygen consumption, but below a critical level of delivery oxygen consumption also started to fall. The delivery value at which this occurred was termed the critical point (Cain 1986). At this point oxygen consumption becomes dependent on supply. In the initial stages of each experiment an early plateau phase was clearly demonstrated during which oxygen consumption remained constant even though oxygen delivery was reduced but there was an abrupt reduction in oxygen consumption when delivery fell below the critical point. It is clear that consumption becomes dependent on delivery when the amount delivered fails to match demands (Nelson et al 1988). As delivery decreases below this critical point lactic acidosis develops, reflecting the onset of significant anaerobic metabolism (Fig. 4.5).

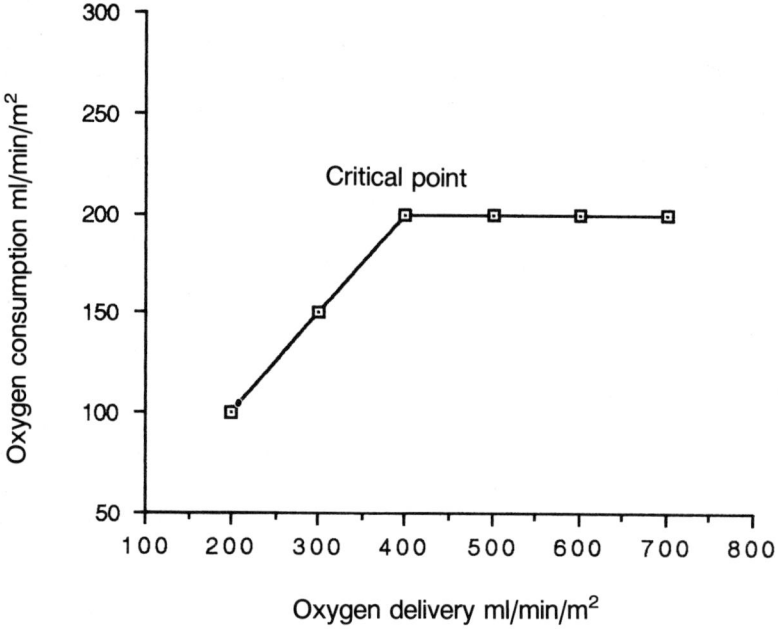

Fig. 4.5   Classical oxygen delivery consumption graph demonstrating the plateau.

It is assumed that the observations associated with a normal delivery falling should be the mirror image of a low delivery rising. At low oxygen delivery any increase in delivery will be matched by an increase in oxygen consumption — supply-dependence — but when the critical point of adequate delivery is reached oxygen consumption will plateau despite further increases in oxygen delivery. In many sick patients this plateau cannot be achieved and oxygen consumption continues to rise even when a normal or greater oxygen delivery has been achieved. This has been termed pathological supply-dependence (Bihari et al 1987) and implies that in these patients the delivery was still inadequate. It is of interest that in many of these patients it appears impossible to increase the extraction ratio above 0.3 (Danek et al 1980).

The conclusions to be drawn from this appraisal would appear simple. In critically ill patients with low oxygen consumption, low delivery and with evidence of anaerobic metabolism, the uptake of oxygen is inadequate for normal aerobic cellular function. Therefore if improvements in delivery can be achieved with a resultant increase in consumption this should be beneficial (Astiz et al 1987). This is supported by a positive correlation between oxygen delivery and survival (Tuchschmidt et al 1989) and evidence that tissue hypoxia is a major factor in the development of multiorgan system failure (Sibbald et al 1989).

When oxygen delivery is considered inadequate there are many methods for increasing oxygen delivery and consumption. Raising the haemoglobin from less than 10 g/dl to between 10 and 12 g/dl increases oxygen delivery but only if lactate was high (Gilbert et al 1986; Table 4.5). Fluid administration is widely used to improve cardiac output and thereby oxygen delivery (Rackow et al 1988, Edwards et al 1989). In one study comparing septic and non-septic patients an increase in oxygen delivery was achieved in both, but only the septic group increased their consumption (Wolf et al 1987). In patients with raised plasma lactate (>2.2 mmol/l) fluid loading with colloid resulted in raised oxygen delivery and consumption. By contrast, those with normal lactates demonstrated a rise in delivery but no change in consumption. Catecholamines can be, and often are, used to increase delivery but in the study mentioned, when catecholamines were used, consumption and delivery increased regardless of lactate levels. This implied that catecholamines themselves raise oxygen consumption (Haupt et al 1985, Gilbert et al 1986, Dhainaut et al 1991). It is therefore possible to postulate that driving the oxygen delivery up may inevitably lead to supply-dependence, with the resultant increased oxygen consumption reflecting not the tissue oxygen use, but the cost of the increased delivery. This is potentially an excellent example of how the physiology of an intervention must be carefully considered and also how the apparent benefits need to be assessed.

Other non-inotropic agents such as prostacyclin may effectively improve delivery but also influence blood flow distribution in a useful fashion (Bihari et al 1987). It is clear that the mechanism for improving delivery must be evaluated in context.

This is an extremely attractive conceptual approach to the management of shock. Assess the adequacy of delivery and, if inadequate, increase it. There are some problems with the application of the concept. The measurement systems employed are open to criticism. Oxygen consumption and delivery employing an indirect Fick method use common components, raising the question of linkage — see equations below:

Oxygen delivery = cardiac index × arterial oxygen content
Oxygen consumption = cardiac index × (arterial − mixed venous) oxygen content

Linkage is a mathematical phenomenon when 'independent' values are derived using common 'dependent' components, in this case cardiac index. If coupling, linkage, is present then apparent relationships between consumption and delivery may merely reflect changes in cardiac output. Views differ on the relevance of linkage (Powers et al 1970, Archie 1981, Vermeij et al 1990).

Table 4.5 Normal and preferred values of oxygen variables

Variable	Units	Normal values	Preferred values
Cardiac index	l/min per m^2	2.8–3.6	>4.5
Oxygen delivery	l/min per m^2	520–720	>550
Oxygen consumption	l/min per m^2	100–180	>167
Oxygen extraction ratio	%	22–30	<31

Modified with permission from Shoemaker & Kram (1990).

Quite apart from these problems it is difficult to determine what delivery or consumption constitutes an adequate value, and plasma lactate levels which should be helpful can be misleading. The question 'how much is enough?' has yet to be resolved.

The practicalities of therapeutic management can be briefly considered. Basic resuscitation with adequate oxygenation and intravascular volume replacement is fundamental and may produce the important changes in oxygen delivery (Reinhart et al 1990). Lactate may be a helpful marker of anaerobic respiration, aiding a balanced view of the adequacy of delivery. Methods of increasing delivery can then be employed and these include inotropes or vasoactive drugs, although there is uncertainty about the optimal method as well as deciding when a worthwhile goal has been achieved.

Probably of greater consequence is the certainty that it is the oxygenation of individual organs or even cells within those organs which is important rather than global measurements and it is glaringly obvious that total body measurements do not reflect individual organ perfusion.

These conclusions are not intended to undermine the importance of oxygenation in illness nor its role in the development of problems in the critically ill. There is no doubt that the general concept of preventing or relieving tissue hypoxia is important and that this physiological approach has led to improved and more informed management of the critically ill. Having agreed that oxygenation should be optimized, the problems have arisen in determining what the optimum is, what goals we should aim for and how to achieve them. Nevertheless a physiologically guided approach to diagnosis and management has been firmly established.

CONCLUSION

Intensive care of the critically ill is applied physiology, although there are still many aspects of practice and especially of management that have more to do with tradition and hearsay than physiological fact. This is rapidly changing and probably far more in the intensive care environment than in almost any other specialty in medicine. As with the oxygen transport story the establishment of a conceptual approach based on physiology often produces as many questions as answers, and usually demonstrates our level of ignorance of the background pathophysiology. Although frustrating at times, it is also very exciting both now and in the future as our approach to intensive care management moves further into applied physiology.

REFERENCES

Annat G, Viale J, Bui Xuan B et al 1983 Effects of PEEP ventilation on renal function, plasma renin, aldosterone, neurophysins and urinary ADH and prostaglandins. Anesthesiology 58: 136–141
Archie J P 1981 Mathematical coupling of data. A common source of error. Ann Surg 193: 296–303

Astiz M E, Rackow E C, Weil M H 1987 Oxygen delivery and consumption in patients with hyperdynamic septic shock. Crit Care Med 15: 26–28

Bihari D M, Smithies M, Gimson A et al 1987 The effects of vasodilation with prostacyclin on oxygen delivery and uptake in critically ill patients. N Engl J Med 317: 397–403

Blevins L, Wand G 1992 Diabetes insipidus. Crit Care Med 20: 69–79

Brezis M, Rosen S, Silva P et al 1984 Transport activity modifies thick ascending limb damage in isolated perfused kidney. Kidney Int 25: 65–72

Brooks G A 1986 Lactate production under fully aerobic conditions: the lacate shuttle during rest and exercise. Fed Proc 45: 2924–2929

Brown C, Ogg C S, Cameron J S 1981 High dose frusemide in acute renal failure: a controlled trial. Clin Nephrol 15: 90–96

Busa W B, Nuccitelli R 1984 Metabolic regulation via intracellular pH. Am J Physiol 246: R409

Cain S M 1986 Assessment of tissue oxygenation. Crit Care Clin 2: 537

Cousins M J, Skowronski G A 1990 Anaesthesia and the kidney. Scientific foundations of anaesthesia. Heinemann, Oxford, p 420

Danek S J, Lynch J P, Weg J G, Dantzker D R 1980 The dependence of oxygen uptake on oxygen delivery in the adult respiratory distress syndrome. Am Rev Respir Dis 122: 387–395

Denison D 1981 The distribution and use of oxygen in tissues. Scientific foundations of respiratory medicine. Heinemann, London, pp 221–237

Dhainaut J-F, Annat G, Armaganidis A 1991 Oxygen supply dependency in septic shock. Update in intensive care and emergency medicine. Springer-Verlag, Berlin, pp 217–226

Downs J, Stock M 1987 Airway pressure release ventilation: a new concept in ventilatory support. Crit Care Med 15: 459–461

Duke G J, Bersten A D 1992 Dopamine and renal salvage in the critically ill patient. Anaesth Intens Care 20: 277–302

Edwards J D, Nightingale P, Wilkins R G, Faragher E B 1989 Hemodynamic and oxygen transport response to modified fluid gelatin in critically ill patients. Crit Care Med 17: 996–998

Finn W 1990 Prevention of ischemic injury in renal transplantation. Kidney Int 37: 171–182

Finn W F, Hak L J, Grossman S H 1987 Protective effect of prostacyclin on post ischaemic acute renal failure. Kidney Int 132: 479

Gilbert E M, Haupt M T, Mandanas R Y et al 1986 The effect of fluid loading, blood transfusion, and catecholamine infusion on oxygen delivery and consumption in patients with sepsis. Am Rev Respir Dis 134: 873–878

Hanley M D K 1981 Prior mannitol and furosemide infusion in a model of ischemic acute renal failure. Am J Physiol 241: F556–564

Haupt M T, Gilbert E M, Carlson R W 1985 Fluid loading increases oxygen consumption in septic patients with lactic acidosis. Am Rev Respir Dis 131: 912–916

Lundberg J, Lundberg D, Norgren L et al 1990 Intestinal hemodynamics during laparotomy: effects of thoracic epidural anesthesia and dopamine in humans. Anesth Analg 71: 9–15

Marinii J J 1990 Strategies to minimize breathing effort during mechanical ventilation. Critical care clinics. W B Saunders, Philadelphia, 635–663

Nelson D P, Samsel R W, Wood L D H et al 1988 Pathological supply dependence of systemic and intestinal O_2 uptake during endotoxaemia. J Appl Physiol 64: 2410–2419

Nunn J F 1987 Ventilatory failure. Applied respiratory physiology 3rd edn. Butterworths, London, pp 379–391

Oh M, Carroll H 1992 Disorders of sodium metabolism: hypernatraemia and hyponatraemia. Crit Care Med 20: 95–103

Parker S, Carlon G, Isaacs M et al 1981 Dopamine administration in oliguria and oliguric renal failure. Crit Care Med 9: 630–632

Pinsky M R 1990 The effects of mechanical ventilation on the cardiovascular system. Critical care clinics. W B Saunders, Philadelphia, 663–678

Polson R, Park G, Lindop M J et al 1987 The prevention of renal impairment in patients undergoing orthotopic liver grafting by infusion of low dose dopamine. Anaesthesia 42: 15–19

Powers S R, Mannal R, Neclerio M et al 1970 Physiological consequences of positive end expiratory pressure (PEEP) ventilation. Ann Surg 178: 265–272

Rackow E C, Astiz M E, Weil M H 1988 Cellular oxygen metabolism during sepsis and shock. The relationship of oxygen consumption to oxygen delivery. JAMA 259: 1989-1993

Reinhart K, Hannemann L, Kuss B 1990 Optimal oxygen delivery in critically ill patients. Intensive Care Med 16: S149-S155

Rose B 1986 New approaches to disturbances in the plasma sodium concentration. Am J Med 81: 1033-1040

Sassoon C 1991 Positive pressure ventilation, alternate modes. Chest 100: 1421-1429

Schrier R, Arnold P, Van Putten V J et al 1987 Cellular calcium in ischemic acute renal failure: role of calcium entry blockers. Kidney Int 32: 313

Shapiro B A 1981 Airway pressure therapy for acute restrictive pulmonary pathology. Critical care state of the art. Society of Critical Care Medicine, Fullerton, pp C1-45

Shoemaker W, Kram H B 1990 Pathophysiology, monitoring, outcome prediction and therapy of shock states. In: Scow C, Feldman S A, Soni N (eds) Scientific foundations of anaesthesia, 4th edn. Heinemann, Oxford, pp 216-232

Sibbald W J, Bersten A, Rutledge F S 1989 The role of tissue hypoxia in mutiple organ failure. Clinical aspects of O_2 transport and tissue oxygenation. Springer, Berlin, pp 102-114

Stern L, Ramos A, Outeridge E W 1970 Negative pressure artificial respiration: use in respiratory failure in the newborn. Can Med Assoc J 102: 595-601

Sterns R, Riggs J, Scochet S S 1986 Osmotic demyelination syndrome following correction of hyponatraemia N Engl J Med 314: 1535-1542

Tuchschmidt J, Fried J, Swinney R et al 1989 Early hemodynamic correlates of survival in patients with septic shock. Crit Care Med 17: 719-723

Vermeij C G, Feenstra B W, Bruining H A et al 1990 Oxygen delivery and oxygen uptake in postoperative and septic patients. Chest 98: 415-420

Wagner K A S, Neumayer H H 1987 Prevention of posttransplant acute tubular necrosis by the calcium antagonist diltiazem: a prospective randomised study. Am J Nephrol 7: 287

Wasserman K 1986 The anaerobic threshold: definition, physiological significance and identification. Adv Cardiol 35: 1-23

Wolf Y G, Cotev S, Perel A et al 1987 Dependence of oxygen consumption on cardiac output in sepsis. Crit Care Med 15: 198-203

5. EDRF – its role in vascular tone and pharmacological manipulation

A. J. Pittard   N. R. Webster

Normal blood pressure is a product of cardiac output and total peripheral resistance. There are very sensitive control mechanisms that maintain blood pressure within strict limits. There are central and peripheral components involved in blood pressure control as well as locally acting mechanisms which alter tissue perfusion over small areas. In this review we aim to examine the biochemical mechanisms underlying the control of vascular tone during health and in disease and the modes of action of vasoactive drugs. This is clearly of importance in the pathogenesis of hypertension as well as in the understanding of the mechanisms involved in tissue blood flow.

BLOOD PRESSURE CONTROL

The most important area of the central nervous system with regard to blood pressure is in the medulla and involves the vasomotor centre. In the periphery, sensory receptors known as baroreceptors are situated in the carotid body and aortic arch. These receptors are stimulated by distention and their discharge rate increases when the pressure within the vessel wall rises. Afferent fibres pass via the glossopharyngeal and vagus nerves to the medulla. Most fibres end in the nucleus of tractus solitarius but some pass directly to the cardioinhibitory centre. From the nucleus tractus solitarius inhibitory neurons pass to the vasomotor centre in the ventrolateral medulla. Impulses generated in baroreceptors inhibit discharge of vasoconstrictor nerves and excite the cardioinhibitory centre producing vasodilation, venodilation, hypotension, bradycardia and a reduction in cardiac output (Fig. 5.1).

As well as central control of blood pressure there are local autoregulatory mechanisms that compensate for changes in tissue perfusion pressure by altering vascular resistance. Two theories explaining how this local control is exerted are the myogenic and metabolic theories. An increase in blood pressure stretches blood vessels and causes a compensatory contraction of the vascular smooth muscle therefore maintaining a normal perfusion pressure — *the myogenic theory*. A fall in blood pressure and tissue blood flow will allow vasodilator metabolites to accumulate which will then cause a vasodilation in an attempt to preserve tissue blood flow — *the metabolic theory*.

73

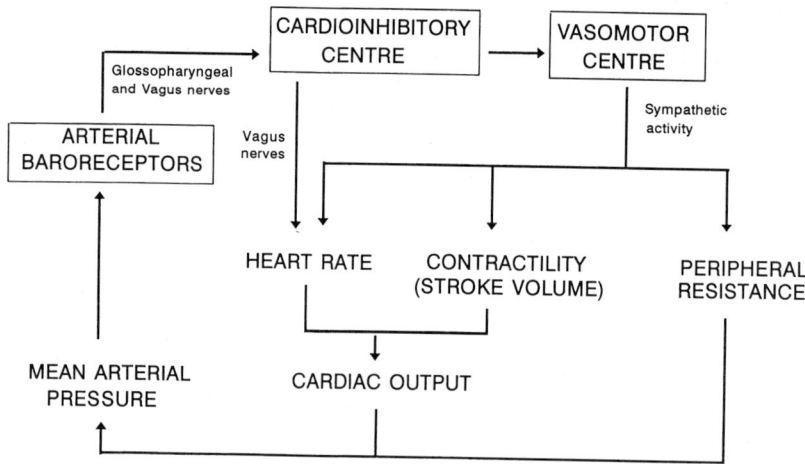

Fig. 5.1 The physiological control of blood pressure

This local regulation of vascular smooth muscle tone plays an integral role in the control of total peripheral resistance. Many endogenous substances have been identified as playing a part in this control. Substances such as bradykinin, acetylcholine and adenosine which relax vascular smooth muscle depend on the release of a relaxing factor from endothelial cells and are therefore known as endothelium-dependent vasodilators. This endothelial-derived relaxing factor (EDRF) was identified by Furchgott & Zawadski in 1980. It is now known that the effects of EDRF are mediated via nitric oxide (NO; Palmer et al 1987). The endothelial-dependent vasodilators release EDRF via a calcium-dependent process in the endothelial cell and ultimately relax vascular smooth muscle.

There are endogenous vasoactive agents that do not act via this mechanism. Noradrenaline, which is an endogenous vasoconstrictor, acts at alpha-receptors.

The endothelium also releases a 21 amino acid vasoconstrictor peptide known as endothelin. This produces severe vasoconstriction resulting in elevation of blood pressure and reduction in renal blood flow but without affecting coronary flow. EDRF may be a natural antagonist inhibiting its synthesis. The hypertensive response to endothelin is more marked when given intra-arterially rather than intravenously, suggesting inactivation or uptake by the pulmonary circulation. Studies have shown a basal endothelin release from arteries. The role of this endogenous endothelin release and the mechanisms involved are unclear but again changes in the second messenger, cyclic guanosine monophosphate (GMP), are thought to be important.

Endothelial cells are thought to release a hyperpolarizing factor acting directly on vascular smooth muscle. By activation of the sodium/potassium pump this factor causes relaxation of the blood vessel.

CONTRACTILE ELEMENTS

The contractile proteins actin and myosin and their interactions are ultimately responsible for the force generated in vascular smooth muscle. The myosin heads bind to actin filaments. A configurational change in the myosin head causes the filaments to slide over each other, increasing overlap and producing shortening. This cross-bridging occurs when the myosin light chain is phosphorylated by the enzyme myosin light chain kinase. Calcium activates this enzyme in the presence of calmodulin. This basic process is identical in smooth muscle taken from both normal and hypertensive subjects.

The intracellular calcium concentration is an important regulator on smooth muscle contraction. It is controlled by calcium channels in the plasma membrane through which calcium enters the cell down a 10 000-fold concentration gradient. There are four different types of channel:

1. Calcium leak channel — continuous activity.
2. Voltage — gated calcium channel.
3. Receptor — gated calcium channel.
4. Stretch — activated calcium channel.

In hypertensive subjects it has been found that there is a greater calcium influx through channel types 1–3. Because of the diversity of the integral proteins involved in these channels there may be a generalized abnormality of the membrane in hypertension that affects protein and hence channel function.

The calcium extrusion pump maintains the normally low intracellular calcium concentration. This is an energy-dependent pump requiring the enzyme calcium and magnesium-dependent adenosine triphosphate. This pump is less active in hypertension. Impaired relaxation secondary to slow extrusion of calcium contributes to the raised total peripheral resistance in hypertension (Dominiczat & Bohr 1989, Rau 1990).

THE GUANYLATE CYCLASE–CYCLIC GMP SYSTEM

Binding of agonist and receptor is the initial step in vascular smooth muscle contraction, each agonist having a specific receptor. The signal generated by receptor occupancy is transmitted to a group of guanine nucleotide binding proteins (G proteins). The G proteins transmit the signal to membrane-associated phospholipases which are activated resulting in phospholipid hydrolysis. Activated phospholipase C hydrolyses phosphatidyl inositol bisphosphate to inositol triphosphate in the cytosol and diacylglycerol in the membrane. Both of these substances produce smooth muscle contraction. Inhibition of hydrolysis reduces the amount of contraction and therefore produces vasodilatation and hypotension (Fig. 5.2).

In almost all cells at least two isoenzymes of guanylate cyclase have been identified: a membrane-bound particulate and a cytosolic-soluble enzyme. In

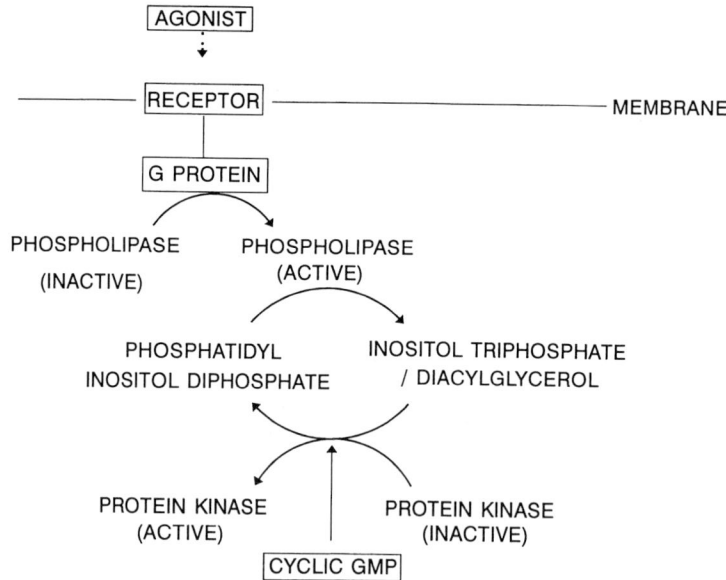

Fig. 5.2   The receptor activation and second messenger pathway involved in local blood pressure control.

vascular smooth muscle each isoenzyme is characteristically regulated by different classes of nitrovasodilators. Endothelium-dependent vasodilators increase cyclic GMP by activating the soluble cytosolic isoenzyme, whilst atrial natriuretic peptides activate the particulate isoenzyme. Although there are different methods of guanylate cyclase activation, the formation of cyclic GMP acts as a common pathway for inducing vascular relaxation (Pou et al 1990).

Relaxation is produced by activation of cyclic GMP-dependent protein kinase. This enzyme alters the phosphorylation state of a variety of proteins including the myosin light chain. It is possible that the protein kinase activates a calcium-dependent adenosine triphosphatase which decreases cytosolic calcium concentration and, therefore, myosin light chain kinase activity (Waldman & Murad 1988).

EDRF/NO

EDRF is a humoral agent whose synthesis and release are dependent upon an intact endothelium. Endothelial cells synthesize NO, which has now been identified as EDRF, from the guanidino nitrogen of L-arginine (Collier & Vallance 1991). This action is both stereoselective and stereospecific, the D isomer having no pharmacological or physiological effect (Fig. 5.3).

Arginine is a nutritionally essential amino acid since it is not synthesized by the human body in sufficient amounts to support growth and must, therefore, be supplied by the diet.

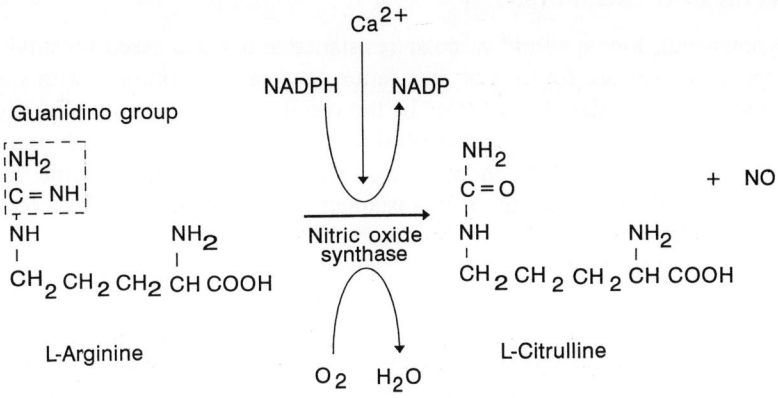

Fig. 5.3 The formation of nitric oxide from L-arginine using nitric oxide synthase.

The action of NO synthase, a soluble enzyme, on L-arginine is dependent on NADPH, requires calcium and is inhibited by L-Ng-monomethyl arginine (LNMMA), an analogue of L-arginine. Release of EDRF can be stimulated by receptor binding, e.g. acetylcholine acting at the muscarinic receptor, and also by increased intracellular calcium concentration (Johns et al 1990). EDRF has a half-life of approximately 6 seconds. It is inactivated by superoxide anion, $O_2^{\cdot-}$ but not other oxygen-derived free radicals. It is thought that the short half life may be a function of the concomitant release of $O_2^{\cdot-}$ by vascular endothelial cells (Cryglewski et al 1987).

NO_2^- and NO_3^- have no relaxant properties on vascular smooth muscle. Haemoglobin inactivates NO probably by binding chemically to it. Superoxide dismutase prolongs the half-life of EDRF by transforming the superoxide anion into hydrogen peroxide (Hong et al 1990).

EDRF activates soluble guanylate cyclase by an interaction between NO and the haem prosthetic group associated with the enzyme. This enzyme catalyses the formation of cyclic GMP from guanosine triphosphate.

Release of EDRF is a calcium-dependent process and activation of phospholipase C, which would ultimately lead to smooth muscle contraction, appears to initiate either the synthesis and/or release of EDRF.

The precise mechanism of vascular relaxation is still controversial. It is known to be mediated via cyclic GMP and it probably acts by inhibiting phosphorylation of myosin light chains. Factors known to enhance the formation and/or release of EDRF include bradykinin, acetylcholine, adenosine triphosphate and the calcium ionophore A23187. It may be that the influx of extracellular calcium is a possible mechanism that couples the interaction of endothelium-dependent vasodilators at endothelial cell surface receptors to the synthesis and/or release of EDRF. Extracellular magnesium inhibits calcium influx at vascular smooth muscle membranes and, therefore, inhibits the synthesis/release of EDRF (Gold et al 1990).

LIVER FAILURE/SEPSIS

Hypotension, low systemic vascular resistance and a decreased sensitivity to vasoconstrictors are features of liver failure and sepsis syndrome with shock. These cardiovascular changes may be the result of an increased production of NO. Studies in humans have suggested that bacterial endotoxin and cytokines induce NO synthase in endothelium. Once induced the enzyme has a prolonged effect and results in a sustained release of NO and hypotension (Munaj et al 1958, Vallance & Moncada 1991).

PULMONARY HYPOXIC VASOCONSTRICTION

The phenomenon of pulmonary hypoxic vasoconstriction was first described in 1946 but its mechanism has yet to be explained. In animal studies the endothelium has been found to be important for the response which may be due to reduced production of EDRF. Hypoxia has been shown in animals to block production of EDRF. It is possible that pulmonary hypertension commonly seen in many chronic lung conditions is due to decreased concentrations of EDRF in the pulmonary vasculature. If this hypothesis proves to be correct then a new and potentially very useful therapeutic intervention may become available (Warren et al 1989).

NITROVASODILATORS

This group of agents includes glyceryl trinitrate (GTN) and sodium nitroprusside (SNP). They activate soluble guanylate cyclase to produce a dose-dependent increase in cyclic GMP and relaxation of vascular smooth muscle. SNP acts directly on guanylate cyclase. Organic nitrates such as GTN require preliminary interactions with tissue sulphydryl groups to be metabolized to NO and hence cause activation of soluble enzyme (Birkenboam et al 1990, Cocks & Angus 1990).

This class of drugs, therefore, acts without causing release of EDRF and they are called endothelium-independent. Several studies have supported the hypothesis that tolerance to organic nitrates is related to oxidation of these sulphydryl groups.

DIRECTLY ACTING VASODILATORS

Agents in this class include diazoxide and hydralazine. Their action is both endothelium-dependent and independent but which of the two mechanisms is the most important is not known.

CALCIUM CHANNEL BLOCKERS

Using calcium channel blockers it has been demonstrated that influx of extracellular calcium couples EDRF release with receptor binding. Nifedipine, a dihydropyridine derivative, diltiazem, a benzothiazepine derivative, and verapamil, a phenylalkyalmine compound, are all calcium channel blockers. None of these structurally different compounds affect the synthesis and/or release of EDRF. The movement of calcium that occurs during EDRF release and relaxation by EDRF is not blocked by these agents. It is probable that all three have the majority of their activity at the voltage-gated calcium channels. The relaxation produced by these compounds is, therefore, endothelium-independent (Jayatody et al 1987, Peterson & Harrison 1991).

ANGIOTENSIN CONVERTING ENZYME (ACE) INHIBITORS

Captopril and enalapril are both ACE inhibitors. Bradykinin is a powerful agonist for the release of EDRF and since ACE also plays a role in the inactivation of bradykinin, it was thought that this was the mechanism by which inhibitors produced their vasodilation.

Enalapril, which is structurally different from captopril, does not cause endothelium-dependent relaxation. In contrast, a stereoisomer of captopril that is 100-fold less potent in its inhibition of ACE does increase endothelium-dependent relaxation. This suggests that the relaxation caused by captopril is mediated via EDRF and is unrelated to its inhibition of ACE.

It is possible that the sulphydryl group of captopril scavenges oxygen-derived free radicals such as superoxide anion ($O_2^{\cdot-}$). As $O_2^{\cdot-}$ inactivates NO (Fig. 5.4) the relaxant effect of captopril could be due to a prolongation of the half-life of EDRF (Goldschmidt & Tallanda 1991).

CONCLUSIONS

It is cyclic GMP that mediates endothelium-dependent and independent vascular smooth muscle relaxation. Influx of extracellular calcium couples receptor binding at the cell membrane to EDRF synthesis and/or release and there is, therefore, a balance between relaxation and contraction. It is thought that the defect present in essential hypertension may be due to an imbalance of these processes producing increased vascular tone (Tolins et al 1991).

Atherosclerotic vessels have exaggerated responses to vasoconstrictors (possibly due to the reduced half-life of EDRF). In this condition monocytes migrate to the intima of vessels and become foam cells by the uptake of low density lipoproteins. This reduces the release of prostacyclin and NO from the vascular endothelial. In addition activated monocytes release oxygen free

$$2NO + O_2^{\cdot-} \longrightarrow 2NO_2$$

$$2NO_2 + H_2O \longrightarrow NO_2^- + NO_3^- + 2H^+$$

Fig. 5.4   The metabolic inactivation of nitric oxide to nitrite and nitrate using the oxygen-derived free radical superoxide anion.

radicals which shorten the half-life of EDRF. Both factors may be involved in the vasospasm associated with atherosclerosis. Thromboxane is released from monocytes which also contribute to vasoconstriction. Endothelium-dependent relaxations in these vessels were depressed but endothelium-independent relaxations were preserved. In essential hypertension, although both mechanisms were depressed, endothelium-independent relaxations were proportionally less so — a factor which may be of importance in the choice of antihypertensive therapy. In renal failure there is limited excretion of an enzyme which destroys EDRF and therefore this may be a further mechanism of hypertension (Vallance et al 1992).

From the current literature the only vasodilator that has its mechanism of action involving EDRF is the ACE inhibitor captopril. All other vasodilators produce endothelium-independent relaxation of vascular smooth muscle.

In animals, endotoxin and cytokines such as interleukin-1 and tumour necrosis factor cause vascular relaxation and hypotension by producing a sustained release of NO from endothelial cells. Recent studies in both animals and humans have shown that by giving L-NMMA (an inhibitor of endogenous NO synthesis) the hypotension of septic shock can be inhibited (Nava et al 1991, Petros et al 1991). It may, therefore, be more appropriate to reverse the cardiovascular effects of septic shock with a single agent aimed specifically at the NO–cyclicGMP system rather than using less selective vasoconstrictors. This alternative therapeutic approach may be associated with a reduction in the morbidity often seen with the use of vasoconstrictors, such as noradrenaline, and possibly a reduction in mortality.

REFERENCES

Birkenboam G, Fang Z Y, Unger P, Fontaine J 1990. Effects of in-vivo SIN treatment on nitrovasodilators relaxation and on EDRF-mediated responses in rat aorta. J Cardiovasc Pharmacol 16: 636–640
Cocks T M, Angus J A 1990. Comparison of relaxation responses of vascular and non-vascular smooth muscle to EDRF, acidified sodium nitrite (NO) and sodium nitroprusside. Arch Pharmacol 341: 364–372.
Collier J, Vallance P 1991. Physiological importance of nitric oxide. Br Med J 302: 1289–1290.
Cryglewski R J, Palmer R M J, Moncada S 1987 Superoxide, anion is involved in the breakdown of EDRF. Nature 327: 524–526.
Dominiczat A F, Bohr D F 1989 Vascular smooth muscle in hypertension. J Hypertens 7 (suppl 4): S107–S115.
Furchgott R F, Zawadski J V 1980. The obligatory role of endothelial cells in the relaxation of arterial smooth muscle by acetylcholine. Nature 288: 373–376
Gold M E, Buga G M, Wood K S, Byrns R E 1990 Antagonistic modulatory roles of magnesium and calcium on release of EDRF and smooth muscle tone. Circ Res 1990; 66: 355–366
Goldschmidt J E, Tallanda R J 1991 Pharmacological evidence that captopril possesses an endothelium-mediated component of vasodilation: effect of sulphydryl groups on EDRF. J Pharmacol Exp Ther 257: 1136–1145
Hong K W, Rhim B Y, Lee W S et al 1990 Release of superoxide dependent relaxing factor from endothelial cells. Am J Physiol 257: H1340–H1346
Jayatody R L, Kappagoda C T, Senaratne M P J, Sreeharon N 1987 Absence of effect of

calcium antagonists on endothelium-dependent relaxations in rabbit aorta. Br J Pharmacol 91: 155–164.

Johns R A, Peach M J, Linden J, Tichotsky A 1990 n Monomethyl L-arginine inhibits EDRF-stimulated cyclic GMP accumulation in cocultures of endothelial and vascular smooth muscle cells by an action specific to the endothelial cell. Circ Res 67: 979–985.

Joulou-Schaeffer G, Gray G A, Flemming I et al 1990 Loss of vascular responsiveness induced by endotoxin involves the L-arginine pathway. Am J Physiol 259: H1038–H1043.

Munaj J F, Dawson A R, Sherlock S 1958 Circulatory changes in chronic liver disease. Am J Med 32: 358:367

Nava E, Palmer R M, Moncada S 1991 Inhibition of nitric oxide synthesis in septic shock: how much is beneficial? Lancet 338: 1555–1556

Palmer R M J, Ferrige A G, Moncada S 1987 Nitric oxide release accounts for the activity of EDRF. Nature 327: 524–526

Peterson T, Harrison D G 1991 Release of nitrogen oxides from cultured bovine aortic endothelial cells is not impaired by calcium channel antagonists. Circulation 83: 1404–1490

Petros A, Bennett D, Vallance P 1991 Effect of nitric oxide synthase inhibitors on hypotension in patients with septic shock. Lancet 338: 1557–1558

Pou W S, Pou S, Rosen G M, El-Fatahany E T 1990 EDRF release is a common pathway in the activation of guanylate cyclase by receptor agonists and calciumionophores. Pharmacology 182: 393–39

Rau L 1990 Hypertension, endothelium and cardiovascular risk factors. Am J Med (suppl 2A): 13–18

Tolins J P, Shultz P J, Ray L 1991 Role of EDRF in regulation of vascular tone and remodelling. Update on humoral regulation of vascular tone. Hypertension 17: 909–916

Vallance P, Moncada S 1991 Hyperdynamic circulation in cirrhosis: a role for nitric oxide? Lancet 337: 776–778

Vallance P, Leone A et al 1992 Accumulation of an endogenous inhibitor of nitric oxide synthesis in chronic renal failure. Lancet 339: 572–575

Waldman S A, Murad F 1988 Biochemical mechanisms underlying vascular smooth muscle relaxation: The guanylate cyclase–cyclic GMP system. Cardiovasc Pharmacol 12 (suppl): 115–118

Warren J B, Maltby N H, MacCormack D, Barnes P J 1989 Pulmonary endothelium-derived relaxing factor is impaired in hypoxia. Clin Sci 77: 671–676

6. Perioperative hypoxaemia

P. S. Mangat   J. G. Jones

The problem of hypoxaemia occurring in the perioperative period has provided a stimulus for research since Bendixen et al (1963) and Nunn (1964) independently described impaired pulmonary gas exchange during anaesthesia nearly 30 years ago. For many years it was thought that the underlying cause of this abnormality of gas exchange was due to closure of airways in the dependent lung. This was confirmed by Hedenstierna and co-workers in the 1980s using computed tomography (CT) scanning techniques; these authors showed that intraoperative impairment of gas exchange is due to dependent lung atelectasis. In the postoperative period this abnormality may persist for hours or even days and provides a background of ventilation to perfusion (V/Q) mismatch which, when combined with impaired ventilatory control due to opioid administration, may cause both profound and prolonged hypoxaemia.

This chapter summarizes current thinking on the pulmonary effects of anaesthesia, discusses the impact of predisposing factors on perioperative hypoxaemia, describes the patterns of oxygen saturation seen in the postoperative period and discusses the clinical significance of hypoxaemia.

PULMONARY CHANGES WITH ANAESTHESIA

Changes in lung volume

Bergman (1963) was the first to show that there was a decrease in functional residual capacity (FRC) of about 20% after induction of anaesthesia. This decrease in FRC was later shown to be closely correlated with an increase in alveolar-arterial Po_2 (A-aPo_2) difference (Hickey et al 1973, Hewlett et al 1974); an extraordinary finding was that the fall in FRC and the increase in A-aPo_2 difference occurred to the same extent whether the anaesthetized patients were breathing spontaneously or were paralysed and ventilated (Hewlett et al 1974). Some years later Heneghan et al (1984) showed that if the FRC of anaesthetized subjects was increased, using positive end expiratory pressure (PEEP), to the value seen in the awake subject, the A-aPo_2 difference did not return to normal. They concluded that a decrease in lung volume by itself was not the cause of impaired gas exchange and reasoned that the fall in FRC caused a V/Q abnormality which was not reversed by PEEP. In a later study Heneghan and Jones (1985) showed that if FRC was increased by phrenic nerve stimulation there was a greater improvement in gas exchange than if the same increase in lung volume was achieved by PEEP alone. They explained these findings as follows: the fall in FRC led to a reduction of alveolar volume in the dependent part of the lung which was not reversed by PEEP. Phrenic nerve stimulation caused a much greater movement of the dependent part of the diaphragm than that seen with PEEP, and therefore a greater improvement in gas exchange by expansion of the alveoli in the dependent lung.

The fall in FRC during anaesthesia implies a change in diaphragm and/or ribcage position; a cranial shift of the diaphragm was demonstrated by Froese & Bryan (1974), though no change was seen in ribcage dimensions. There followed considerable speculation whether a reduction in tone of the chest wall fully explained the fall in FRC or whether there was also a change in thoracoabdominal blood volume (Jones 1987). Subsequent work by Hedenstierna et al (1985) using CT scanning, central blood volume measurement and FRC recordings confirmed the cranial shift of the diaphragm and noted a slight reduction in transverse cross-sectional area of the thorax. These changes are consistent with a reduction in respiratory muscle tone due to the effects of anaesthesia. They also showed that diversion of blood occurred away from the thorax, probably with pooling in the abdomen, with consequent reduction in intrathoracic volume by 0.8 l.

The reduction in FRC invites the hypothesis that *airway closure* in the dependent lung occurs during anaesthesia and more so in those patients in whom closing volume was very near the end expiratory point (Jones 1982). Patients susceptible to this type of airway closure would be the very young, the elderly, smokers and the obese. In such patients any FRC reduction would result in airway closure during tidal breathing. If this occurred, increased right-to-left shunt and impaired V/Q ratios would explain intraoperative hypoxaemia. This prediction was confirmed when Dueck et al (1988) showed that if the FRC *during* anaesthesia was less than *awake* closing capacity, then the shunt increased to a much greater extent than if the FRC during anaesthesia exceeded the awake closing capacity. This increase in shunt was greater in patients who were smokers.

Opinions vary regarding the airway closure theory and on the effects of different types of general anaesthesia. Attempts have been made to simulate the effects of anaesthesia by reducing FRC by thoracoabdominal restriction using a corset in awake healthy volunteers. However this method also reduced closing capacity (CC) so that the difference between FRC and CC remained relatively unaltered (Tokics et al 1988). This is a poor model of the effects of anaesthesia on pulmonary function because chest wall restriction has long been known to increase lung recoil pressure and thus to reduce closing volume.

Overall, there is poor correlation between degree of airway closure, as measured from changes in expired gas concentration, and the extent of impaired gas exchange during anaesthesia. However, it must be pointed out that airway closure is inferred from measurements of *expired* tracer gas concentration and this technique may not accurately reflect the tendency to dependent airway closure *within* the lungs.

It is of interest that different anaesthetics may have different effects on pulmonary function. Whereas volatile agents and/or neuromuscular blockade cause a fall in FRC and an impairment in gas exchange, Bickler et al (1987) showed that a fall in FRC and airway closure were unlikely during methohexitone anaesthesia where patients were spontaneously ventilating and suggested that intubation itself was somehow related to subsequent changes in pulmonary function. Furthermore Tokics et al (1987a) showed that ketamine anaesthesia was not associated with development of dependent atelectasis. This may be due to the preservation of diaphragmatic tone with this agent.

Hypoxic pulmonary vasoconstriction

Hypoxic pulmonary vasoconstriction (HPV) is a mechanism by which blood is directed away from regions which have low V/Q ratios. Inhibition of HPV by several inhalational anaesthetic agents has been suggested as the cause of impaired gas exchange during anaesthesia, although intravenous agents do not appear to inhibit HPV (Eisenkraft 1990).

All manner of ingenious preparations, methods and species have been used to examine the effect of anaesthetics on HPV. Because of compensatory mechanisms which may be difficult to measure accurately, particularly in humans, *the inhibition of HPV is usually of little clinical consequence in terms of worsening hypoxaemia.*

For HPV to have any significant effect, an underlying disturbance of lung function is required for arterial oxygenation to be impaired. However, abolition of HPV alone does not produce impairment of gas exchange. The present consensus is that potent inhaled anaesthetic agents are not contraindicated for thoracic surgery requiring one-lung ventilation when active HPV is most desirable. Indeed, their use has been advocated because of their salutary effect on bronchomotor tone, high potency (allowing high inspired concentrations of oxygen) and rapid elimination (Eisenkraft 1990).

Atelectasis

Bendixen et al (1963) noticed a progressive decrease in lung compliance during anaesthesia and postulated, 30 years ago, that atelectasis developed following anaesthetic induction. Conventional radiography has repeatedly failed to demonstrate such pulmonary changes. However several factors predispose to atelectasis: decreased lung volume with consequent airway narrowing; marked volume reduction in dependent regions of the lung; proportionally greater impairment of movement of the dependent part of the diaphragm; and inability of PEEP or positive pressure ventilation to overcome reduced movement of dependent lung and diaphragm.

The work by Brismar et al (1985) comparing CT scans in awake patients with scans on the same patients following induction of anaesthesia (Fig. 6.1) has demonstrated regions of dependent lung atelectasis which occur within 15 min of induction in 90% of subjects with normal lungs. Atelectasis develops whether the patient is breathing spontaneously or is paralysed and ventilated mechanically (Strandberg et al 1986). For many years atelectasis has been attributed to absorption collapse of lung units, particularly when insoluble gases such as nitrogen are replaced by more soluble gases such as nitrous oxide or oxygen. Browne et al (1970) have shown that there is a 50% reduction in the area of radiographic atelectasis during one-lung anaesthesia if nitrogen is included in the anaesthetic mixture. The effect of nitrogen in reducing the collapse of alveoli distal to closed airways was first shown by Green and Burgess (1962) who demonstrated that 20% nitrogen added to inspired oxygen markedly reduced lung collapse in RAF jet fighter pilots following high G turns. Furthermore Dantzker et al (1975) have shown that the time to atelectasis depends not only on the V/Q ratio of the region but also the solubility of the gas contained in the alveoli. In contrast to these examples of absorption atelectasis Hedenstierna (1990) stated that the dense regions in the dependent lung developed even when the fractional inspired oxygen (Fio_2) was changed between 0.4 and 1.0 — a finding at variance with the theory of absorption atelectasis.

Work in the sheep lung showed that the dense regions induced by anaesthesia in dependent zones were microscopically completely collapsed

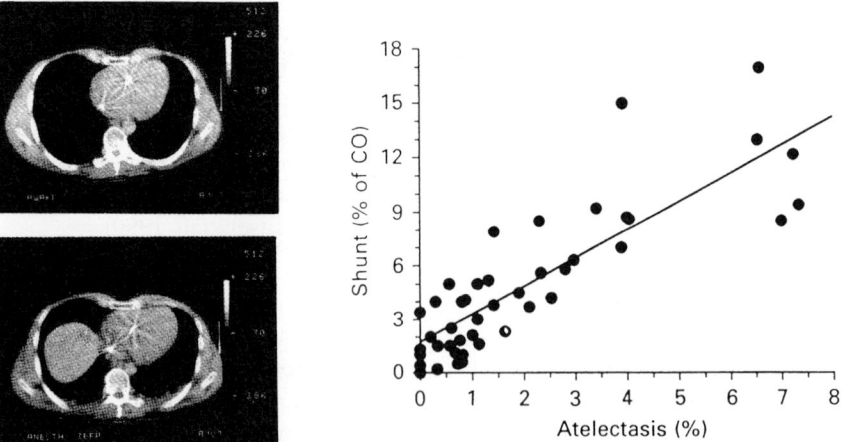

Fig. 6.1   Left: The computed tomography (CT) scans show the change from awake (top) to anaesthetized (bottom) where extensive atelectasis appears in the dependent parts of the lung bilaterally. **Right**: the relationship between the area of atelectatic lung and shunt during anaesthesia. (CT scans courtesy of Dr Hedenstierna; shunt diagram reproduced from Hedenstierna 1990 with permission of *Br J Anaesth*.)

lung units — that is, atelectasis with moderate vascular congestion but no interstitial oedema. Hedenstierna et al (1989) termed these dense areas *compression atelectasis*. An important finding is that the size of the dependent lung densities correlated closely with the degree of intrapulmonary shunt (Hedenstierna et al 1986; Fig. 6.1). The administration of 10 cm H_2O PEEP reduced the volume of the densities on CT scans but did not decrease the shunt (Tokics et al 1987b). The authors postulated that PEEP may have redistributed pulmonary blood from high to low V/Q regions. The type of anaesthetic regimen also affects the regions of compression atelectasis. Both intravenous (barbiturate or propofol) and inhalational anaesthesia result in regions of compression atelectasis. Addition of neuromuscular blockade induces a further (though small) increase in the atelectatic areas (Hedenstierna et al 1986). In contrast ketamine has been found to produce atelectasis, though subsequent paralysis in patients receiving ketamine caused atelectatic areas to appear (Tokics et al 1987a). This confirms the concept that the tone of the chest wall is a major determinant of atelectasis.

Recently Lindberg et al (1992) found that atelectasis persisted for at least 4 days into the postoperative period. They suggested that following the initial *compression* atelectasis, absorption of soluble gases may well occur behind closed-off airways to produce further regions of *absorption* atelectasis during anaesthesia. These effects will persist even after termination of anaesthesia and return of chest wall tone. Gunnarsson et al (1991) showed no significant correlation between the development of atelectasis and increasing age. A curious finding is that after a patient is anaesthetized the densities are relatively resistant to changes in posture. A patient moved from the supine to the lateral position loses the densities from the upper lung, and the densities in the lower lung enlarge, *but remain in the previously dependent aspect of the lung.* There is no information available on the prone position following induction of anaesthesia in the supine position. This work may be even more interesting.

In summary, Hedenstierna's work has confirmed the original hypothesis of Bendixen et al (1963) that impairment of gas exchange during anaesthesia is largely due to atelectasis in the dependent part of the lung. The decrease in FRC and compliance are explained by the loss of tone in the muscles of the ribcage and diaphragm with anaesthesia. The fact that ketamine anaesthesia preserves respiratory muscle function and results in normal gas exchange suggests that a loss of tone in the chest wall causes a fall in lung volume which results in *compression* atelectasis. It is also likely that additional regions of *absorption* atelectasis develop during prolonged anaesthesia which persist for at least 4 days into the postoperative period.

PREOPERATIVE RISK FACTORS

In normal young people breathing air at sea level the oxygen saturation is about 97% but with increasing age there is a progressive fall in oxygen saturation to about 95% in subjects between 70 and 80 years of age (Blom et al 1988; Fig. 6.2). This effect of age on oxygen saturation is similar to the effect on closing volume where the difference between FRC and closing capacity gets progressively smaller with age (Jones 1982). Based on prolonged monitoring of normal young subjects (Wheatley et al 1990), we defined hypoxaemia as an arterial oxygen saturation of less than 94% for >4 min/h. It is evident from the shape of the oxyhaemoglobin dissociation curve that when oxygen saturation falls below 94%, small changes in alveolar Po_2 will cause very large changes in oxygen saturation.

With increasing altitude the inspired partial pressure of oxygen (Pio_2) falls, so that, for example, in Mexico City, Denver or Harare, the altitude is about 5000 ft (1400 m) above sea level and the Pio_2 will be about 16 kPa. Commercial aircraft are pressurized to approximately 8000 ft with a Pio_2 of about 15 kPa. It is not easy to predict the arterial oxygen saturation (Sao_2) under these conditions because Sao_2 is determined both by the Pio_2 as well as pulmonary factors (shunt, V/Q and diffusion) and circulatory factors (cardiac output, position of the oxyhaemoglobin dissociation curve and metabolic rate). The effect of increasing shunt and contribution of low V/Q on the relationship between Pio_2 and Sao_2 is shown in Figure 6.3. This representation is a useful method for predicting the effects of changing Pio_2 on SaO_2. Increasing shunt moves the upper part of the curve downwards, whereas increasing the low V/Q contribution moves the curve to the right (Sapsford & Jones 1992). In this figure, data from a normal subject are compared with an obese patient with an abnormally low V/Q ratio. Also a patient with adult respiratory distress syndrome is shown; this patient had both a large shunt and an abnormally low V/Q contribution. The importance of a shift in curve position to the right is shown in the obese patient. Here the steep part of the curve lies on the 21 kPa line (air) and *a small further shift to the right will produce a very large fall in oxygen saturation.*

While the majority of patients presenting for anaesthesia may have normal pulmonary function, many patients present with abnormal lung function which may exaggerate the effects of anaesthesia in producing hypoxaemia. A

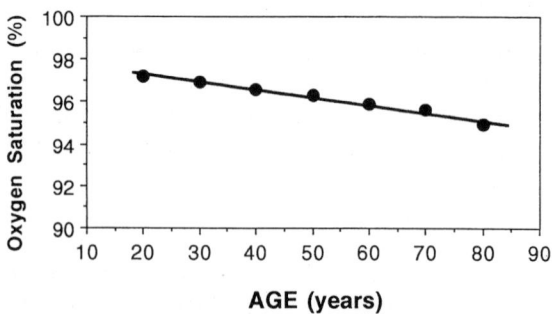

Fig. 6.2   The effect of age on oxygen saturation in healthy subjects.

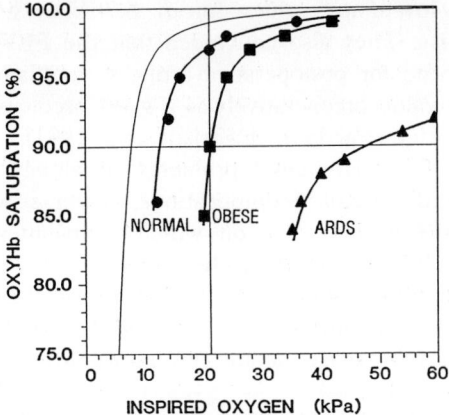

Fig. 6.3 The effect of changing inspired oxygen (P_{IO_2}) on oxygen saturation. A normal anaesthetized subject (circles) is compared with a morbidly obese subject (squares) and a patient with adult respiratory distress syndrome (triangles). The line on the left shows the haemoglobin dissociation curve (the ordinate for this curve is P_{aO_2}). Note that in the obese patient the curve is shifted to the right of normal and is very steep as it crosses the P_{IO_2} line at 21 kPa (air). (See text.)

prospective study of over 7000 patients undergoing a variety of surgical procedures examined the risk factors for postoperative pulmonary complications (Pedersen et al 1990). Factors likely to increase the incidence of hypoxaemia were chronic obstructive pulmonary disease, age >70 years, general anaesthesia involving muscle relaxation and thoracoabdominal surgery. Upper abdominal surgery resulted in a 33% incidence of pulmonary complications. The recent availability of pulse oximeters for long-term postoperative monitoring has provided evidence that hypoxaemia may occur in most patients for prolonged periods postoperatively. This will be discussed below.

This next section reviews some pulmonary risk factors and their management.

Chronic obstructive pulmonary disease (COPD)

A history of dyspnoea on exertion and orthopnoea together with impaired pulmonary function tests may be good predictors of postoperative complications. A retrospective analysis was carried out by Milledge and Nunn (1975) and by Nunn et al (1988) in 42 patients with severe obstructive airway disease (FEV_1 0.3–1 l). In the former paper, they concluded that a high arterial carbon dioxide tension indicated a poor prognosis, whereas, in the second paper (which included the patients from the original study), the authors proposed that a *low arterial oxygen tension* and *dyspnoea at rest* were best predictors of a need for postoperative mechanical ventilation. It was unclear from their paper what should be regarded as a low P_{aO_2}, although 4 patients with particularly low Pa_{O_2} values (mean 6.7 kPa) had an uneventful postoperative course. They also concluded that the FEV_1 was not a good predictor of the need for postoperative artificial ventilation. Clearly a low oxygen saturation value preoperatively is a good predictor of postoperative hypoxaemia (Wheatley et al 1990, Entwistle et al 1991).

In addition to the well-known problems of airway obstruction, V/Q mismatch and cardiovascular complications, patients with COPD have impaired respiratory muscle function which contributes to postoperative hypoxaemia. The hyperinflation of the ribcage and particularly the flat diaphragm seen in emphysema renders inspiratory muscles mechanically disadvantaged. The respiratory-depressant effects of drugs commonly used during anaesthesia may exaggerate any respiratory difficulty in the postoperative period.

Preoperative treatment of COPD may include bronchodilators, physiotherapy, (Selsby & Jones 1990), continuous oxygen therapy, correction of malnutrition and antibiotics. Malnutrition is common in emphysematous patients and is associated with a poor prognosis. Enteric feeding (1000 kcal above normal intake for 16 days) has been shown to increase body weight and improve respiratory muscle strength and endurance (Whittaker et al 1990). Hypophosphataemia is common (20%) among COPD patients and is associated with respiratory muscle weakness. The use of frusemide and steroids may exacerbate hypophosphataemia by decreasing renal reabsorption of phosphate. Since phosphorus is a key element in respiratory muscle function, replacement therapy should be instituted prior to elective surgery. Supplemental oxygen therapy with correction of hypoxaemia has been shown to induce a sodium diuresis and reduction of oedema (Mannix et al 1990). Thus preoperative and postoperative controlled oxygen therapy may be of benefit in chronically hypoxaemic patients.

The place of central respiratory stimulants is now being re-examined in the context of postoperative respiratory function. Doxapram has been claimed to decrease postoperative pulmonary complications (Jansen et al 1990). Almitrine bismezylate, a respiratory stimulant acting directly on the carotid body, has recently been developed. In addition to its effect on the carotid body it also improves V/Q distribution. Unfortunately, side-effects may limit its use (Roe and Jones 1991).

Asthma

The incidence of asthma has increased over recent decades and the rising mortality rates have raised the profile of the disease, culminating in the publication of Guidelines for Management of Asthma in Adults (British Thoracic Society 1990a,b). This recommends a more liberal use of steroids with peak flow monitoring. The place of methylxanthines in the treatment of asthma must now be seriously questioned. Their life-threatening side-effects, small therapeutic window and inferior efficacy in treating bronchoconstriction (compared with β_2-stimulants) renders them unsuitable as front-line treatment (Jones et al 1987, Lam & Newhouse 1990). While the recent introduction of long-acting β-stimulants (salmeterol and formoterol) has provided improved control in asthmatics, and they are claimed to have an anti-inflammatory action, they cannot be used as an alternative to inhaled steroid therapy.

Bronchospasm during anaesthesia is rare, presumably because inhalational agents are bronchodilators (Jones et al 1987). However, light levels of anaesthesia, which may occur during induction or emergence, and the presence of tracheal tubes can precipitate bronchospasm. Premedication with inhaled β_2-stimulants may attenuate this response.

Cystic fibrosis

The recent identification and sequencing of the cystic fibrosis gene has provided an explanation of the chloride channel defect that characterizes the condition (Riordan et al 1989). How decreased chloride permeability leads to suppurative lung disease is uncertain but it is thought that viral infection predisposes to bacterial colonization. *Pseudomonas aeruginosa* is present in a form unique to cystic fibrosis and is responsible for the production of alginate which combines with mucus to produce the highly viscid secretions typical of cystic fibrosis.

With progressive tissue damage, bronchiectatic regions develop which impair gas exchange and cause worsening hypoxaemia. Current treatment includes antibiotics, postural drainage and physiotherapy. Oxygen therapy has been used to treat pulmonary hypertension and sodium retention. Anti-inflammatory agents and nebulized amiloride have been shown to be beneficial (see Roe & Jones 1991 for review).

Pulmonary complications in the acquired immune deficiency syndrome (AIDS)

Pneumocystis carinii is the commonest pathogen in a wide spectrum of respiratory infections that can occur in AIDS. *P. carinii* pneumonia (PCP) is the presenting disease in two-thirds of AIDS patients. PCP indicates a poor prognosis with mortality rates of up to 85%. Diagnoses have been made until recently by fibreoptic bronchoalveolar lavage providing direct samples from lungs. O'Doherty et al (1989) have described aerosol transfer of ^{99m}Tc DTPA (diethylenetriaminepentaacetic acid) as a diagnostic test of PCP. This is very useful in clearly differentiating between PCP and other pneumonias which may develop in the perioperative period. Treatments of PCP consist of high-dose co-trimoxazole or pentamidine. Prophylactic antibiotics in patients with human immunodeficiency virus may be justified, though the place of steroids in these patients is controversial.

Bleomycin

Bleomycin is a cytotoxic agent which is used primarily for treating lymphomas, testicular tumours and squamous cell carcinomas (Cooper et al 1986). The use of this drug has been limited by adverse pulmonary complications, including chronic progressive fibrosis and hypersensitivity pneumonitis in 10% of recipients (Blum et al 1973). Work by Goldiner et al (1978) based on retrospective experience in 5 patients has led to the assertion that patients previously treated with bleomycin were more susceptible to lung damage if high inspired oxygen concentrations were administered. Review of this paper reveals that these patients received Fio_2 concentrations of less than 0.45 but they were all subject to massive fluid overload. Other workers have found that high intraoperative Fio_2 does not necessarily result in an increased incidence of pulmonary complications (Lamartia et al 1984). Prior or concomitant thoracic radiotherapy definitely increases the incidence of severe bleomycin pulmonary toxicity (Rosenow 1988). This will cause hypoxaemia and the treatment of this disorder with oxygen in the perioperative period will need caution. It is probably wise to use continuous pulse oximeter monitoring and to maintain an oxygen saturation between 90 and 94% using less than 30% inspired oxygen.

Obesity

Obese patients often present multisystem risk factors to the anaesthetist, including airway difficulty, hypertension, diabetes and gastro-oesophageal reflux. Obesity is defined as body mass index of 27–35 kg/m^2 (which is weight/height^2). Morbid obesity is defined as body mass index >35 kg/m^2. The effects of obesity on pulmonary mechanics are well-known. Decreased compliance, total lung capacity (TLC), FRC and expiratory reserve volume are all caused by diaphragmatic splinting due to the increased mass of the chest wall tissue. The low FRC has been proposed as the reason for hypoxaemia which arises from a mismatching of V/Q. The well-perfused lung bases are underventilated due to airway closure and alveolar collapse (Holley et al 1967). Even with a 3-min period of preoxygenation, morbidly obese patients have a significantly shorter period of adequate oxygenation during apnoea compared with patients of normal body weight (Berthoud et al 1991).

Sleep apnoea (SA)

Interest in SA has increased in the last decade, though the picture of the sleepy, snoring, obese, oedematous individual was described by Charles Dickens in the 19th century. SA has relevance to the anaesthetist for several reasons. An increasing number of patients will present for surgery to correct their obstructive apnoea. More importantly perhaps is the increased number of patients who will be recognized as having obstructive apnoea presenting for other surgical procedures. There is a spectrum of severity of obstructive apnoea along which people move depending on the degree of sedation with anaesthetic agents, opioid analgesics, alcohol or benzodiazepines. The hypoxaemia associated with anaesthesia will be exacerbated by postoperative obstructive SA (OSA). Patients with obstructive apnoea have been shown to have increased opioid activity in cerebrospinal fluid and this regressed after successful treatment of the underlying cause (Gislason et al 1989). This may explain the increased sensitivity of such patients to opioid administration.

Sleep apnoea is invariably associated with hypoxaemia and has been demarcated into central SA (CSA) or OSA types. It is unlikely however that these two conditions are mutually exclusive. The pathophysiological mechanisms of SA result in cardiovascular complications, respiratory insufficiency and an increased mortality (Ancoli-Israel et al 1989). Features of OSA include snoring (due to upper airway collapse), excessive daytime sleepiness and periods of apnoea or hypopnoea. Patients with OSA suffer airway collapse during sleep because of a combination of several factors: pharyngeal structural abnormality, increased collapsibility of the upper airway and inadequate response of the muscles of the upper airway to mechanical, chemical and proprioceptive stimuli (Hoffstein & Zamel 1990).

Sleep *apnoea* can be defined as cessation of breathing for greater than 10 s. Sleep *hypopnoea* is a reduction in tidal volume of greater than 50% for more than 10 s. Both of the above should be accompanied by a 4% fall in oxygen saturation. The apnoea or hypopnoea index (AHI) is the number of episodes of sleep apnoea or hypopnoea per hour. Some workers define SA as an AHI of 10 episodes/h (Hoffstein & Zamel 1990), though others use an AHI of 5 episodes/h (Lindholm et al 1990). Aber et al (1989) found that a third of elderly men may be classified differently on different nights if a strict cut-off point is adhered to. Since SA in the elderly can be as high as 70% if an AHI of 5 episodes/h is accepted as the cut-off point for positive diagnosis (Ancoli-Israel et al 1989), it may be that different AHI values should apply to different age groups.

A variety of diagnostic tools have been advocated to diagnose SA. Cine-CT images one slice of the airway every 24 ms, which allows visualization of the airway during apnoeic episodes and determines the site of obstruction. The acoustic reflection technique (Hillberg et al 1989) has successfully diagnosed airway abnormalities from mouth to carina, although it was most sensitive to defects in the trachea (see review by Hoffstein & Zamel 1990).

The site of obstruction can be at several places between the nares and trachea. The localization of the site is therefore important if treatment is to be directed to the specific abnormality. A variety of medical treatments have been tried including respiratory, carotid body and central stimulants as well as drugs which improve activity in the upper airway muscle. The only useful measures however have been nasal continuous positive airway pressure (NCPAP) and treatment of underlying conditions such as acromegaly, hypothyroidism, obesity and allergic rhinitis. Sullivan et al (1981) showed that NCPAP abolishes sleep apnoea in most patients and improves the clinical symptoms of SA. NCPAP splints the upper airway during inspiration but may also cause either reflex activation of pharyngeal muscles or direct dilatation of the upper airway. Long-term NCPAP has also been shown to improve daytime oxygenation by increasing FRC and hence alveolar ventilation (Sforza et al 1990). NCPAP also improves CSA which may be the result of improved alveolar ventilation (Guilleminault et al 1989). A recent study (Sanders & Kern 1990) has considered airway collapse during expiration. The authors were able to adjust inspiratory and expiratory positive airway pressure and found that positive expiratory airway pressure and PEEP eliminated OSA more efficiently compared with NCPAP.

Surgical correction 15 years ago was limited to tracheostomy and has been shown to have a high technical success rate in treating OSA. There are side-effects related to excessive secretions, the tracheostomy itself, the social stigma and inadequate humidification. The most common surgical procedure currently performed is uvulopalatopharyngoplasty (UPPP). However this is a controversial procedure because the problems of criteria for diagnosis and outcome of OSA make UPPP difficult to evaluate.

Prediction of outcome

There is certainly a requirement for an index of pulmonary insufficiency. This needs to be simple, universally applicable and correlated to outcome. Difficulties arise because many extrapulmonary factors such as myocardial function, intravascular volume, extent of surgery and haemoglobinopathy have a bearing on postoperative respiratory function. Seymour et al (1990) applied a system described by Knill-Jones (1987) to predict postoperative respiratory complications. This method evaluates the severity of given preoperative factors in predicting postoperative respiratory compromise. It allowed for the variability and interdependence of symptoms and conditions. Preoperative respiratory pathology, surgical incision site, smoking in the 6 weeks preceding surgery and circulating volume depletion were the features examined. Curiously the factor which was the strongest predictor of pulmonary outcome in this study was hypovolaemia! This may well have reflected the poor overall condition of these patients.

Gass & Olsen (1986) reviewed the use of pulmonary function tests in preoperative prediction of outcome, but the complexity of tests made them appear impractical. The respiratory reserve has been promulgated as an important predictor of a patient's ability to tolerate the physiological defects induced by anaesthesia. Beachey & Olsen (1990) quantified respiratory reserve by the difference between maximum sustainable ventilation and the degree of ventilation required to produce an arteriolar pH of 7.3. Their reasoning was that the respiratory system is dependent on the cardiovascular system which in turn is dependent on the degree of respiratory acidosis in COPD and cor pulmonale patients. Their index was able to discriminate between those patients who progressed to respiratory failure and those who did not.

The search for a single preoperative index which can reliably predict perioperative hypoxaemia continues. The studies by Seymour et al (1990) and Beachey & Olsen (1990) however are very useful in helping to resolve this issue.

POSTOPERATIVE HYPOXAEMIA

Hypoxaemia in the postoperative period is of particular concern due to its possible contribution to postoperative morbidity and mortality. As pointed out in the introduction, the cause of postoperative hypoxaemia is likely to be a combination of impaired gas exchange (atelectasis), impaired control of breathing (sleep, analgesia) and other factors associated with anaesthesia. Intraoperative atelectasis with associated impaired gas exchange persists for at least 4 days into the postoperative period (Lindberg et al 1992) and is often exacerbated by incisional pain and reflex diaphragmatic dysfunction. A recent review by Wahba (1991) makes the important point that diaphragmatic contractility is also decreased for several postoperative days, though phrenic nerve stimulation restores normal diaphragmatic movement (Dureuil et al 1987). This suggests that the diaphragmatic dysfunction is likely to be of a reflex nature rather than due to pain, and is supported by the findings that epidural bupivacaine (Mankikian et al 1988) but not fentanyl (Simonneau et al 1983) seems to improve diaphragmatic function. This diaphragmatic dysfunction encourages further atelectasis, hypoxaemia and a shift from abdominal to ribcage breathing, which explains the rapid shallow breaths associated with abdominal surgery.

Early-phase hypoxaemia

Craig (1981) described an early and late phase of postoperative hypoxaemia. The early phase of postoperative hypoxaemia is most likely to be due to central or obstructive apnoea. Central apnoea and hypoxaemia are caused by a low Pa_{CO_2} in sedated postoperative patients (Northwood et al 1991). Anaesthetized and sedated patients behave differently from awake subjects. Thus ventilation ceases if the Pa_{CO_2} falls below the apnoeic threshold in anaesthetized or sedated patients. In contrast, in fully conscious subjects, breathing continues if Pa_{CO_2} falls below this threshold. Added to central apnoea is episodic obstructive apnoea due to the residual effects of anaesthesia in impairing control of patency of the upper airway. This is a very important cause of postoperative hypoxaemia. N_2O washout is not an important cause of hypoxaemia. Lampe et al (1990) found that when N_2O was added to isoflurane it failed to increase the incidence of early or late postoperative hypoxaemia compared with just oxygen and isoflurane. This supports the assertion of Jones et al (1990) that diffusion hypoxia during N_2O elimination is unimportant. Other factors contributing to early postoperative hypoxaemia include small systemic concentrations (0.1 MAC) of inhalational agents which abolish hypoxic ventilatory drive.

Incomplete reversal of neuromuscular blockade is a common postoperative complication. A number of studies (Viby-Mogensen et al 1979, Beemer & Rozental 1986, Bevan et al 1988) reported 42, 21 and 36% incidences of inadequate reversal. This high incidence has persisted for over 10 years despite the increased use of neuromuscular monitoring. The incidence appears to be less in those patients receiving atracurium and vecuronium. The development of shorter-acting agents such as mivacurium and rocuronium and modern neuromuscular monitoring systems with double-burst stimulation may further decrease this problem.

Late-phase hypoxaemia

While early-phase hypoxaemia may be acute and dramatic during the immediate postoperative period, late-phase hypoxaemia may be very prolonged and profound, with oxygen saturation as low as 60%. Factors affecting the late phase of postoperative hypoxaemia are dominated by the combined effects of atelectasis and opioid-induced abnormalities of respiratory control; the latter is exacerbated by the effect of sleep. Continuous respiratory monitoring techniques showed that opioid analgesia caused short periods of respiratory obstruction (Catling et al 1980). These abnormalities were not noticed during intermittent observation by nursing or medical staff and were later shown to be accompanied by episodes of profound hypoxaemia with $Sao_2 < 70\%$ (Catley et al 1985). It follows that patients with conditions that predispose to respiratory disturbances (obesity, sleep apnoea) or to hypoxaemia (lung disease, pulmonary infection, upper abdominal or thoracic surgery) may suffer prolonged and profound periods of oxyhaemoglobin desaturation.

In a pioneering study, the effects of sleep and of different postoperative analgesic regimens on breathing patterns and oxygenation were examined in two groups of patients monitored continuously overnight following surgery (Catley et al 1985). Each patient had received a standardized general anaesthetic and was recovering from either cholecystectomy or hip replacement. The patients received either regional anaesthesia with bupivacaine or an intravenous infusion of morphine.

There was a considerable reduction in arterial saturation after operation in both groups and this recovered towards normal over the subsequent 16 h. The Sao_2 in the regional anaesthesia group was higher than in the morphine group but the most remarkable difference between the two groups was the frequency of episodes of profound oxygen desaturation in the morphine group. During a 16 h period patients who received morphine had almost 500 episodes of marked oxygen desaturation ($Sao_2 < 80\%$) which occurred only when the ventilatory pattern was disturbed. In contrast, no patient in the postoperative regional anaesthesia group showed SaO_2 less than 87%, despite the fact that patients in this group also had apnoeic episodes. There was a strong association between obstructive apnoea and hypoxaemia, and no episode of hypoxaemia was seen in association with central apnoea. *All the hypoxaemic episodes (SaO_2<80%) occurred during sleep and all in patients who received morphine.*

Effects of sleep and analgesia on upper airway patency

The combined effects of sleep and opioid analgesia closely simulate SA. Obstructive apnoea is caused by closure of the upper airway, which may remain closed despite increased breathing effort. The oropharynx is the only collapsible segment of the upper airway because its walls are too compliant to resist the effects of a negative transmural pressure. Reduced patency is promoted by negative airway pressure, neck flexion and abnormal anatomy.

A large negative pressure (as much as 8 kPa) is needed to close the upper airway completely in normal awake humans whereas a pressure of <1 kPa is required during sleep or sedation. The large mechanical forces that oppose collapse when awake are due to the tone in the airway muscles. This tonic activity dilates the airway, decreases its compliance and increases its resistance to collapse.

In awake subjects all the muscles of the upper airway also exhibit phasic activation which just precedes activation of the diaphragm. In this way the upper airway suddenly becomes highly resistant to the collapsing pressure induced in the airway lumen during activation of the diaphragm. However, when the neural control of the upper airway is impaired or abolished (as in rapid eye movement sleep, during anaesthesia or postoperatively during sleep after morphine administration), the phasic activation of the upper airway musculature may be reduced, become synchronous with, or follow diaphragmatic activation, when oropharyngeal collapse ensues.

Presentation of data from long-term pulse oximetry

The availability of the pulse oximeter for postoperative monitoring presents problems in data management. The conventional method of presenting these data is where the SaO_2 is plotted against time. This is useful particularly for short periods of data collection. A more convenient method is a cumulative plot of SaO_2 for epochs of up to 1 h. This may be a useful way of presenting data so that the patterns of SaO_2 during long periods of monitoring can be displayed more readily.

The pattern of oxygen saturation in 5-min epochs is shown in a preoperative patient in Figure 6.4. Each epoch displays a distribution curve of oxygen saturation during the 5-min data collection period. Note that the peaks tend to be superimposed during the first 15-min. When a morphine premedication is given, the subsequent peaks move gradually to the left.

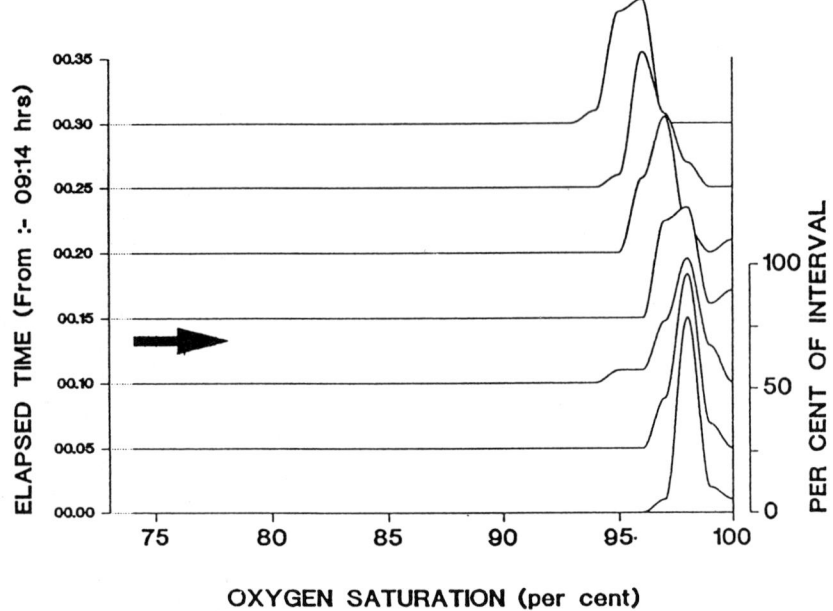

Fig. 6.4 Continuous monitoring of oxygen saturation (Spo2) with data divided into 5-min periods starting at 09.14 h. A premedication dose of morphine is given at the arrow. Note the gradual fall in oxygen saturation after morphine.

In a study of patients immediately following thoracotomy, four patterns of oxygen saturation with subjects breathing air were seen (Fig. 6.5; Entwistle et al 1991). This figure shows epochs of 1 h for either an 18-h or 24-h data collection period. Of the four patterns of oxygen saturation seen there was a stable pattern without hypoxaemia (A), a stable but hypoxaemic pattern where there is a gradual improvement during the 18-h monitoring period (B), a stable but hypoxaemic pattern throughout the study (C), or an entirely unstable pattern (D). The advantage of this type of display is that artefacts can be identified and the underlying cause of hypoxaemia (whether shunting or abnormality of ventilatory control, as well as the response to oxygen) can be ascertained. This approach can also be used to examine the changes in consecutive nights before and after surgery (Fig. 6.6). This shows the pattern with the patient breathing air on the preoperative nights and compares this with monitoring periods on the first (I), second (II), third (III) and fourth (IV) postoperative nights. Note that this patient was most hypoxaemic on the second postoperative night and had not recovered to preoperative values even by the fourth night. *All these patients were studied breathing air.*

The patterns of oxygen saturation described above (stable or unstable) are determined by the position of the P_{IO_2} vs Spo_2 curve. In Figure 6.7 the curve is shifted to the right of normal so that the steep part of the curve lies on the ine marking a P_{IO_2} at 21 kPa (air). Note the unstable pattern seen when the

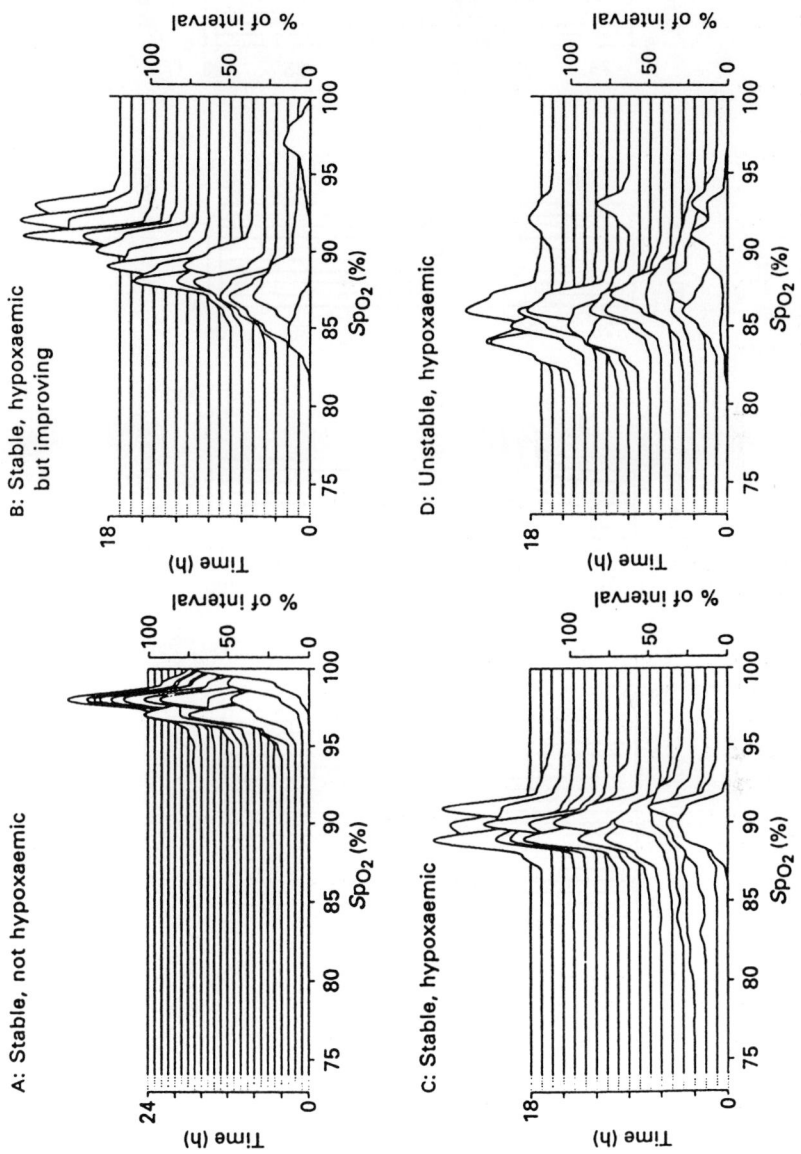

Fig. 6.5 Patterns of oxygen saturation (Sp_{O_2}) plotted in 1-h intervals. (See text.) (Reproduced from Entwistle et al 1991 with permission of *Br J Anaesth.*)

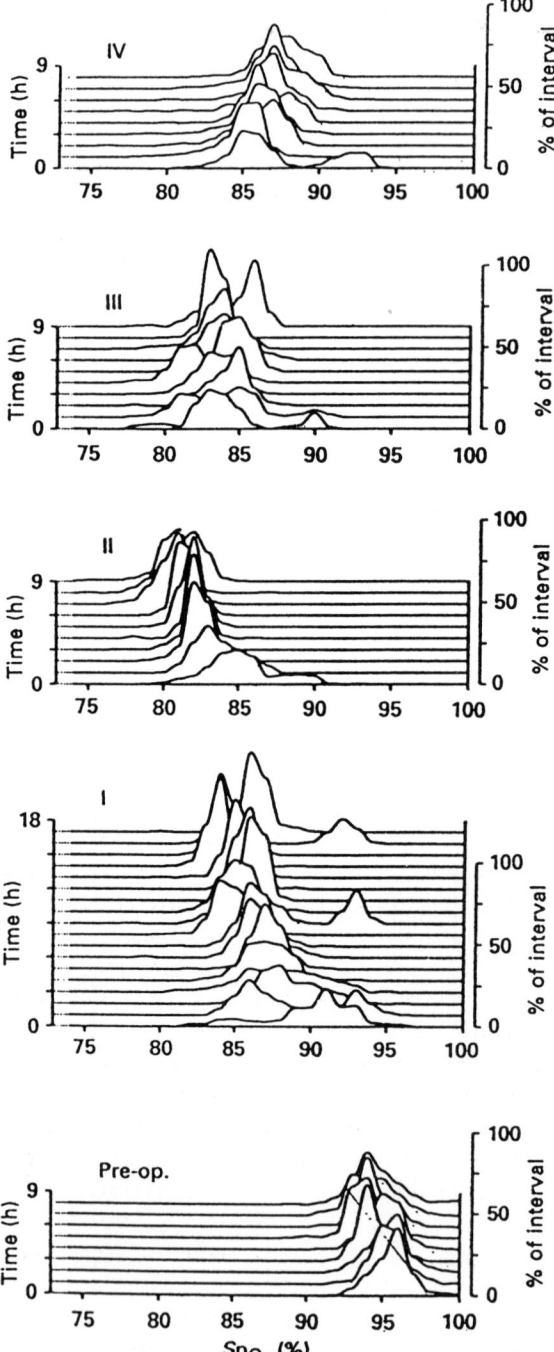

Fig. 6.6 The change in pattern of oxygen saturation (Spo₂) during a 5-night study period before and after surgery. (See text.) (Reproduced from Entwistle et al 1991 with permission of *Br J Anaesth*.)

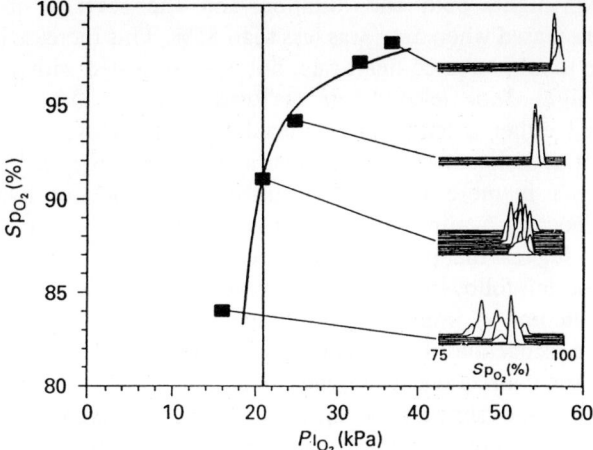

Fig. 6.7 The pattern of oxygen saturation is determined by the P_{IO_2} and position of the curve relating P_{IO_2} to oxygen saturation (Sp_{O_2}). When the inspired P_{O_2} lies on the steep part of the curve there is a very unstable pattern of Sp_{O_2}. (Reproduced from Jones et al 1992 with permission of *Br J Anaesth.*)

patient breathes air or a reduced F_{IO_2} (0.16 kPa) compared to the stable pattern when $P_{IO_2} > 25$ kPa (Jones et al 1992).

Significance of hypoxaemia

A recent editorial (Hanning 1992) urges the use of oxygen administration for postoperative hypoxaemia despite the fact that there are few clear indications for oxygen therapy. It seems likely that patients with vascular disease would be at risk during prolonged hypoxaemia and it has long been standard practice to administer increased oxygen in the immediate postoperative period. However there is no agreement about why, how much or for how long. Certainly it is very unusual to administer oxygen routinely for 5 nights postoperatively despite the fact that we now know that in some patients hypoxaemia may persist for this period of time. Nevertheless, the routine administration of oxygen for up to 5 nights postoperatively is costly, inconvenient and illogical if there are no clear indications.

What evidence links hypoxaemia to exacerbations of cardiac or cerebral disease? A recent review article on perioperative cardiac morbidity does not mention hypoxaemia as a risk factor (Mangano 1990). However, following major vascular surgery some patients show ischaemic changes in the electrocardiogram which are associated with a fall in oxygen saturation and are reversed by the administration of oxygen (Reeder et al 1991, 1992). In other postoperative patients frequent, and often prolonged, periods of myocardial ischaemia have been reported during the first 2 postoperative nights *even when the Sa_{O_2} was in the normal range.* However on the third postoperative night, both the duration and the severity of myocardial ischaemia increased when Sao_2 was less than 85%. This increase in ischaemia was not due to an increased heart rate, but was associated with a much lower mean overnight Sao_2 level (Muir & Reeder 1991). Other studies have demonstrated either a temporal relationship between hypoxaemia and the development of ischaemia (Rosenberg et al 1990) or suggested that myocardial ischaemia is more likely to occur if an episode of hypoxaemia is prolonged (beyond 5 min) and severe ($Sao_2 < 85\%$; Gill et al 1992). These observations suggest that patients may benefit from efforts to reduce their total ischaemic burden following surgery. However direct evidence is still unavailable that outcome is improved by reducing the duration and severity of perioperative ischaemia in a general surgical population.

What are the consequences of hypoxaemia on cerebral function? Hornbein et al (1989) have shown that normal volunteers exposed to profound hypoxaemia (Sao_2 50–60%) for several days show some mild cognitive deficits but there was no evidence that older subjects were more susceptible to the effects of hypoxaemia than younger volunteers. Deleterious effects of hypoxaemia on cerebral function in the immediate postoperative period have not been extensively documented and reliable data which clearly identify patients at risk are not yet available. Little is known whether prolonged postoperative hypoxaemia has a long-term effect on cerebral function and performance in patients with cerebrovascular disease. It is a matter of some urgency that this issue is resolved.

The benefits of supplementary oxygen in the postoperative period have not been extensively investigated. There is some evidence that hypoxaemia may delay wound healing as well as predispose to wound infection (Knighton et al 1984, Jonsson et al 1988) and that the administration of oxygen may be of benefit. As postoperative cardiac ischaemia has been shown to occur while patients are receiving supplementary oxygen with levels of Sao_2 in the normal range, it would appear that hypoxaemia is only one of many potential causes of postoperative myocardial ischaemia (Reeder et al 1992). Thus myocardial ischaemia should be viewed in terms of a balance between supply and demand. In this way hypoxaemia will either tip the balance in favour of ischaemia, or by acting synergistically with other insults, serve to worsen the duration and severity of any ischaemia that ensues. Though it would seem sensible to administer supplementary oxygen to all patients who may be at high cardiovascular or cerebrovascular risk, we must still await well-controlled studies before we can definitely say that the administration of oxygen postoperatively reduces the amount of ischaemia and improves outcome.

REFERENCES

Aber W R, Block A J, Hellard D W, Webb W B 1989 Consistency of respiratory measurements from night to night during the sleep of elderly men. Chest 96: 747–751

Ancoli-Israel S, Klauber M R, Kriphe D F, Parker L, Cobarrubias M 1989 Sleep apnoea in female patients in a nursing home. Chest 96: 1054–1058

Beachey W D, Olsen D E 1990 Quantifying ventilatory reserve to predict respiratory failure in exacerbations of COPD. Chest 97: 1086–1097

Beemer G H, Rozental P 1986 Postoperative neuromuscular function. Anaesth Intensive Care 14: 41–45

Bendixen H H, Hedley-Whyte J, Laver M B 1963 Impaired oxygenation in surgical patients during general anaesthesia with controlled ventilation. A concept of atelectasis. N Engl J Med 269: 991–996

Bergman N A 1963 Distribution of inspired gas during anaesthesia and artificial ventilation. J Appl Physiol 18: 1085–1089

Berthoud M C, Peacock J E, Reilly C S 1991 Effectiveness of preoxygenation in morbidly obese patients. Br J Anaesth 67: 464–466

Bevan D R, Smith C E, Donati F 1988 Postoperative neuromuscular blockade: a comparison between atracurium, vecuronium and pancuronium. Anesthesiology 69: 272–276

Bickler P E, Dueck R, Prutow R J 1987 Effects of barbiturate anaesthesia on functional residual capacity and ribcage/diaphragm contributions to ventilation. Anesthesiology 66: 147–152

Blom H, Mulder M, Verwei J W 1988 Arterial oxygen tension and saturation in hospital patients: effect of age and activity. Br Med J 297: 720–721

Blum R H, Carter S, Agre K 1973 A clinical review of bleomycin, a new antineoplastic agent. Cancer 31: 903–914

Brismar B, Hedenstierna G, Lungquist H, Strandberg A A, Svensson L, Tokics L 1985 Pulmonary densities during anaesthesia with muscular relaxation — a proposal of atelectasis. Anesthesiology 62: 422–428

British Thoracic Society, Research Unit of the Royal College of Physicians of London, Kings Fund Centre, National Asthma Campaign 1990a Guidelines for management of asthma in adults I: chronic persistent asthema. Br Med J 301: 651–653

British Thoracic Society, Research Unit of the Royal College of Physicians of London, Kings Fund Centre, National Asthma Campaign 1990b Guidelines for management of asthma in adults II: acute severe asthma. Br Med J 301: 797–800

Browne D R G, Rochford J, O'Connell W, Jones J G 1970 The incidence of postoperative atelectasis in the dependent lung following thoracotomy: the value of added nitrogen. Br J Anaesth 42: 340–346

Catley D M, Thornton C, Jordon C, Lehane J R, Royston D, Jones J G 1985 Pronounced episodic oxygen desaturation in the postoperative period: its association with ventilatory pattern and analgesic regimen. Anesthesiology 63:20–28

Catling J A, Pinto D M, Jordan C, Jones J G 1980 Respiratory effects of analgesia after cholecystectomy in comparison of continuous and intermittent papaveretum. Br Med J 281: 478–480

Cooper J A D Jr, White D A, Matthay R 1986 Drug induced pulmonary disease. Part I. Cytotoxic drugs. Am Rev Respir Dis 133: 321–340

Craig D B 1981 Postoperative recovery of pulmonary function. Anaesth Analg 60: 46–52

Dantzker D R, Wagner P D, West J B 1975 Instability of lung units with V/Q ratios during O_2 breathing. J Appl Physiol 38: 886–895

Dueck R, Prutow R J, Davies N J H, Clausen J L, Davidson T M 1988 The lung volume at which shunting occurs with inhalational anaesthesia. Anesthesiology 69: 854–861

Dureuil B, Cantineau J P, Desmonts J M 1987 Effects of upper or lower abdominal surgery on diaphragm function. Br J Anaesth 59: 1230–1235

Eisenkraft J B 1990 Effects of anaesthetics on the pulmonary circulation. Br J Anaesth 65: 63–78

Entwistle M D, Roe P G, Sapsford D J, Berrisford R G, Jones J G 1991 Patterns of oxygenation after thoracotomy. Br J Anaesth 67: 704–711

Froese A B, Bryan C H 1974 Effects of anaesthesia and paralysis on diaphragmatic mechanics in man. Anesthesiology 41: 242–255

Gass G D, Olsen G N 1986 Preoperative pulmonary function testing to predict postoperative morbidity and mortality. Chest 81: 127–135

Gill N P, Wright B, Reilly C S 1992 Relationship between hypoxaemic and cardiac ischaemic events in the perioperative period. Br J Anaesth 68: 471–473

Gislason T, Almqvist M, Boman G, Linholm C E, Terenius L 1989 Increased CSF opioid activity in sleep apnoea syndrome. Chest 96: 250–254

Goldiner P L, Carlon G C, Cvitrovic E, Schwizet O 1978 Factors influencing post operative morbidity and mortality in patients treated with bleomycin. Br Med J 1: 1664–1667

Green I D, Burgess B F 1962 An investigation into the major factors contributing to post flight chest pain in fighter pilots. Flying Personnel Research Committee report no 1182. Ministry of Defence, London

Guilleminault C, Stools R, Schneider H, Podszuz T, Peter J H, Von Wickert P 1989 Central alveolar hypoventilation and sleep. Treatment by intermittent positive pressure ventilation through nasal mask in an adult. Chest 96: 1210–1212

Gunnarsson L, Tokics L, Gustavsson H, Hedenstierna G 1991 Influence of age on atelectasis formation and gas exchange impairment during general anaesthesia. Br J Anaesth 66: 423–432

Hanning C D 1992 Prolonged postoperative oxygen therapy. Br J Anaesth 69: 115–116

Hedenstierna G 1990 Gas exchange during anaesthesia. Br J Anaesth 64: 507–514

Hedenstierna G, Strandberg Å, Brismar B, Lundquist H, Svenson L, Tokics L 1985 Functional residual capacity, thoraco-abdominal dimensions and central blood volume during general anaesthesia with muscle paralysis and mechanical ventilation. Anesthesiology 62: 247–254

Hedenstierna G, Tokics L, Strandberg Å, Lundquist H, Brismar B 1986 Correlation of gas exchange impairment to development of atelectasis during anaesthesia and muscle paralysis. Acta Anaesthesiol Scand 30: 183–191

Hedenstierna G, Tokics L, Lund B et al 1989 Pulmonary densities during anaesthesia. An experimental study on lung histology and gas exchange. Eur Respir J 2: 528–535

Heneghan C P H, Jones J G 1985 Pulmonary gas exchange and diaphragmatic position. Effect of tonic phrenic stimulation compared with that of increased airway pressure. Br J Anaesth 57: 1161–1166

Heneghan C P H, Bergman N A, Jones J G 1984 Changes in lung volume (PaO_2-PaO_2) during anaesthesia. Br J Anaesth 56: 437–445

Hewlett A M, Hulands G H, Nunn J F, Milledge J S 1974 Functional residual capacity during anaesthesia III: artificial ventilation. Br J Anaesth 46: 495–503

Hickey R F, Visick W D, Fairley H B, Fourcade H E 1973 Effects of halothane anaesthesia on functional residual capacity and alveolar-arterial oxygen tension difference. Anaesthesiology 38: 20–24

Hillberg O, Jackson A C, Swift D L, Pederson O F 1989 Acoustic rhinometry: evaluation of nasal cavity by acoustic reflection. J Appl Physiol 66: 295–303

Hoffstein V, Zamel N 1990 Sleep apnoea and the upper airway. Br J Anaesth 65: 139–150

Holley H, Milic-Emili J, Becklare M, Bates D 1967 Regional distribution of pulmonary investigation and perfusion in obesity. J Clin Invest 46: 475–481

Hornbein T F, Townes B D, Schoene R B, Sutton J R, Houston C S 1989 The cost to the central nervous system of climbing to extremely high altitude. N Engl J Med 321: 1714–1719

Jansen J E, Sorensen A I, Naesh O, Grichsen C J, Pedersen A 1990 Effect of doxapram on postoperative pulmonary complications after upper abdominal surgery in high risk patients. Lancet 335: 936–938

Jones J G 1982 Closing volume. In: Kaufman L (ed) Anaesthesia review 1. Churchill Livingstone, London, pp 43–54

Jones J G 1987 Anaesthesia and atelectasis: the role of VTAB and the chest wall. Br J Anaesth 59: 949–953

Jones J G, Jordan C, Slavin B, Lehane J R 1987 Prophylactic effect of aminophylline and salbutamol on histamine induced bronchoconstriction. Br J Anaesth 59: 498–502

Jones J G, Sapsford D J, Wheatley R G 1990 Post operative hypoxaemia: mechanisms and time course. Anaesthesia 45: 566–573

Jones J G, Roe P G, Sapsford D J 1992 Postoperative hypoxaemia: an analysis of causative factors. Br J Anaesth 68(4): 435 P

Jonsson K, Hunt T K, Mathes S J 1988 Oxygen as an isolated variable influences resistance to infection. Ann Surg 208: 783–787

Knighton D R, Halliday B, Hunt T K 1984 Oxygen as an antibiotic. Arch Surg 119: 199–204

Knill-Jones R P 1987 Diagnostic systems as an aid to clinical decision making. Br Med J 295: 1392–1396

Lam A, Newhouse M 1990 Management of asthma and chronic airflow limitation. Chest 98: 44–52

Lamartia K R, Glick J H, Marshall B E 1984 Supplemental oxygen does not cause respiratory failure in bleomycin treated surgical patients. Anesthesiology 60: 65–67

Lampe G H, Wauk L Z, Whitendale P et al 1990 Post operative hypoxaemia after nonabdominal surgery: a frequent event not caused by nitrous oxide. Anaesth Analg 71: 597–601

Lindberg P, Gunnarsson L, Tokics L et al 1992 Atelectasis and lung function in the post operative period. Acta Anaesthesiol Scand 36: 546–553

Lindholm C E, Hillerdahl G, Hultcrantz E 1990 Sleep apnoea and airway surgery. Curr Opin Anaesthesiol 3: 916–919

Mangano D T 1990 Perioperative cardiac morbidity. Anesthesiology 72: 153–184

Mankikian B, Cantineau J P, Bertrand M et al 1988 Improvement of diaphragmatic function by a thoracic extradural block after upper abdominal surgery. Anesthesiology 68: 379–386

Mannix E T, Dowdeswell I, Carlone S, Palange P, Aronoff G, Farber M 1990 The effect of oxygen on sodium excretion on hypoxaemic patients with chronic obstructive lung disease. Chest 97: 840–844

Milledge J S, Nunn J F 1975 Criteria of fitness for anaesthesia in patients with chronic obstructive lung disease. Br Med J 3: 670–673

Muir A D, Reeder M K 1991 Postoperative oxygen desaturation and myocardial ischaemia in patients presenting for vascular surgery. Br J Anaesth 66: 369 P

Northwood P, Sapsford D J, Jones J G, Griffiths D, Wilkins C 1991 Nitrous oxide sedation causes post-hyperventilation apnoea. Br J Anaesth 67: 7–12

Nunn J F 1964 Factors influencing the arterial oxygen tension during halothane anaesthesia with spontaneous respiration. Br J Anaesth 36: 327–341

Nunn J F, Milledge J S, Chen D, Dove C 1988 Respiratory criteria of fitness for surgery and anaesthesia. Anaesthesia 43: 543–551

O'Doherty M J, Page C J, Bradbeer C S 1989 The place of lung ^{99mTc}DTPA aerosol transfer in the investigation of lung infarctions in HIV positive patients. Respir Med 83: 395–401

Pedersen T, Eliasen K, Henriksen E 1990 A prospective study of risk factors and cardiopulmonary complications associated with anaesthesia and surgery: risk indicators of cardiopulmonary morbidity. Acta Anaesthesiol Scand 34: 144–155

Reeder M K, Muir A D, Foex P, Goldman M D, Loh L, Smart D 1991 Postoperative myocardial ischaemia: temporal association with nocturnal hypoxaemia. Br J Anaesth 67: 626–631

Reeder M K, Goldman M D, Loh L, Muir A D, Casey K R, Lehane J R 1992 Late postoperative nocturnal dips in oxygen saturation in patients undergoing major abdominal vascular surgery. Anaesthesia 47: 110–115

Riordan J F, Rommens J M, Kerem B et al 1989 Identification of the cystic fibrosis gene. Cloning and characterisation of complementary DNA. Science 245: 1066–1073

Roe P G, Jones J G 1991 Pulmonary disease. Curr Opin Anaesthesiol 4: 853–859

Rosenberg J, Rasmussen V, van Jensen F, Ullstad T, Kehlet H 1990 Late postoperative episodic and constant hypoxaemia and associated ECG abnormalities. Br J Anaesth 65: 684–691

Rosenow III E C 1988 Drug-induced pulmonary disease. In: Murray J F, Nadal J A (eds) Textbook of respiratory medicine. W B Saunders, Philadelphia pp 1681–1702

Sanders M H, Kern N 1990 Obstructive sleep apnoea treated by independently adjusted inspiratory and expiratory positive airway pressure via nasal mask. Physiological and clinical implications. Chest 98: 317–324

Sapsford D J, Jones J G 1992 The derivation of V_A/Q from the position of P_{IO_2} versus Sp_{O_2} cure. Br J Anaesth 69: 541P

Selsby D, Jones J G 1990 Some physiological and clinical aspects of chest physiotherapy. Br J Anaesth 64: 621–631

Seymour D G, Green M, Vaz F G 1990 Making better decisions: construction of clinical scoring systems by the Spiegelhalter–Knill–Jones approach. Br Med J 300: 223–226

Sforza E, Kreiger J, Weitzenblum E, Appriu M, Lampert E, Ratamaro J 1990 Long term effects of treatment with nasal or continuous positive airway pressure on daytime lung function and pulmonary haemodynamics in patients with obstructive sleep apnoea. Am Rev Respir Dis 141: 866–870

Simonneau G, Vivien A, Sartene R et al 1983 Diaphragmatic dysfunction induced by upper abdominal surgery: role of postoperative pain. Am Rev Resp Dis 128: 899–903

Strandberg A A, Tokics L, Brismar B, Lundquist H, Hedenstierna G 1986 Atelectasis during anaesthesia and in the postoperative period. Acta Anaesthesiol Scand 30: 154–158

Sullivan C E, Issa F G, Berthon-Jones M, Eves L 1981 Reversal of obstructive sleep apnoea by continuous positive pressure applied through the nares. Lancet 1: 862–865

Tokics L, Strandberg Å, Brismar B, Lundquist H, Hedenstierna G 1987a Computerised tomography of the chest and gas exchange measurements during ketamine anaesthesia. Acta Anaesthesiol Scand 31: 684–692

Tokics L, Hedenstierna G, Strandberg Å, Brismar B, Lundquist H 1987b Lung collapse and gas exchange during general anaesthesia — effects of spontaneous breathing, muscle paralysis and positive expiratory pressure. Anesthesiology 66: 157–167

Tokics L, Hedenstierna G, Brismar B, Strandberg Å, Lundquist H 1988 Thoracoabdominal restriction in supine men: computerised tomography and lung function measurements. J Appl Physiol 64: 599–604

Viby-Mogensen J, Jorgensen B C, Ording H 1979 Residual curarization in the recovery room. Anesthesiology 50: 539–541

Wahba R W M 1991 Perioperative functional residual capacity. Can J Anaesth 38: 384–400

Wheatley R G, Somerville I D, Sapsford D J, Jones J G 1990 Postoperative hypoxaemia: comparison of extradural, i.m. and patient-controlled opioid analgesia. Br J Anaesth 64: 267–275

Whittaker J S, Ryan C F, Buckley P A, Road J D 1990 The effect of refeeding on peripheral and respiratory muscle function in malnourished chronic obstructive pulmonary disease patients. Am Rev Respir Dis 142: 283–288

7. Information processing during sleep and anaesthesia

R. Munglani   J. G. Jones

What? Asleep? Did all I say go in one ear and out the other? *Peer Gynt Act 4 Henrik Ibsen.*

It is consciousness, not behaviour without consciousness which remains completely inexplicable *(Dixon 1981)*.

The possibility of information processing by anaesthetized patients has been ignored on the grounds that adequately anaesthetized patients are unconscious by definition (Prys-Roberts 1987). Anaesthetists tend to become defensive when it is intimated that their patients may be able to process and remember intraoperative events. This view excludes the growing evidence that conscious awareness is not necessary to process and respond to stimuli (Griffiths & Jones 1990, Jessop & Jones 1991, Ghoneim & Block 1992). We use the term conscious awareness to indicate that the brain monitors the environment with explicit recall of events. However the brain may also monitor the environment without explicit recall but instead with implicit memory of events. This chapter presents evidence from psychological studies from normal awake and brain-damaged patients and during sleep, showing that information can be processed without conscious awareness. Such evidence enables us to construct a model of information processing during general anaesthesia. The literature concerning information processing during anaesthesia is reviewed and the implications for anaesthetic practice are discussed.

The issue of conscious awareness during anaesthesia caused by faulty technique or equipment malfunction will not be addressed directly as this implies inadequate anaesthesia. This latter topic has been reviewed (Rosen & Lunn, 1987); it has also been a subject of a Medical Defence Union report (Hargrove 1987) and a recent editorial in the *British Medical Journal* (Brighouse & Norman 1992).

EVIDENCE FOR INFORMATION PROCESSING OUTSIDE OF AWARENESS (Fig. 7.1)

Short-term or working memory is responsible for a variety of control processes such as the rapid encoding of stimuli, decision-making and retrieval. It is flexible but of limited capacity and only able to hold a few items

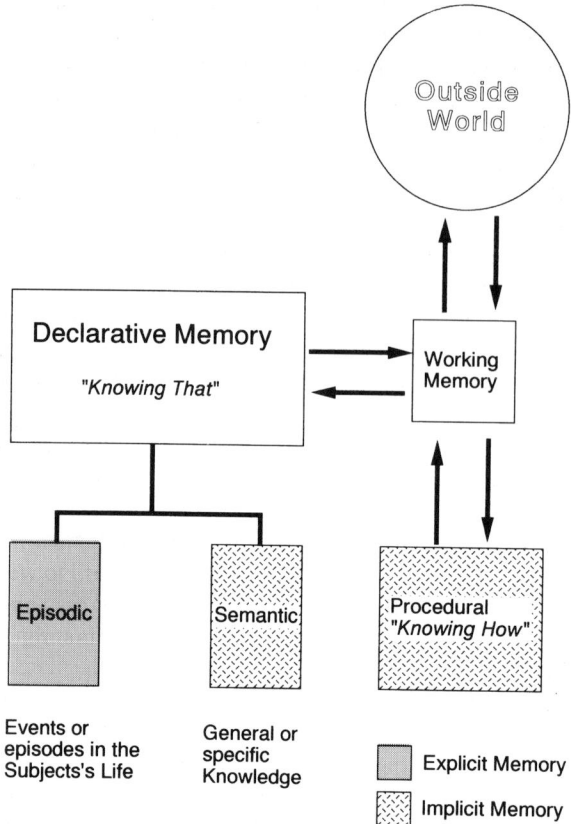

Fig. 7.1 The structure of human memory: see text for details. Adapted from Richardson (1989).

within it (Baddeley 1986). Working memory has a number of systems within it such as the visual spatial sketch pad. The latter is responsible for the construction and manipulation of spatial and pictorial representations which are important components in the utilization of mental imagery (Baddeley 1988). The limited capacity of working memory means that there exists large capacity stores divided into 'knowing how' and 'knowing that'. The former is known as procedural memory and is concerned with the memory of how to perform actions. It is an implicit process in that it does not require effort; for example it is effortless to recall how to walk or to ride a bicycle. 'Knowing that' or declarative memory is the store for knowledge and is further subdivided into episodic and semantic memory. Semantic memory is simply factual knowledge *without* recollection of the circumstances of learning (for example, oranges and apples are fruits), and is also an implicit function of memory because no effort is required to retrieve it. Episodic memory, in contrast, includes details of when the fact was learnt and so requires effortful or explicit recall (The weather at our wedding was sunny). Implicit memory can be revealed by a change in experience, thought, or action that is attributable to an event, without that event being consciously remembered. Note that implicit and explicit are descriptive terms which are primarily concerned with a person's psychological experience *at the time of retrieval*. They do not imply two independent memory systems* (Schacter 1987, Khilstrom 1992). Evidence will be presented to show that anaesthesia tends selectively to impair episodic or explicit memory.

There is evidence that certain attributes of a stimulus are encoded into memory automatically when it is presented to a subject. These attributes include temporal and spatial information as well as the frequency coding of events. The latter is tested by presenting subjects with long lists of words in which certain words are repeated and asking subjects to remember which words were repeated and how many times (Zacks et al 1982). Using effortful or explicit recall of the words alone, there is a positive practice effect and large and reliable individual differences. In contrast, performance in the frequency coding of the words does not increase with practice, showing no reliable individual differences and is not hindered by competing demands. The implications are that there are *basic memory processes* which are automatic or 'hardwired', i.e. they are virtually independent of the attentional level. Indeed they show limited developmental trends and are completed at an early age. Frequency encoding has been shown to be no different in mentally disabled children compared with normal schoolchildren. An auditory divided-attention task has been used to test the effect of reduced attention on implicit memory tasks (Eich 1984). In this test, homophones (words with the same sound but different spelling, e.g. *mail* or *male*) were presented to one ear within a phrase intended to bias the low-frequency interpretation of the homophone, for example, 'daily *mail*'. To the other ear, an essay was presented on which the subject had to concentrate. Subsequently subjects showed no explicit memory for the homophones, but when asked to spell the target words, they provided the low-frequency spelling of the homophone more often than under baseline conditions. Thus they demonstrated implicit memory for the unattended information. Zacks et al (1982) comment that:

these *basic memory processes* drain minimal energy from our limited-capacity attentional mechanism, do not interfere with other on going cognitive activities, function at a constant level *in all circumstances*, occur without intention and do not benefit with practice [our italics].

Stimuli can have an impact on subjective performance even though the stimulus may not be consciously perceived. For example, the effect of subliminal Oedipal messages on dart-throwing performance was tested by

---

*It would be prudent here to state that there are other views of the implicit/explicit distinction. Crowder (1989) prefers the concept of modules within memory rather than distinct systems. Sherry & Schacter (1987) provide an evolutionary argument for the development of two separate parallel memory systems. See also Wolters & Phaf (1990).

Silverman et al (1978). After baseline dart-throwing measurements, male sub-jects were presented subliminally with one of the following phrases; *'Beating Dad is wrong'*; *'Beating Dad is OK'*, or *'People are standing'*. The subjects then competed in a dart-throwing competition. Exposure to the subliminal message that reduced anxiety resulted in an improved score whilst exposure to the anxiety-producing message resulted in reduced performance. Presentation of the neutral message had no effect. Other work on blind sight and dichotic listening suggests that information processing occurs unconsciously and can influence behaviour (Dixon 1981, Marcel 1983, Eich 1984, Bornstein 1989).

Stimuli can be processed to quite a complex level before entering consciousness. This is known as preconscious processing (Dixon 1981, 1989). A typical example is driving a car. After the initial learning phase, a person can drive whilst doing other things and yet respond quickly when, for example, a pedestrian steps into the road. Another example includes the 'cocktail party phenomenon' of ignoring background chatter and yet imme-diately paying attention when one's name is mentioned across the room. Even during sleep this process continues to occur; it is well-known that a mother will waken to the sounds of her baby yet ignore the louder traffic outside.

There are two distinct information processing systems within the brain. The first is a large-capacity system and most of the information it deals with never enters our consciousness. This receives an input and determines and executes an appropriate response. The second is associated with formulating new ideas and plans for action; it is verbal and of limited capacity. This second system is associated with our conscious experience. Much stimulus process-ing, including learned behaviour such as driving a car, may be left to the primary system. Thus consciousness sits above a complex system dedicated to receiving and processing huge amounts of data from without and within (Fig. 7.2). Some yet undefined system regulates the entry of information into conscious experience.

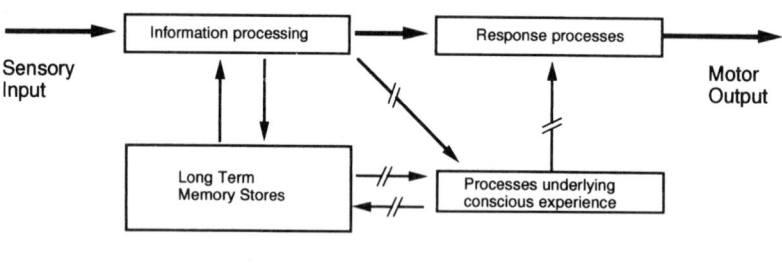

—//▶   = May represent interruption of the pathway by anaesthesia

Fig. 7.2   Organization of sensory processing. Incoming stimuli may initiate physiological and psychological effects, leading to responses with or without part of this traffic being represented in consciousness. Adapted from Dixon (1981).

EXPLICIT AND IMPLICIT MEMORY SYSTEMS IN BRAIN-DAMAGED PATIENTS

The altered behaviour seen in brain-damaged patients sheds light on the basic memory systems in normal subjects. Amnesic patients with Korsakoff's syndrome and anoxic encephalopathy were asked to memorize word lists (Graf et al 1984). The amnesic patients performed very badly on memory tests which examined free recall, recognition and cued recall. These tests require *effortful (or explicit) recall* of the subject matter that was presented during the study. However in a different test, word completion, *the amnesic patients did as well as the controls*. This was surprising because the test is similar to the cued recall in that the first three letters were given, but in contrast to the latter, the instructions directed patients away from the effortful memory aspect of the test, and the patients were asked instead to write down *any word* that came to mind which began with those letters. The word completion test does not require effort and is a known test for implicit recall of information. Similar results are reviewed by Schacter (1987) and Richardson (1989).

Brain-damaged patients show implicit knowledge of stimuli that they cannot perceive explicitly or process semantically. For example, patients with lesions to the primary visual projection areas and who have no conscious perceptual experiences within that visual field can nevertheless correctly guess what may lie in that field. This is known as blindsight. A similar phenomenon occurs with patients with facial recognition deficits who show stronger galvanic skin responses to familiar than to unfamiliar faces though they do not explicitly recognize any faces as familiar (Popper & Eccles 1977, Schacter 1987).

Thus mechanisms exist within human cognition that may explain why information may be processed without conscious awareness in states such as anaesthesia and sleep, where attentional levels are lower. The lack of responsiveness during anaesthesia and inability to remember these events postoperatively (source amnesia) do not necessarily mean that these experiences have not been processed, and they may also influence thought and action postoperatively (Khilstrom 1991).

THE NEUROPHYSIOLOGICAL AND METABOLIC COMPARISONS OF SLEEP AND ANAESTHESIA

Sleep and anaesthesia show remarkable parallels. An appreciation of these will allow us to understand the continued information processing seen in both sleep and anaesthesia. For many years it was thought that inhibition in the ascending reticular activating system (RAS) led to both sleep and anaesthesia. The observations firstly that transection of the brainstem produced a state indistinguishable from sleep (Bremer 1935), and secondly that stimulation of the brainstem reticular formation produced arousal in an otherwise sleeping animal (Moruzzi & Magoun 1949) supported this RAS-based model. Similarly anaesthesia was thought to be produced by depression of the RAS (French et al 1953).

The observations that removal of sensory inputs to the reticular formation does not increase sleep or prevent sleep/wake cycles and that rapid eye movement (REM) sleep* occurred illustrated the fact that the simple RAS-based model was inadequate. REM and non-REM sleep have very different electroencephalogram (EEG) characteristics and these can be used to define the neuronal sites associated with particular stages of sleep (Siegal 1990). The slow-wave activity of non-REM sleep is seen in separate neuronal groups in the basal forebrain, hypothalamus, midbrain and the brainstem. The most caudal structure involved is the nucleus tractus solitarius (NTS). Stimulation of the NTS leads to rapid sleep onset whereas cooling the medulla leads to *arousal* as this cooling inhibits a hypnogenic area contained within. Lesion of the sleep centre in the hypothalamus region produces profound insomnia with a permanent reduction in sleeping time. REM sleep production has been localized to a small region within the pontine reticular formation whose neurons have a high rate of discharge in REM sleep. Lesions of the pons will produce REM sleep without atonia.

The rest of the brain is not a passive responder to REM-associated neuronal discharge, but modulates the pontine–geniculo–occipital spikes which drive the eye movements and are thought to be related to the dream imagery in humans. Compared with wakefulness, information entry into the cortex is known to be reduced at the thalamocortical junction during non-REM sleep and this is due to hyperpolarization of the neurons. In REM sleep, however, information transfer is increased. Upon wakening there is a *reduction* in the spontaneous discharge of some cortical neurons, but an enhanced probability of responding to an external stimuli This has been interpreted as increasing the signal to noise ratio of the system at the same time as the locus coeruleus seems to suppress weak stimuli but enhance strong ones, this may be a feature extracting process (Steriade 1989).

The site of action of anaesthetic agents is still not known. Recently a model has been proposed in which general anaesthetics interfere with the inward transmission of sensory information at the thalamus (Angel 1991). Normally, stimulation of the peripheral receptors causes impulses to pass up the dorsal columns to the first synapse which occurs in the cuneate nucleus. From here secondary fibres ascend to the contralateral ventrobasal thalamic complex where they synapse. The afferents from these cells then ascend to layers IV and VI of the cerebral cortex (Fig. 7.3).

---

*All the phases of sleep are distinguished on EEG criteria. Non-REM (non-rapid eye movement sleep), otherwise known as slow wave sleep (SWS), is divided into four stages on EEG criteria. The deepest (stage 4) sleep has the largest proportion of low-frequency (delta) waves. REM sleep was first described by Askerinsky & Kleitmann (1953). It is the stage of sleep associated with dreaming. Pontine–geniculo–occipital (PGO) spikes are produced and characterize REM sleep. The mind seems to be more perceptive during REM sleep than at other times (Bootzin et al 1990).

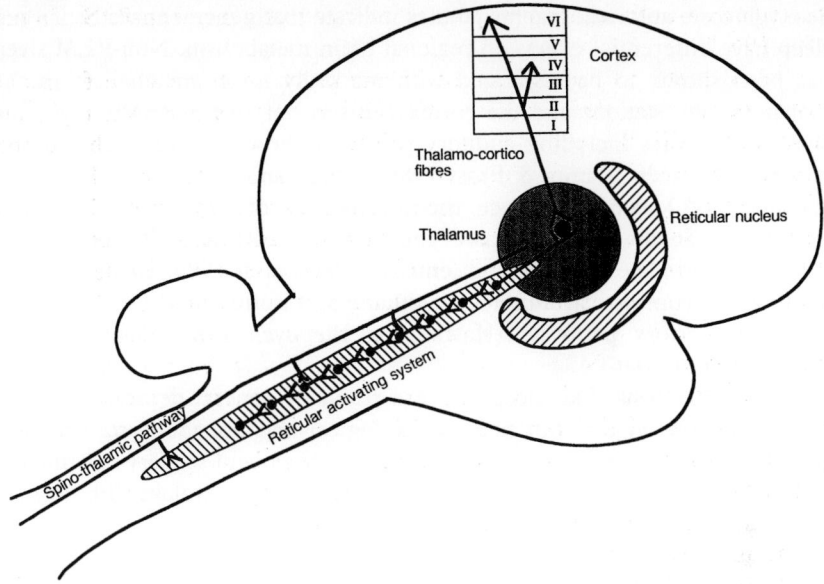

Fig. 7.3 Pathway for sensory stimuli reaching the brain. Gating of information occurs at the thalamus. Sleep and anaesthesia increase this gating. For clarity, only some pathways are shown. Adapted from Stockard & Bickford (1981).

Anaesthesia has little effect on the cuneate nucleus but, in contrast, the thalamic cells show graded decreases in their response to peripheral stimulation with increasing depth of anaesthesia. This gating at the thalamus is seen with a wide variety of anaesthetic agents. The reduced discharge frequency of cells in cortical layers IV and VI is due to this thalamic gating but layers IV and VI are in themselves not sensitive to anaesthetic agents. However layers II, III and V of the cortex are more susceptible to anaesthetics and show various types of spontaneous activity — either a high-voltage low-frequency wave (HVLF) or a low-voltage high-frequency wave (LVHF). Simultaneous recording of cortical and thalamic cells shows that the spontaneous change in HVLF to LVHF is accompanied by increased synaptic transmission through the ventrobasal thalamus. Thus there is cortical control over the thalamic sensory input. This effect is mediated through and supplemented by the reticular nucleus. There is also a feedback loop between the reticular nucleus and the cortex which gates the input of information through the ventrobasal thalamus. Anaesthetics have very complex actions on the hippocampus, the site intimately associated with encoding of memories. In general, however, they do not inhibit long-term potentiation (LTP); this electrophysiological event is associated with memory formation (Pearce et al 1989, Krnjevic 1991).

Metabolic studies using the uptake of radioactive deoxyglucose also reveal the extent of regional brain activity in sleep and anaesthesia. Using [^{14}C] deoxyglucose, autoradiographic studies indicate that general anaesthetics and sleep have differential effects on regional brain metabolism. Non-REM sleep has been shown to be associated with markedly lower metabolism in the thalamic relay stations and the cortex. This is not so for REM sleep. The sensory pathways including auditory pathways show little or no significant change with sleep (Ramm & Frost 1986). All general anaesthetics (with the exception of ketamine) reduce the metabolism of the cortex but some anaesthetic agents tend to spare the auditory pathways. These include Althesin, etomidate propofol and fentanyl (Davis et al 1984, 1986, Samra et al 1984). In contrast barbiturates, halothane and isoflurane cause depression of these auditory pathways (Hawkins & Biebuyck 1980, Sokoloff 1981, Maekawa et al 1986).

Thus anaesthesia, like sleep is not a result of general depression of the central nervous system but neurophysiological and metabolic studies have clearly shown that there is an interruption of the flow of sensory information through the thalamus in both states, which may explain the loss of consciousness seen.

Cognition during sleep

The phenomenon of sleep learning was generally dismissed for many years after it was shown that information presented during sleep could not be recalled upon awakening unless presentation coincided with EEG alpha activity (Emmons & Simon 1956, Eich 1990). The revival of interest in the subject followed reports that using auditory evoked responses (AER), subjects could discriminate between presented sounds even in the deepest stages of sleep (Oswald et al 1960, Kutas 1990). The brainstem evoked potentials (BER) provide information about the integrity of the sensory pathway and do not show any changes with the different stages of sleep.

The auditory evoked response is shown in Fig. 7.4 (Jones 1988). Components of the AER between 10 and 100 ms are known as the middle latency responses (MLR), and those occurring after 100 ms are known as the cognitive event-related potentials. The MLR is initially similar in awake and sleeping subjects, indicating that information must be reaching the primary auditory cortex. However with increasing non-REM sleep, the MLR is of reduced amplitude but reappears with REM sleep (Erwin & Buchwald 1986). The late cognitive evoked responses have been studied in more detail. In general, sleep produces an overall reduction in amplitude of the evoked response. During sleep, in response to an abrupt change in auditory stimuli there is a large negative wave at 300–500 ms (known as N_2), occasionally followed by a wave at 800 ms latency (P_3 or P_{300}; Kutas 1990). In the awake subjects these waves have been associated, attending to changes within the stimulus (Regan 1990). Recently Nielsen-Bohlman et al (1991) presented auditory stimuli to sleeping subjects whilst monitoring the EEG to define the stage of sleep. They recorded the AER of the subject to occasional tones

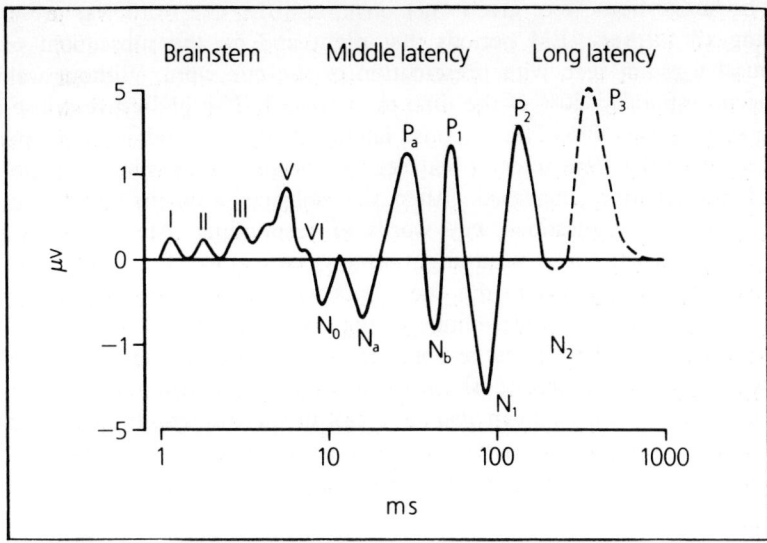

Fig. 7.4   The auditory evoked response. The early cortical waves are also referred to as the middle latency waves. Adapted from Jones (1988).

presented on a background of regular clicks. At specific stages of sleep, subjects showed specific changes in the evoked responses.

Auditory presentation of stimuli during REM sleep can cause it to be incorporated into dreams in 50% of cases (Dement and Wolpert 1958, Berger 1963). The stimulus was found to be incorporated into the dream in three ways:

1. Assonance or 'clang association', such as presenting the name '*An*d*rew*' caused the subject to dream of h*and* and l*and*.
2. Association and representation; for example, a subject who was given the name Richard dreamt about shopping in Edinburgh where she had been to on the previous day and the name of the shop visited included the name Richard.
3. Direct insertion of the subject matter into the dream. One subject was sprayed with water during REM sleep. He had been dreaming of acting in a play when suddenly he and the leading lady were both covered with water and looked up to see a hole in the hall roof.

Stimulus presentation can also alter behaviour during sleep. During REM sleep, verbal suggestions were presented to the subjects (Evans 1990). Typical suggestions included:

'Whenever I say the word *itch*, your nose will feel itchy until you scratch it'.
'Whenever I say the word *pillow*, your pillow will feel uncomfortable until you move it'.

The suggestions were given only once, and the cue word was presented during all further REM periods that night and on the subsequent night. Arousal was not seen with presentation of the cue word. Without waking, subjects responded 20% of the time to cue word. The highest response rate by a subject was 48%. The response latency was 32 seconds and this period increased as the time interval between the original suggestion and the cue word presentation increased. After the subjects awakened, none could remember the suggestions, cue words or responding. After 5 months, 6 subjects returned for a third night in the laboratory. Four out of the 6 responded appropriately to the cue words without being given the suggestions. None had any intervening waking memory for the procedure. The subjects who had the highest response rates also were the most hypnotizable, indicating there is a predisposition to respond in this manner.

Learning during sleep can also aid recall in wakefulness. In another study pictures of common items were presented to subjects just before bedtime (Tilley 1979). When asleep in either REM or stage 2 sleep, a tape containing half the items was repeatedly played to the subjects. The next morning, the subjects were asked which pictures they could (explicitly) recall. There was a significantly better recall of items which were named during sleep — interestingly more so if presentation took place during stage 2 rather than REM sleep. Unlike Evans (1990), other studies have shown a relationship between the duration of cortical activation at the time of stimulus presentation and extent of recall (Koukkou & Lehmann 1968). Eich (1990) reviews the literature in this field and comments that:

1. Subjects learn items better during sleep if they have had prior exposure to the stimuli.
2. Repetition of the material is vital.
3. Recognition seems to be a more sensitive test of memory than recall.
4. Certain subjects are more likely to show sleep learning than others; these include those who are good hypnotic subjects.

Eich (1990) also points out that there are no studies yet published testing for *implicit* memory in sleep learning.

Conclusions from the studies in sleep and of brain-damaged subjects

Evidence has been presented to show that:

1. Multiple functional memory systems exist, consisting of explicit and implicit units.
2. Damage to one system (such as explicit memory functions in the case of Korsakoff's syndrome) may leave the other intact.
3. Many functions of memory processing are automatic and *effortless*.
4. Information may be preconsciously processed.
5. Such information may alter performance in a task without any conscious awareness.

6. To look for evidence of information processing one may need to use tests of implicit memory (that is, tests of word completion or change in task performance) rather than tests of explicit memory (forced recall and recognition).

INFORMATION PROCESSING DURING ANAESTHESIA

Any study looking for evidence of intraoperative perception of events by an anaesthetized patient has to make two assumptions: that memory is formed for the perceived event and that the tests used are appropriate and sensitive enough to identify the memory. If one sets aside the cases of conscious awareness during anaesthesia due to inadequate doses of anaesthetic agent either because of faulty technique or equipment failure (Hargrove 1987), one is left looking for evidence of information processing during 'adequate' anaesthesia; where adequacy is defined as a lack of response to surgical events, and no postoperative explicit recollection of these events, i.e. the patient to all intents and purposes appears unconscious (Khilstrom et al 1990).

The effect of anaesthesia on cognitive function

Cognitive function in patients during the lightest stage of ether analgesia were studied by Artusio (1955). The results are shown in Table 7.1. Very light anaesthesia produced analgesia and total (explicit) amnesia for perioperative events, and yet patients continued to respond to verbal stimuli, showing that anaesthetics have differential effects on brain functions.

Dose-related impairment in short-term memory has been shown with enflurane and halothane (Cook et al 1978) and with isoflurane (Newton et al 1988). The effect of controlled subanaesthetic concentrations of enflurane on learning and on the ability to change previously developed decision strategies was examined by Bentin et al (1978). They showed that 0.25% enflurane slowed the rate of learning and increased the number of trials required for

Table 7.1 Differential effect on cognitive function with increasing concentrations of ether anaesthesia

	Stage of anaesthesia		
Cognitive function	Plane 1	Plane 2	Plane 3
Subsequent recall	FR	O	O
Response to spoken voice	FR	FR	FR→O
Memory for recent events	FR	FR	SR→O
Memory for past events	FR	FR	FR→O
Distinguish colour	FR	FR	SR→O
Pain perception	FR	SR	SR→O

FR = Full response: SR = some response; O = no response.
Adapted from Artusio (1955)

readjusting the prediction strategy to the new situation. Similar effects have also been shown for other agents. Adams (1979) comments that subanaesthetic doses of volatile agents caused normal subjects to behave like patients suffering from alcoholism and Korsakoff's syndrome, i.e. adopting a rigid pattern of behaviour. A *similar* pattern of behaviour was seen in rats after hippocampal lesions. Adams (1979) also reported that low concentrations of isoflurane produce state-dependent memory (in which memories formed in one state may be better recalled in the same state rather than a different one). Another finding was that verbal memory was more impaired than non-verbal memory and that retrieval of information learned during the administration of the volatile agent was better at 1 week compared with 2 hours.

General anaesthetics affect copying of light sequences, a task sensitive to left hemisphere deficits in right-handed individuals. Cyclopropane affects facial recognition in low concentrations, a task said to test right hemisphere functions. Together, these studies indicate that left hemisphere functions may be impaired before right hemisphere functions and developmentally later functions are impaired before earlier ones. All memory functions, including the retrieval of old memories, are impaired with subanaesthetic concentrations of nitrous oxide (Ghoneim et al 1981), but implicit memory functions are more resistant to impairment by nitrous oxide than either explicit or short-term memory (Block et al 1988). Jessop et al (1991) showed that subjects inhaling 60% nitrous oxide could complete a task with 100% accuracy whilst having no (explicit) recollection of the event. Rapid (within a few hours) tolerance develops to the sedative and analgesic effects of nitrous oxide in volunteers (Ruprecht and Dzoljic 1990). There also seems to be a continual fluctuation in the conscious level during nitrous oxide anaesthesia. McMenemin and Parbrook (1988) have shown that for equianalgesic concentrations of isoflurane and nitrous oxide, isoflurane produces more cognitive impairment. Ghoneim & Block (1992) have commented that in addition to minimum alveolar concentration (MAC) for analgesia, MAC for cognitive processing and learning need to be defined.

Drugs such as hyoscine (scopolamine) and atropine have dose-dependent transient effects on human learning and memory. Hyoscine especially interrupts the encoding of new information into long-term memory (Kopelman 1986). The retrieval of old episodic memories and retention of information in working memory are not impaired. Thus a situation reminiscent of Korsakoff's syndrome is induced by these drugs. Benzodiazepines facilitate transmission at the gamma-aminobutyric acid (GABA) receptors. There are high concentrations of GABA receptors within the hippocampus, a structure known to be involved in memory encoding. Like hyoscine, the benzodiazepines tend to have a specific effect upon the encoding of new episodic memories into long-term storage. Retrieval of semantic or episodic memory was not affected (Curran 1986). Both diazepam and scopolamine reduce performance in recall and recognition but have little or no effect on repetition priming. Some studies, however, show a weak relationship between

Table 7.2 Responses with the isolated forearm technique during general anaesthesia

Type of response	Technique				
	N_2O–fentanyl	Air–etomidate–fentanyl	Thiopentone–N_2O	Ketamine–thiopentone–N_2O	Ketamine–N_2O
Response to command (%)	44	7	58	36	8
Purposive movement (%)	72	43	69	72	0
Postoperative recall (%)	4	0	8	18	0

Data from Russel (1986) and Schultetus et al (1986).

attention and implicit memory performance, indicating larger doses of these sedative drugs may be required to obtund implicit memory effects.

The effect of surgery as well as the anaesthetic must be taken into account when studying memory and cognitive function. It has been known for some time that conditioning can take place in a rat model during barbiturate anaesthesia if a catecholamine is infused (Weinberger et al 1984). It was postulated that surgically induced catecholamine release during anaesthesia may promote learning and memory of intraoperative events. Adrenaline may be the 'chemical tap on the shoulder which says pay attention!' (Goldmann 1990). Similarly neuropeptides such as vasopressin and adrenocorticotrophic hormone can enhance learning in volunteers, probably as a result of increased attention (Beckwith et al 1990). Surgical stress and some anaesthetic agents are known to stimulate their release (see Richardson 1989, Block & Ghoneim 1992 for further discussions).

Special tests are needed to investigate cognitive processes during light general anaesthesia with neuromuscular blockade. The isolated forearm technique (IFT)* was described by Tunstall (1977) for this purpose. With 0.4% halothane and nitrous oxide it was shown that all patients responded to the incision but response to verbal commands only occurred in the low nitrous oxide concentration group. No patient had any recall. The responsiveness of the patient, varies according to the anaesthetic technique (Table 7.2).

The notable findings are that a large proportion of patients respond purposefully with most techniques, but there is usually no explicit recall. The IFT was also used by Millar & Watkinson (1983), who found the results difficult to interpret, as there was so much hand movement in response to

---

*The technique should be familiar to most readers. In brief, however, one forearm is protected from neuromuscular blockade with a tourniquet and at intervals the patient is asked to squeeze the anaesthetist's hand in a specified way. The problems are firstly, that the patient's arm can interfere with surgery, especially if the anaesthetic is light enough for spinal reflexes to be preserved; and secondly, that there are documented cases of false negatives where the patient was aware but did not respond. Nevertheless the IFT is a direct attempt to deal with intraoperative awareness as it does not rely on postoperative recall. See Jessop & Jones (1991) and Russell (1989) for a discussion.

intubation and surgery! Goldmann and Levy (1986) used a galvanic skin response (GSR) as a sign of responsiveness in patients receiving general anaesthesia for elective arthroscopies. They found that patients responded to the name of Arthur Scargill, the coal miners' leader, but hardly at all to their own name or that or the surgeon or anaesthetist. As this study took place during the coal miners' strike, the authors comment that the salience of the stimulus is important when looking for information processing. They also found that some jokes elicited a response when others did not, implying that a sense of humour may also be retained.

Memory formation during general anaesthesia

A number of surgical patients who had experienced a poor course of postoperative recovery were hypnotized by Cheek (1959, 1964). He showed that they recalled negative or life-threatening statements that had been made about them during surgery but ignored the banter and jokes that had also taken place. In another study, a mock crisis was staged during deep anaesthesia, as defined by the EEG (Levinson 1965). The anaesthetist said the following words: 'Stop the operation. I don't like the patient's colour. His/her lips are too blue. I'm going to give a little oxygen', followed by: 'There, that's better. Now, you can carry on with the operation'.

One month later under hypnosis, 4 out of 10 patients recalled verbatim everything the anaesthetist had spoken, and another 4 patients had partial recall. All 8 became anxious during the recollection process. These early studies demonstrated that salient intraoperative events could be explicitly recalled postoperatively.

Millar & Watkinson (1983) played a list of words to patients undergoing gynaecological surgery. The patients received a variety of anaesthetics but all received on average 0.5% halothane in 66% nitrous oxide in oxygen for maintenance. Afterwards, though none of the patients had any conscious recollection of the perioperative events, the experimental group were more likely to choose with fewer errors the words they were presented with. This study was replicated with isoflurane (Stolzy et al 1986) but not fentanyl (Stolzy et al 1987).

Goldmann (1986) gave a preoperative general information questionnaire to two groups of patients. One group were played the answers during anaesthesia. Postoperatively none recalled being played the answers but the experimental group performed better on a postoperative recognition test (explicit recall). Millar (1987) also presented word lists intraoperatively and showed that words presented during anaesthesia were more likely to be recalled earlier in the retrieval sequence during postoperative free recall (implicit recall). Recently Jelicic et al (1992) presented patients with exemplars of word categories during nitrous oxide/narcotic general anaesthetic. No volatile agent was used. Four exemplars were then repeatedly presented (known as repetition priming). Postoperatively, there was an increased chance of those particular exemplars being generated. Other studies replicated these results with isoflurane (Khilstrom et al 1990, Roorda-Hrdlicková et al 1990). In a remarkable study, using four different anaesthetic techniques (opioid/nitrous oxide alone and with the addition of isoflurane at three concentrations: 1, 1.3 and 1.5 MAC), Block (1991) showed that implicit learning took place and was *independent of the depth of anaesthesia*. A different study did not find any evidence of intraoperative memory using a homophone test (Eich 1984). However in the study, information was only presented once during anaesthesia and precise details of the anaesthetic techniques were not given. Later, in fact, 6 out of the 48 patients recollected something of the surgery, of which 2 gave details which were corroborated.

The use of repetition priming seems particularly successful in causing memory formation in the absence of attentional processing. The nature of the process can best be described as the automatic activation and strengthening of pre-existing memory representations (Jelicic et al 1992). Implicit memory seems to be less sensitive to manipulation of the attentional level than explicit memory tests.

Information processing during general anaesthesia affects postoperative behaviour

It may be of considerable therapeutic benefit if the postoperative course could be influenced by intraoperative suggestion and a number of studies support this possibility. Bennet et al (1985) showed that patients touched their ears more in the course of a postoperative interview when asked to do so by means of a tape played intraoperatively. No patient had any recall of the intraoperative suggestion even by hypnosis but this study has received criticism on methodological grounds*. However another study did show evidence of patients responding to intraoperative suggestions while undergoing cardiopulmonary bypass (Goldmann et al 1987). In this study there was increased incidence of chin touching in the experimental group. Anaesthetic technique was not a significant factor for awareness in this last study. Block et al (1991) also showed increased chin and ear touching in their study, and, as previously mentioned, anaesthetic depth did not influence the results (see also Ghoneim & Block 1992).

Patients undergoing major biliary tract surgery who were played a tape containing positive suggestions had fewer prolonged stays in hospitals if they were over 55 years of age (Bonke et al 1986). The explanation offered by the authors is that younger patients tend to spend less time in hospital, thus any difference in stay would be minimized. In another study, no difference was seen in outcome in patients undergoing simple cholecystectomy (Boeke et al 1988). These authors comment that perhaps the nature of the operation may

---

*The correspondence over this point in the pages of the *British Journal of Anaesthesia* (1987; 59: 1333–1337) is highly informative!

be important, with a greater effect for intraoperative suggestion being seen in more major operations where the potential for longer stays in hospitals is present. Woo et al (1987) found no effect on postoperative outcome in women undergoing hysterectomy. The EEG was monitored to ensure no arousal did occur. However the authors did not state how many times they played the tape and whether they used any tests of implicit memory. Evans & Richardson (1988) showed that positive intraoperative suggestion reduced the postoperative stay in hysterectomy patients. Surprisingly they also found a reduced duration of postoperative pyrexia. The experimental group also had a 23% reduction in their morphine requirements compared to controls; however this did not reach significance. McClintock et al (1989) and Furlong (1990) both showed statistically significant reduced analgesia requirements in groups of patients given intraoperative suggestions. The pain scores were similar in both experimental and control groups. Both studies had used patient-controlled analgesia to assess the amount of opioid required, unlike the study by Evans & Richardson (1988).

These studies illustrate that appropriate methods must be used to detect evidence of intraoperative memory formation. Millar & Watkinson (1983) combined the chance of choosing the right word with the lower error of choosing the wrong word into a single measurement before getting a significant result. The signal detection theory used here adds considerable sensitivity to the assessment (see Millar 1987), though Stolzy et al (1986) did not have to use it to achieve significance. Another problem in such studies is to know whether verbal or non-verbal retrieval methods should be used. Lack of verbal retrieval (verbal amnesia) does not necessarily indicate lack of learning (Squire 1982). Goldmann et al (1987) used ideometer signalling, in which the subject is asked to choose one finger to signal 'yes' and another for 'no'. On many occasions the verbal and non-verbal responses contradict each other (Cheek and Le Cron 1968). Khilstrom & Schacter (1989) point out that since verbal material is effective in establishing and retrieving memory for anaesthesia, ability to process language must be present during anaesthesia and argue that both methods should be used concurrently.

Cognitive processing during anaesthesia and the 40 Hz steady-state response

Of all the monitoring equipment generally available to the anaesthetist in the theatre, none directly measures cognitive function during general anaesthesia. The methods of monitoring depth of anaesthesia have been reviewed (Jones 1989, Thornton 1991, Munglani et al 1992b). The most promising indicator of conscious awareness was the MLR of the AER, more specifically the N_b latency. In a comparison with the isolated forearm, in 5 out of 7 patients the N_b latency decreased to less than 44.5 ms if they were responding with the IFT. Increasing the anaesthetic dose increased the latency to greater than 44.5 ms and abolished the responses of the IFT (Thornton et al 1989).

The problems with using the N_b latency as a monitor of depth of anaesthesia is that it takes 5 min to average the signal, is insensitive to opioid anaesthesia (Kileny et al 1983) and, as shown, does not work in everybody. If the auditory stimulation is presented at a higher frequency than 6 Hz, the evoked response rapidly appears (within seconds rather than minutes), with a stimulating frequency of 40 Hz. This is known as the steady-state response (SSR; Galambos et al 1981). The wave seems to be produced by superimposition of the MLR which was discussed earlier (Fig. 7.5).

This wave can be analysed by fast Fourier transform (FFT). The FFT spectra provide information on both phase and amplitude of the signal. The 40 Hz SSR and the EEG were examined in patients who received a thiopentone, fentanyl and isoflurane anaesthetic (Plourde & Picton 1990). The patients were asked to press a button to indicate changes in the tone of auditory clicks used to elicit the SSR. With induction of anaesthesia they continued with the task until they lost consciousness, when there was a dramatic reduction in the amplitude of the 40 Hz SSR. The button-pressing response only reappeared during emergence and recovery, at which time the amplitude of the 40 Hz SSR had increased. The EEG, however, showed little variation during the same recovery period. The 40 Hz SSR was studied with high-dose sufentanil anaesthesia during cardiac surgery and it was found to be sensitive to the level of consciousness, disappearing during induction and reappearing on recovery (Plourde & Boylan 1991). The EEG and MLR are not useful during opioid anaesthesia, as the former induces a persistent delta rhythm with the EEG and the MLR shows no change (Kileny et al 1983).

The 40 Hz SSR seems to have a close link with cognitive processing. Sleep is associated with a 50% decrease in the amplitude of the 40 Hz SSR

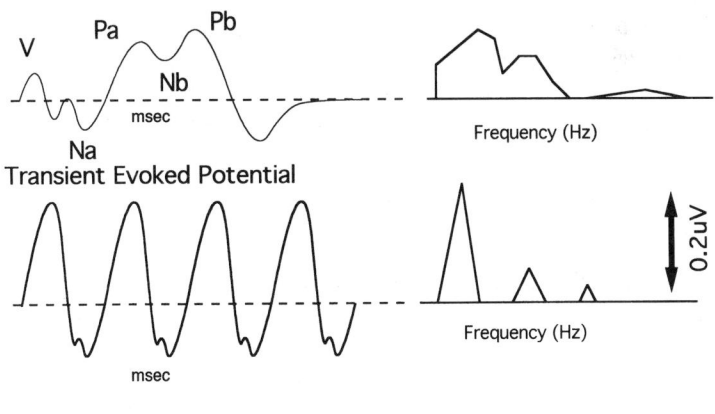

Fig. 7.5 Analysis of transient and steady-state evoked potentials by fast Fourier analysis. Modified from Plourde & Picton (1990).

compared to the awake subject (Galambos et al 1981), though the SSR is insensitive to changes between different sleep stages (Linden et al 1985). Recordings of single cells in the brain indicate that there seems to be an intrinsic 30–60 Hz oscillatory frequency. However these cells usually oscillate out of phase but when an appropriate visual stimulus appears they oscillate in phase (Gray & Singer 1989, Gray et al 1989). The synchronized oscillation of cells in the visual cortex leads to perception of an object (Echkhorn et al 1988). An analysis of the interpeak latencies of the auditory, somatosensory and visual evoked responses gives evidence of three oscillatory brain networks with its own dominant discharge frequency; the response of each system is governed by this dominant frequency (Deshmukh 1988). Both the reaction times of a button press to an indicator lamp and eye movements show evidence of a basic 40 Hz rhythm in the cortex (Poppel 1989; Fig 7.6).

The relationship between the SSR and consciousness is not straightforward, as the SSR can be recorded from comatose patients (Firsching et al 1987). Synchronized but transient oscillations may explain how short-term memory exists, since no anatomical site has been found for it. Whether or not a stimulus enters consciousness may be determined by the presence of synchronized oscillations, and perhaps consciousness itself is simply a process of feature-linking (Crick & Koch 1990). In fact these neuronal oscillations can be seen clearly in the middle latency or $N_a/P_a/N_b$ complex of the AER (see Fig 7.4 and 7.5). A method of eliciting the neuronal oscillations in the AER is to present clicks at 10 Hz and use an autoregressive moving average (ARMA) model to look at the frequency spectra obtained from the EEG. This method has a greater frequency resolution than the FFT (Keller et al 1990). Anaesthesia reduces the frequency (and amplitude) of the neuronal oscillations from that seen in wakefulness (Fig 7.7).

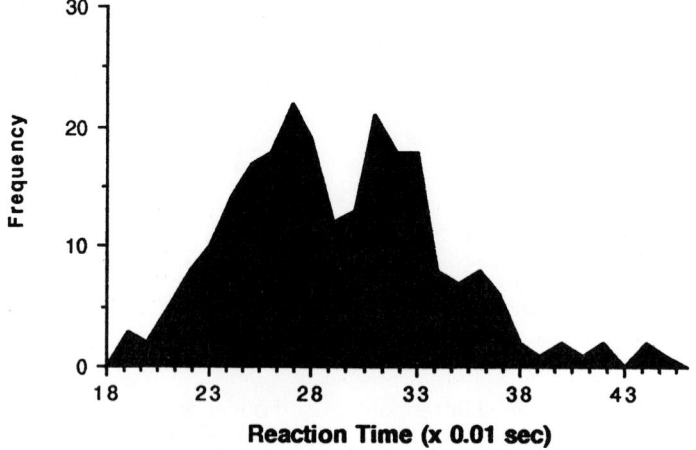

Fig. 7.6 Histogram of auditory reaction time of a subject, showing the bimodal distribution of the response times. Adapted from Poppel (1989).

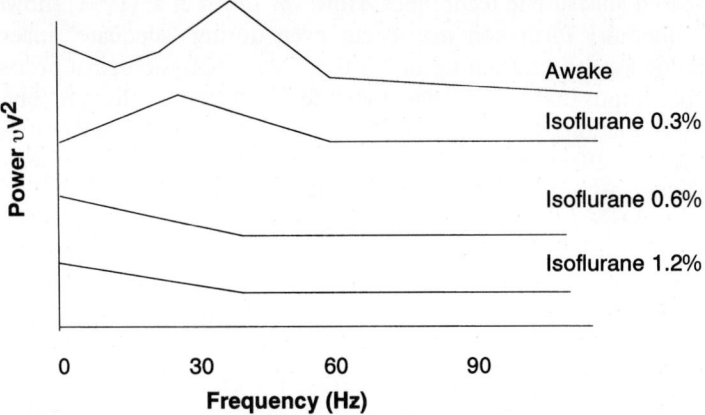

Fig. 7.7 Shift in neuronal oscillation frequency with anaesthesia. Modified from Madler et al (1991).

The reduction of this frequency may be a more appropriate measure of loss of consciousness than loss of power of the 40 Hz SSR and clearly a reduction in the 40 Hz SSR amplitude with anaesthesia is due to power shifting down the frequency band. This is similar to the observations with the raw EEG and anaesthesia. However the frequency changes within the EEG are anaesthetic agent-specific. These frequency changes described with the neuronal oscillations have also been shown to be similar with etomidate and enflurane (Madler & Pöppel 1987, Schwender et al 1992a). The relationship between explicit/implicit memory formation and neuronal oscillations has been examined using two techniques, high-dose opioid and isoflurane for cardiac surgery (Schwender et al 1992b). No explicit memory was found in either group. However the presence of the neuronal oscillation in the opioid group was associated with implicit memory formation. In contrast, the isoflurane group showed no neuronal oscillation and no implicit memory formation.

CONCLUSIONS

These studies indicate that information can be processed without awareness and that memory of an event can exist and affect behaviour without it ever reaching consciousness. Both anaesthesia and sleep alter the way the mind interacts with the environment; both demonstrate reversible loss of consciousness, stimulation causing arousal, and processing of sensory information during the sleeping or anaesthetized state.

These findings can be summarized as follows:

1. Processing of information during general anaesthesia is a real phenomenon. Factors associated with information processing include the lack of or inadequate doses of volatile agents; no premedication, and unsupplemented

opioid-based anaesthetic techniques. However Block et al (1991) showed that implicit memory formation may occur even during 'adequate' anaesthesia. Anaesthetic agents tend not to inhibit those electrophysiological processes in the hippocampus that are associated with learning (see Griffiths & Jones 1990 for an introduction), but ketamine, a weak antagonist at the NMDA receptor, does have an effect. Studies examining implicit learning in humans with low-dose ketamine have not been done as far is known.

2. Certain anaesthetic agents spare metabolically the auditory pathway, these include opioids and some intravenous induction agents except thiopentone or the volatile agents (Jones 1988). However it is not known whether this is the cause of the increased perception of stimuli when volatile agents are not used.

3. Salient and repetitive stimuli increase the chances of recall.

4. Psychological studies indicate that there may be subgroups of patients who might be more prone to process information. The ability to be hypnotized is correlated with this. The relevance of this finding to anaesthesia is not known.

5. The information *is* retrievable, but as general anaesthesia dissociates explicit and implicit memory, tests of the latter must be used along with both verbal and non-verbal methods of retrieval.

6. Information presented intraoperatively can certainly alter performance in psychological tasks postoperatively and may also alter postoperative outcome.

7. The SSR and the related neuronal oscillations of the MLR seem to be promising monitors of cognitive function during anaesthesia. Further studies of the link between these monitors and implicit memory are required.

The evidence to show that information processing occurs under adequate general anaesthesia is convincing. Anaesthetists rather than the press or legal profession should take the lead in modifying anaesthetic techniques to minimize information processing. Studies to examine whether the addition of other agents to our anaesthetic, such as the NMDA antagonists, may prevent information processing, as well as further development of monitors of the anaesthetic state, are required. Until then we should make sure that we are doing no harm to our patients by careless remarks — and perhaps do some good instead.

REFERENCES

Adams N 1979. Disruption of memory functions associated with general anaesthetics. In: Khilstrom J F, Evans F J (eds) Functional disorders of memory. LEA, New Jersey, pp 218–238
Angel A 1991 The G L Brown lecture. Adventures in anaesthesia. Exp Physiol 76: 1–38
Artusio J F 1955 Ether analgesia during major surgery. JAMA 157: 33–36
Askerinsky E, Kleitmann N 1953 Regularly occurring periods of ocular motility and concomitant phenomena during sleep. Science 118: 361–375
Baddeley A D 1986 Working memory. Oxford University Press, Oxford pp 289

Baddeley A D 1988 Imagery and working memory. In: Denis M, Engelkemp J, Richardson J T E (eds) Cognitive and neuropsychological approaches to mental imagery. Martinus Nijholt, Dordrecht, pp 169–180

Beckwith B E, Petros T V, Couk D I, Tinius T P 1990 The effects of vasopressin on memory in healthy young volunteers. Ann N Y Acad Sci 57: 215–226

Bennet H L, Davis H S, Gianni J A 1985 Non-verbal response to intraoperative conversation. Br J Anaesth 57: 174–179

Bentin S, Collins G I, Adam N 1978 Effects of low concentrations of enflurane on probability learning. Br J Anaesth 50: 1179–1183

Berger R J 1963 Experimental modification of dream content by meaningful verbal stimuli. Br J Psychiatr 109: 722–740

Block R I, Ghoneim M M, Pathak D et al 1988 Effects of a subanaesthetic concentration of nitrous oxide on overt and covert assessments of memory and associative processes. Psychopharmacology 96: 324–331

Block R I, Ghoneim M M, Sum Ping S T, Ali M A 1991 Human learning during general anaesthesia and surgery. Br J Anaesth 66: 170–178

Boeke S, Bonke B, Bouwhuis-Hoogerwerf M L et al 1988 The effects of sounds presented during general anaesthesia on postoperative course. Br J Anaesth 60: 697–702

Bonke B, Schmitz P I M, Verhage F, Zwaveling A 1986 Clinical study of so called unconscious perception during general anaesthesia. Br J Anaesth 58: 957–964

Bootzin R R, Khilstrom J F, Schacter D L 1990 Sleep and cognition. American Psychological Association, Washington

Bornstein R F 1989 Subliminal techniques as propaganda tools. J Mind Behav 10: 231–262

Breckenridge J L, Aitkenhead A R 1983 Awareness during general anaesthesia: a review. Annals of the Royal College of Surgeons of England. 65: 93–96.

Brighouse D I, Norman J 1992 To wake in fright. Br Med J 304: 1327–1328

Bremer F 1935 Quelques propriétés de l'activité électrique du cortex cérébrale 'isolé'. C R Soc Biol (Paris) 118: 1241

Cheek D B 1959 Unconscious perception of meaningful sounds during surgical anaesthesia as revealed under hypnosis. Am J Clin Hypn 1: 101–113

Cheek D B 1964 Surgical memory and reaction to careless conversation. Am J Clin Hypn 6: 237

Cheek D B, Le Cron L M 1968 Clinical hypnotherapy. Grune & Stratton, New York

Cook T L, Smith M, Starkweather J A, Eger E I II 1978 Effect of subanaesthetic concentrations of enflurane and halothane on human behaviour. Anaesth Analg 57: 434–440

Crick F, Koch C 1990 Towards a neurobiological theory of consciousness. Semin Neurosci 2: 263–275

Crowder R G 1989 Modularity and dissociations in memory systems. In: Roediger H L, Craik F I M (eds) Varieties in memory and consciousness. Erbaulm, Hillsdale, N J, pp 271–294

Curran H V 1986 Tranquillising memories: a review of the effects of benzodiazepines on human memory. Biol Psychol 23: 179–213

Davis D W, Hawkins R A, Mans A M et al 1984 Regional cerebral glucose utilization during Althesin anaesthesia. Anaesthesiology 61: 362

Davis D W, Mans A M, Biebuyck J F, Hawkins R A 1986 Regional brain glucose utilization in rats during etomidate anaesthesia. Anesthesiology 64: 751

Dement, W, Wolpert E A 1958 The relation of eye movement, bodily motility and external stimuli to dream content. J Exp Psychol 55: 543–553

Deshmukh V D 1988 A chain of suprasegmental neuroscillatory circuits: a human brain theory. Clin Electroencephalogr 19: 7–14

Dixon N F 1981 Preconscious processing. Wiley, Chichester

Dixon N F 1989 Unconscious perception and general anaesthesia. In: Jones J G (ed) Depth of Anaesthesia. Baillière Tindall, London, pp 473–486

Echkhorn R, Bauer R, Jordon W et al 1988 Coherent oscillations: a mechanism of feature linking in the visual cortex? Biol Cybern 60: 121–130

Eich E 1984 Memory for unattended events: remembering with and without awareness. Mem Cognition 12: 105–111

Eich E 1990 Learning during sleep. In: Bootzin R R, Khilstrom J F, Schacter D L (eds) Sleep and cognition. American Psychological Association, Washington, pp 88–108

Emmons W H, Simon C W 1956 The non-recall of material presented during sleep. Am J Psychology 69: 76–81

Erwin R, Buchwald J S 1986 Midlatency auditory evoked responses: differential effects of sleep in the human. Electroencephalogr Clin Neurophysiol 65: 383

Evans F J 1990 Sleep suggestion. In: Bootzin R R, Khilstrom J F, Schacter D L (eds) Sleep and cognition. American Psychological Association, Washington, pp 77–87

Evans C, Richardson P H 1988 Improved recovery and reduced postoperative stay after therapeutic suggestions during general anaesthesia. Lancet ii: 491–493

Firsching R, Luther J, Eidelerg E et al 1987 40-Hz middle latency evoked response in comatosed patients. Electroencephalogr Clin Neurophysiol 67: 213–216

French J D, Verzeano M, Magoun H W 1953 A neural basis of the anaesthetic state. Arch Neurol Psychiat 69: 519–529

Furlong M 1990 Positive suggestion presented during anaesthesia. In: Bonke B, Fitch W, Miller K (eds) Awareness and memory in anaesthesia. Swets, Amsterdam, pp 170–175

Galambos R, Makieg S, Talamachoff P J 1981 A 40-Hz auditory potential recorded from the human scalp. Proc Natl Acad Sci USA 78: 2643–2647

Ghoneim M M, Block R I 1992 Learning and consciousness during general anaesthesia. Anaesthesiology 76: 279–305

Ghoneim M M, Mewaldt S P, Petersen R C 1981 Subanaesthetic concentration of nitrous oxide and human memory. Progr Neuropsychopharmacol 5: 395–402

Goldmann L 1990 Cognitive processing and general anaesthesia. In: Bootzin R R, Khilstrom J F, Schacter D L (eds) Sleep and cognition. American Psychological Association, Washington, pp 127–138

Goldmann L, Levy A B 1986 Orientating under anaesthesia. Anaesthesia 41: 1056–1057

Goldmann L, Shah M V, Hebden M W 1987 Memory of cardiac anaesthesia. Anaesthesia 42: 596–603

Graf P, Squire L R, Mandler G 1984 The information that amnesic patients do not forget. J Exp Psychol 10: 164–178

Gray C M, Singer W 1989 Stimulus-specific neuronal oscillations in orientation columns of the cat visual cortex. Proc Natl Acad Sci USA 86: 1698–1702

Gray C M, Känig P, Engel A K, Singer W 1989 Oscillatory responses in cat visual cortex exhibit inter-columnar synchronization which reflect global stimulus properties. Nature 338: 334–337

Griffiths D, Jones J G 1990 Awareness and memory in anaesthetized patients. Br J Anaesth 65: 603–606

Hargrove R L 1987 Awareness under anaesthesia. J Med Defence Union 3: 9

Hawkins R A, Biebuyck J F 1980 Regional brain function during graded halothane anaesthesia. In Fink B R (ed) Molecular mechanisms in anaesthesia Raven Press, New York

Jelicic M, Bonke B, Wolters G, Hans Phaf R 1992 Implicit memory for words presented during general anaesthesia. Eur J Cognitive Psychology 4: 71–80

Jessop J, Jones J G 1991 Conscious awareness during general anaesthesia — what are we attempting to monitor? Br J Anaesth 66: 635–637

Jessop J, Griffiths D E, Furness P et al 1991 Changes in amplitude and latency of the P300 component of the auditory evoked potential with sedative and anaesthetic concentrations of nitrous oxide. Br J Anaesth 67: 524–531

Jones J G 1988 Awareness under anaesthesia. Anaesthesia rounds no 21. ICI Pharmaceuticals, Alderley Park, Macclesfield, Cheshire

Jones J G (ed) 1989 Depth of anaesthesia. In: Clinical anaesthesiology. Baillière Tindall, London

Keller I, Madler C, Scwender S, Poppel E 1990 Oscillatory components in perioperative AEP-recordings: a non parametric procedure for frequency measurements. Clin Electroencephalogr 21: 88–92

Khilstrom J F, Couture L J 1992 Awareness and information processing in general anaesthesia. J Psychopharmacol 6: 410–417

Khilstrom J F, Schacter D L 1989 Anaesthesia, amnesia and the cognitive unconscious. In: Bonke B, Fitch W, Miller K (eds) Awareness and memory in anaesthesia. Swets, Amsterdam, pp 21–44

Khilstrom J F, Schacter D L, Cork R C et al 1990 Implicit and explicit memory following surgical anaesthesia. Psychol Sci: 303–306

Kileny P, Dobson D, Gelf E T 1983 Middle latency auditory evoked responses during open heart surgery with hypothermia. Electroencephalogr Clin Neurophysiol 55: 268–276

Kopelman M D 1986 The cholinergic neurotransmitter system in human memory and dementia: a review. Q J Exp Psychol 38A: 535–573

Koukkou M, Lehmann D 1968 EEG and memory storage in sleep experiments with humans. Electroencephalogr Clin Neurophysiol 25: 455–462

Krnjevic K 1991 Cellular mechanisms of anaesthesia. Annals NY Acad Sci 625: 1–17

Kutas M 1990 Event related brain studies of cognition during sleep. In: Bootzin R R, Khilstrom J F, Schacter D L (eds) Sleep and cognition. American Psychological Association, Washington, pp 88–108

Levinson B W 1965 States of awareness during general anaesthesia: preliminary communication. Br J Anaesth 37: 544–546

Linden R D, Campbell K B, Hamel G, Picton T W 1985 Human auditory steady state evoked responses during sleep. Ear Hearing 6: 167–174

McClintock T, Aitken H, Kenny G 1989 Effect of intraoperative suggestions on postoperative analgesics requirements. In: Bonke B, Fitch W, Miller K (eds) Awareness and memory in anaesthesia. Swets, Amsterdam

Madler C, Keller I, Schwender D, Pöppel E 1991 Sensory information processing during general anaesthesia: effect of isoflurane on auditory neuronal oscillations. Br J Anaesth 66: 81–87

Madler C, Pöppel E 1987 Auditory evoked potentials indicate the loss of neuronal oscillations during general anaesthesia. Naturwissenschaften 74: 42–43

Maekawa T, Tommasino C, Shapiro H M et al 1986 Local cerebral blood flow and glucose utilization during isoflurane anaesthesia in the rat. Anaesthesiology 65: 152

Marcel A J 1983 Conscious and unconscious perception: an approach to the relations between phenomenal experience and perceptual processes. Cognitive Psychol 15: 238–300

McMenemim I M, Parbrook C D 1988 Comparison of the effects of subanaesthetic concentrations of isoflurane or nitrous oxide in volunteers. Br J Anaesth 60: 56–63

Millar K 1987 Assessment of memory for anaesthesia. In: Hindmarch I, Jones G J, Moss E (eds) Aspects of recovery from anaesthesia. Wiley, Chichester

Millar K, Watkinson N 1983 Recognition of words presented during general anaesthesia. Ergonomics 26: 585–594

Moruzzi G, Magoun H W 1949 Brainstem reticular formation and activation of the EEG. Electroencephalogr Clin Neurophysiol 1: 455–473

Munglani R, Andrade J, Sapsford D J, Baddeley A, Jones G J 1993 Validation of coherent frequency of the brain as a measure of consciousness during anaesthesia. Br J Anaesth (in press)

Newton D E F, Thornton L, Roneiczko K et al 1988 Levels of consciousness in volunteers breathing sub-MAC concentrations of isoflurane. Br J Anaesth 60: 56–63

Nielsen-Bohlman L, Knight R T, Woods D L, Woodward K 1991 Differential auditory processing continues during sleep. Electroencephalogr Clin Neurophysiol 79: 281–290

Oswald I, Taylor A M, Treisman M 1960 Discriminitive responses to stimulation during human sleep. Brain 83: 440–453

Pearce R A, Stringer J L, Lothman E W 1989 Effect of volatile anaesthetics on synaptic transmission in the rat hippocampus. Anesthesiology 71: 591–598

Plourde G, Boylan J F 1991 The auditory steady state response during sufentanil anaesthesia. Br J Anaesth 66: 683–691

Plourde G, Picton T W 1990 Human auditory steady-state response during general anaesthesia. Anesth Analg 71: 460–468

Poppel E 1989 Taxonomy of the subjective. In: Brown J W (ed) Neuropsychology of visual perception. Lawrence Erbaulm Associates, Hillsdale, pp 219–232

Popper K R, Eccles J C 1977 The Self and its brain. Springer Verlag, London

Prys-Roberts C 1987 Anaesthesia: a practical or impractical construct? Br J Anaesth 59: 1341–1345

Ramm P, Frost B J 1986 Cerebral and local cerebral metabolism in the cat during slow wave and REM sleep. Brain Res 365: 112–124

Regan D 1990 Electrophysiology of the human brain. Elsevier, Amsterdam

Richardson J T E 1989 Human memory: psychology, pathology and pharmacology. In: Jones

J G (ed) Depth of anaesthesia. Bailliere Tindall, London

Roorda-Hrdličková, Wolters G, Bonke B, Phaf P 1990 Unconscious perception during general anaesthesia demonstrated by an implicit memory task. In: Bonke B, Fitch W, Miller K (eds) Awareness and memory in anaesthesia. Swets, Amsterdam, pp 150–156

Rosen M, Lunn J N (eds) 1987 Conscious awareness and pain in general anaesthesia. Butterworth, London

Ruprecht J, Dzoljic M 1990 Tolerence to the effect of nitrous oxide. A cause of awareness. In: Bonke B, Fitch W, Miller K (eds) Awareness and memory in anaesthesia. Swets, Amsterdam, pp 296–299

Russell I F 1986 Comparison of wakefulness with two anaesthetic regimens. Br J Anaesth 58: 965–968

Russell I F 1989 Conscious awareness during general anaesthesia: relevance of autonomic signs and isolated arm movements as guides to depth of anaesthesia. In: Jones J G (ed) Depth of anaesthesia. Baillière Tindall, London, pp 511–532

Samra S K, Lilly D J, Rush N L, Kirsh M M 1984 Fentanyl anesthesia and human brain stem auditory evoked potentials. Anesthesiology 61: 261

Schacter D L 1987 Implicit memory: history and current status. J Exp Psychol Learning Mem Cognition 13: 501–518

Schulteus R R, Hill G R, Dharamraj C M et al 1986 Wakefulness during cesarean section after anaesthetic induction with ketamine, thiopentone or thiopentone and ketamine combined. Anesth Analg 65: 723

Schwender D, Madler C, Klasing S, Peter K 1992 Enflurane and Isoflurane cause a dose dependent decrease of neuronal oscillations in auditory evoked potentials. Anesth Analg 74: S1–S368

Schwender D, Kaiser A, Klasing S 1992b Explicit and implicit memory and mid-latency auditory evoked potentials during cardiac surgery. Anesth Analg 74: S1–S368

Sherry D F, Schacter D L 1987 The evolution of multiple memory systems. Psychol Rev 94: 439–454

Siegel J M 1990 Mechanisms of sleep control. J Clin Neurophysiol. 7: 49–65

Silverman L H, Ross D, Adler J, Lustig D 1978 A simple research paradigm for demonstrating subliminal psychodynamic activation. J Abnormal Psychol 87: 341–357

Sokoloff L 1981 Localization of functional activity in the central nervous system by measurement of glycose utilization with radioactive de-oxyglucose. J Cerebral Blood Flow Metab 1: 7

Squire L R 1982 The neuropsychology of human memory. Annu Rev Neurosci 5: 241

Steriade M 1989 Brain electrical activity and sensory processing during waking and sleeping states. In: Kryger M H, Roth T, Dement W C (eds) Principles and practice of sleep medicine. Saunders, Philadelphia, pp 86–103

Stockard J, Bickford R 1981 The neurophysiology of anaesthesia. In: Gordon E (ed) A basis and practice of neuroanaesthesia. Biomedical Press, Amsterdam. pp 3–46

Stolzy S, Couture L J, Edmonds H L 1986 Evidence of partial recall during general anaesthesia. Anesth Analg 65: S1–S170

Stolzy S, Couture L J, Edmonds H L 1987 A postoperative recognition test after balanced anaesthesia. Anesth Analg 67: A377

Thornton C 1991 Evoked potentials in anaesthesia. Eur J Anaesthesiol 8: 89–107

Thornton C, Barrowcliffe M P, Konieczko K M et al 1989 The auditory evoked response as an indicator of awareness. Br J Anaesth 63: 113–115

Tilley A J 1979 Sleep learning during stage 2 and REM sleep. Biol Psychol 9: 155–161

Tunstall M E 1977 Detecting wakefulness during general anaesthesia for caesarian section. Br Med J i: 1321

Weinberger N M, Gold P E, Sternberg D B 1984 Epinephrine enables Pavlovian fear conditioning under anaesthesia. Science 223: 605

Wolters G, Phaf R H 1990 Explicit and implicit measures of memory: evidence for two learning mechanisms. In: Bonke B, Fitch W, Miller K (eds) Awareness and memory in anaesthesia. Swets, Amsterdam, pp 57–63

Woo R, Seltzer J L, Marr A 1987 The lack of response to suggestion under controlled surgical anaesthesia. Acta Anaesthesiol Scand 31: 567–571

Zacks R T, Hasher L, Sanft H 1982 Automatic encoding of event frequency: further findings. J Exp Psychol: Learning, Mem Cognition 8: 106–116

8. Endocrine response to surgery

J. P. Desborough   G. M. Hall

The endocrine response to surgery is one component of a systemic reaction to the physiological disturbance which follows tissue injury, infection and inflammatory disorders. This systemic response to injury is known in a broad sense as the acute-phase response, and in addition to alterations in endocrine activity, it includes fever, leukocytosis, complement activation, manufacture of new proteins in the liver, and fluid and electrolyte changes (Table 8.1).

The endocrine response to surgical trauma and the metabolic consequences of the hormonal changes have been extensively investigated in recent years. This subject has been of interest for more than half a century (Cuthbertson 1932) and the development of sensitive radioimmunoassays for the measurement of hormones has allowed detailed examination of the endocrine response. The effects of different anaesthetic regimens on the response has also been comprehensively studied with the aim of suppressing the increase in catabolic hormone secretion and preventing the metabolic changes which follow. With the advances in immunology during the past 10 years there has also been a vast increase in the understanding of the links between the neuroendocrine and immune systems.

INITIATION OF THE RESPONSE

The endocrine response is initiated by afferent nerve impulses, both somatic and autonomic, from the site of surgery. Increased neuronal input to the hypothalamus causes an increased secretion of hypothalamic-releasing

Table 8.1 Components of the acute-phase response

Hypothalamic–pituitary–adrenal axis activation
Increased sympathetic autonomic activity
Hyperglycaemia and negative nitrogen balance
Fever
Leukocytosis
Acute-phase protein production
Water retention
Mineral and electrolyte imbalance

hormones which in turn stimulate secretion of hormones from both the anterior and posterior lobes of the pituitary gland. Increased efferent sympathetic autonomic neuronal activity results in release of noradrenaline at presynaptic nerve endings and a rise in circulating concentrations of catecholamines secreted from the adrenal medulla. Noradrenaline is primarily a neurotransmitter, but there is some spill-over of noradrenaline released from nerve terminals into the circulation. This augmented sympathetic activity results in the well-recognized cardiovascular effects which are seen as tachycardia and hypertension. In addition, there are direct hormonal effects of adrenergic stimulation of a number of visceral organs, including the pancreas and the kidney.

The pituitary response is characterized by an increase in the secretion of adrenocorticotrophic hormone (ACTH), growth hormone (GH), beta-endorphin and prolactin from the anterior lobe of the pituitary. The secretion of luteinizing hormone (LH) and follicle-stimulating hormone (FSH) also changes, as does thyroid-stimulating hormone (TSH), but less information is available on the changes of these anterior pituitary hormones during surgery. Arginine vasopressin (AVP) is released from the posterior pituitary and causes an increase in water reabsorption by the kidney.

Subsequent to the alterations in pituitary hormone secretion there are secondary effects on secretion from target organs. Adrenocortical secretion (mainly cortisol) is stimulated as a result of increased release of ACTH. Sympathetic adrenergic stimulation of the pancreas causes an increased secretion of glucagon and reduction in the release of insulin. Renin is secreted from the kidney in response to a variety of stimuli, including sympathetic stimulation, and promotes the conversion of angiotensinogen to angiotensin I, which is then converted into angiotensin II. This peptide stimulates the secretion of the mineralocorticoid aldosterone from the adrenal cortex. Aldosterone acts on the epithelium of the distal tubule and collecting duct of the kidney to increase the reabsorption of sodium from the urine.

The overall effects of these alterations in hormone secretion are a relative increase in catabolic hormone concentrations which promote mobilization of substrates to provide energy sources, and a mechanism to retain salt and water in order to maintain circulating fluid volumes and cardiovascular homeostasis. The hormonal changes are summarized in Table 8.2. In general, the magnitude of the endocrine response is related to the severity of the surgical trauma. For example, the response to major upper abdominal or thoracic surgery is greater than that resulting from minor, peripheral operations. In addition, the hormonal responses can be markedly modified by the anaesthetic regimen.

The importance of the nervous system in the hormonal response has been clearly demonstrated in an early experiment in which the afferent nerves of an animal limb were sectioned; the hormonal responses to subsequent injury were prevented (Hume & Egdahl 1959). In a similar way, blockade of afferent nerve impulses by epidural or spinal analgesia with a local anaesthetic agent

Table 8.2 Hormonal responses to surgery

	Increased secretion	Increased/decreased secretion	Decreased secretion
Pituitary	Adrenocorticotrophic hormone Growth hormone Beta-endorphin Prolactin Arginine vasopressin	Thyroid-stimulating hormone Luteinizing hormone/ follicle-stimulating hormone	
Adrenal	Catecholamines Cortisol Aldosterone		
Pancreas	Glucagon		Insulin
Other organs	Renin		Testosterone/oestradiol Triiodothyronine

can prevent the anterior pituitary and catecholamine response to surgery. In pelvic surgery, an extensive epidural block from dermatomal level T^4 to S^5 can completely inhibit the cortisol and glycaemic response (Engquist et al 1977) and also the increase in GH secretion (Bythell et al 1989).

Cytokines

In addition to the neuronal initiation of the endocrine response, tissue injury results in a local reaction which stimulates the production of cytokines. The cytokines are produced from activated leukocytes, in particular monocytes, and also from activated fibroblasts and endothelial cells. This group of low molecular weight glycoproteins includes the interleukins (IL), tumour necrosis factor (TNF) and the interferons. The cytokines have both local effects and major systemic effects mediated by the activation of specific receptors. There are many interactions between the cytokines; IL-1 can induce IL-6 production and was first suggested as the link between the immune and neuroendocrine systems, as it was shown to stimulate the pituitary adrenal axis in animals in vivo. TNF-α is well-known as a mediator of septic shock, although its precise biological role is not yet clear. Much interest in critical care currently focuses on the use of manufactured antibodies against endotoxins and TNF, in an attempt to reduce the mortality from Gram-negative septicaemia in critical illness.

IL-1 has diverse effects in the body and acts as an endogenous pyrogen. It may produce fever by a direct action on the hypothalamus and in addition may cause local release of prostaglandins and other inflammatory and pyretic mediators. IL-1 also has effects on the immune system and it has been suggested that it may promote proteolysis.

Following surgery, circulating concentrations of IL-6 are raised in proportion to the severity of tissue trauma, although concentrations of the cytokines IL-1β and TNF-α in plasma are not increased. Cruickshank et al (1990) have demonstrated changes in IL-6 values 2–4 hours after the start of surgery with the peak values occurring after 6–12 hours. Laparoscopic surgical techniques led to smaller increases in IL-6 than those following conventional surgery (Joris et al 1992). This study showed that, although the endocrine changes were similar to those in patients having cholecystectomy with a standard surgical technique, the IL-6 responses were significantly lower following laparoscopic surgery. It has also been demonstrated that regional anaesthesia has no impact on circulating concentrations of IL-6 following surgical trauma (Moore et al 1992). Although, as discussed later, regional anaesthetic blockade can effectively inhibit the changes in cortisol and other hormones, it cannot reduce the cytokine production which is initiated by tissue trauma.

IL-6 is however closely associated with the systemic manifestation of the acute-phase response, and may also have a local role within the hypothalamus and pituitary (Imura et al 1991). IL-6 is a prime inducer of the synthesis of acute-phase proteins from the liver, and one of its previous names, hepatocyte-stimulating factor, reflects this role. The acute-phase proteins are produced by hepatocytes, usually at the expense of decreased production of other proteins such as albumin. A large variety of proteins are synthesized in response to tissue trauma. C-reactive protein (CRP) was first identified in patients with infections and inflammatory diseases. It is one of the most easily measured acute-phase proteins; normally serum levels in humans are extremely low. Others include fibrinogen, the proteins of the complement series, haptoglobin, serum amyloid A, α_1-antitrypsin and ceruloplasmin. These proteins have a role in promoting haemostasis, tissue repair and regeneration (Thompson et al 1992). Cruickshank et al (1990) demonstrated a correlation between the increase in circulating IL-6 values and the increase in CRP concentrations which occurred following surgery.

In addition to the production of IL-6 by macrophages and fibroblasts following tissue injury, IL-6 is known to be produced in the hypothalamus and by the folliculostellate cells of the pituitary (Vankelecom et al 1989); IL-6 may have an autocrine action, that is, it acts locally to promote hormone secretion in the hypothalamus and pituitary. For example, in vitro preparations of cultured anterior pituitary cells respond to IL-6 by an increased secretion of prolactin and GH (Spangelo et al 1989). However, it is very unlikely that circulating concentrations of IL-6 produced in response to surgical trauma might be responsible for initiating the endocrine response, since the time-course of the rise in IL-6 is much later than the changes in pituitary hormones (Moore et al 1992). It is likely that the production of IL-6 by macrophages and other cells requires new protein to be synthesized, whereas release of hormones from the pituitary in response to hypothalamic stimulation needs only the secretion of ready synthesized hormone from a releasable pool.

HORMONES

Catecholamines

Noradrenaline, adrenaline and dopamine are secreted into the adrenal vein by the adrenal medulla. In humans adrenaline is the major hormonal output of the adrenal. Most of the noradrenaline released at presynaptic nerve endings is taken back up into the nerve terminal. However, some noradrenaline enters the circulation, although it rarely reaches the threshold value for exerting metabolic effects. Most of the effects of noradrenaline are caused directly by its release from nerve endings as an adrenergic neurotransmitter.

Cardiovascular effects

The effects of increased sympathetic activity during anaesthesia and surgery are assessed indirectly by routine monitoring of the cardiovascular system. Measurements of heart rate and arterial pressure correlate with changes in plasma catecholamines and therefore reflect alterations in sympathetic activity (Derbyshire & Smith 1984). The metabolic activity of the catecholamines includes the breakdown of glycogen in the liver and muscle (glycogenolysis), which results in increased plasma concentrations of lactate and glucose, and also mobilization of free fatty acids from fat stores.

Cortisol

The C^{21} corticosteroid cortisol has both glucocorticoid and mineralo-corticoid effects. Amongst its many glucocorticoid actions, cortisol has complex effects on the intermediary metabolism of carbohydrate, fat and protein. It causes an increase in blood glucose concentrations by stimulating protein catabolism and promoting glucose production in the liver by gluconeogenesis. Cortisol reduces peripheral glucose utilization by an anti-insulin effect. Glucocorticoids also have well-known anti-inflammatory actions mediated by a decrease in the production of inflammatory mediators such as leukotrienes and prostaglandins. Thus, high doses of exogenous glucocorticoids can inhibit the inflammatory response to tissue injury. In addition, there is immunoregulatory feedback between the glucocorticoid hormones and IL-1; the production and action of IL-1 is inhibited by ACTH and cortisol.

Surgery is associated with an increased white cell count with granulocytosis and lymphopenia. These changes may be partially modified during surgery under regional anaesthesia, suggesting that increased secretion of cortisol or other hormones may influence the white cell changes. Indeed, in vitro studies have shown that cortisol and catecholamines modulate neutrophil and lymphocyte activity (Weissman 1990).

Growth hormone

GH is a polypeptide of 191 amino acids. It has both diabetogenic and protein anabolic effects. The anabolic effects on tissue growth are mediated through polypeptides originally known as somatomedins, now more commonly referred to as growth factors. The principal growth factor is somatomedin C, or insulin-like growth factor (IGF-1), so called because of its structural and biological similarities to insulin. IGF-1 is secreted by the liver and other tissues in response to GH stimulation. The major role of IGF-1 is in promoting skeletal and cartilaginous growth.

Recent attention to the role of GH in surgical trauma has focused on the use of recombinant GH or IGF-1 to promote tissue repair and reduce the muscle protein breakdown associated with the catabolic state (Chwals & Bristrian 1991, Ross et al 1991). Exogenous IGF-1 might promote protein anabolic effects without the substrate mobilizing action of GH; indeed an argument has been postulated that the administration of recombinant IGF-1 or of GH together with IGF-1 may be more effective than GH alone in promoting anabolic protein metabolism (Chwals & Bristrian 1991). Recombinant IGF-1 has been given to humans by intravenous infusion, and further studies are in progress to determine whether it may confer beneficial effects on protein metabolism in catabolic states following injury.

Insulin

Insulin is the key anabolic hormone. It is a polypeptide with two chains of amino acids linked by disulphide bridges. It is secreted from the B cell of the islets of Langerhans in the pancreas. Insulin is usually secreted in response to hyperglycaemia, and promotes the uptake of glucose into muscle and adipose tissue, promotes the formation of glycogen from glucose in the liver and prevents lipolysis and protein breakdown. Most studies indicate that there is a failure of insulin secretion in response to the hyperglycaemia associated with surgical trauma. Insulin concentrations in the plasma during and after surgery may be low, normal or raised but are usually low relative to the degree of hyperglycaemia. The apparent reduction in insulin secretion may be caused in part by catecholamine-mediated inhibition of secretion, directly at the B cell. Alpha-adrenergic stimulation inhibits insulin secretion through release of noradrenaline, and this mechanism may be effective when sympathetic activity increases during surgery.

It is frequently stated that insulin resistance following trauma is a factor in the hyperglycaemic response. Insulin resistance is a defect of the insulin receptor, but the details of the mechanisms involved are incompletely understood. Infusions of insulin have been used to counteract the effect of catabolic hormones following trauma and surgery. These studies are in contrast to those which aim to reduce circulating concentrations of catabolic hormones. During gynaecological surgery an infusion of insulin decreased circulating glucose values in addition to a reduction in fatty acids and B-hydroxybutyrate, substrates produced by lipolysis (Hall et al 1983).

Beta-endorphin and prolactin

Beta-endorphin is an opioid peptide of 31 amino acids which is derived when the precursor protein, pro-opiomelanocortin (POMC) is cleaved into ACTH and beta-lipotrophin. Beta-lipotrophin is then partially cleaved to gamma-lipotrophin and beta-endorphin. A small amount of beta-endorphin is derived from peripheral tissues. The secretion of beta-endorphin into the circulation from the pituitary during surgery and other trauma may reflect the increased secretory activity of the pituitary at this time. It has no major metabolic effects. Immunoreactive beta-endorphin can be easily measured by radioimmunoassay. Absolute values of beta-endorphin released during stress are low, and its role remains uncertain, although it has been suggested that it may modulate immune function (Weissman 1990).

Prolactin has 199 amino acid residues and is structurally similar to GH. Secretion of prolactin increases during pregnancy, causes milk secretion from the breast and also increases during exercise and surgical stress. Like beta-endorphin, prolactin has little metabolic activity, but has been shown to affect immune function both in vitro and in vivo (Spangelo et al 1989).

TSH and thyroid hormones

The hormones thyroxine (T_4) and triiodothyronine (T_3) are secreted from the thyroid gland under the influence of TSH from the anterior pituitary. T_3, the more active hormone, is also produced from T_4 in peripheral tissue. Inactive reverse triiodothyronine (r T_3) is formed mainly from deiodination of T_4. The hormones are extensively bound to plasma proteins, albumin, thyroxine-binding prealbumin and thyroxine-binding globulin and have a long half-life (T_4 approximately 6–7 days). The small percentage of free T_3 and T_4 which is unbound in the circulation is in equilibrium with the protein-bound hormones. Any changes in the plasma concentrations of the binding hormones may affect both the total and free plasma concentrations of T_3 and T_4. Free T_3 and T_4 exert a negative feedback effect on TSH secretion from the anterior pituitary.

It has been postulated that in certain circumstances such as trauma and other non-thyroidal illnesses, the specific enzyme which catalyses the formation of T_3 and the metabolism of r T_3 is inhibited. This leads to a decrease in plasma T_3 and an increase in r T_3. This phenomenon has been termed the euthyroid sick syndrome, low T_3 syndrome or non-thyroidal illness (Ziegler et al 1990).

Thyroid hormones increase the metabolic rate, stimulate oxygen consumption and increase heat production. Secondary to the increased metabolic rate, protein and fat stores are mobilized. These effects of thyroid hormones are closely related to those of the catecholamines. In addition, the thyroid hormones increase the sensitivity of the heart to the effects of catecholamines.

Studies of changes in thyroid hormones and TSH following surgery have demonstrated broadly similar results. There is usually a pronounced and prolonged decrease in total and free T_3 concentrations with an increase in r T_3. TSH values have been shown to increase during surgery, or immediately postoperatively, but this change is not prolonged and is an inconsistent finding. It has been suggested that since exogenous glucocorticoids decrease circulating TSH and T_3 concentrations, a rise in serum cortisol values during surgery may influence the changes in the pituitary–thyroid axis. However, a study in which the increase in cortisol concentrations was reduced by extensive epidural blockade showed that the changes in thyroid hormones were similar to those in patients who received general anaesthesia (Brandt et al 1976). The significance of the changes in thyroid hormones following surgery — particularly the decrease in total and free T_3 concentrations — is uncertain, but may represent an adaptive response to minimize the increase in metabolic rate in the presence of increased sympathetic activity.

Pituitary gonadotrophins and testosterone

LH is trophic to the Leydig cells of the testis which produce testosterone. In females LH promotes maturation of ovarian follicles, secretion of oestrogens and the formation of the corpus luteum following ovulation. FSH is responsible, as the name suggests, for the early growth of ovarian follicles. In males, FSH maintains the spermatic epithelium and Sertoli cells which secrete a glycoprotein, inhibin. Testosterone is a C_{19} steroid, synthesized from cholesterol in the Leydig cells of the testis. Small amounts are also produced from the adrenal cortex. Testosterone exerts a negative feedback effect on LH secretion from the pituitary. It is responsible for male secondary sexual characteristics and in addition has important protein anabolic and growth effects and a role in the adolescent growth spurt.

There are few reported investigations of the changes in gonadal function which occur following surgery. Several studies have demonstrated a decrease in testosterone levels which remain suppressed for several days (Wang et al 1978, Woolf et al 1985). However, the cause of this remains uncertain since the decrease in testosterone associated with surgery has been accompanied by LH values which increased to a peak during surgery and then declined after the first postoperative day (Wang et al 1978), although in other major illnesses including surgery, LH values were decreased or remained unchanged (Woolf et al 1985). A recent study (Dong et al 1992) showed that Sertoli cell function characterized by circulating inhibin values was less affected by critical illness than the testosterone-producing Leydig cells.

There is a paucity of data on the effects of surgery on female hormones. Wang et al (1978) demonstrated a decline in oestradiol concentrations which persisted for up to 5 days following surgery. The significance of the changes in pituitary gonadotrophins and gonadal function following surgery remains to be elucidated.

Arginine vasopressin

AVP is a polypeptide of amino acids. In addition to its well-known role as an antidiuretic hormone it has important vasopressor and haemostatic effects and an endocrine function (Philbin 1989).

AVP promotes the release of ACTH through secretion of corticotrophin-releasing factor (CRF) from the hypothalamus. Evidence that AVP may also stimulate the release of other anterior pituitary hormones is conflicting. AVP may have some effect on the regulation of blood glucose by increasing glucagon secretion and by enhancing glycogenolysis and gluconeogenesis in the liver (Philbin 1989).

AVP increases the permeability of the collecting ducts to water and is also released in response to an increase in plasma osmolality and hypovolaemia and hypotension, a homeostatic mechanism to maintain circulating fluid volume.

Anaesthesia itself does not stimulate AVP secretion, although during surgery AVP values are increased, and this increase may be attenuated with opioid anaesthesia (Kono et al 1981). Regional anaesthetic techniques are more effective in blocking the AVP response, but only for lower abdominal surgery.

METABOLIC CONSEQUENCES OF THE ENDOCRINE RESPONSE

The metabolic responses to injury have been extensively reviewed (Frayn 1985, Weissman 1990).

Carbohydrate metabolism

Hyperglycaemia is a prominent feature of the metabolic changes occurring during surgery. It is also one which can be most readily monitored by laboratory methods. During cardiac surgery, blood glucose values can increase up to 8–10 mmol/l during cardiopulmonary bypass in patients anaesthetized with high-dose opioids (Desborough et al 1990) and during upper abdominal surgery the glycaemic response gives rise to blood glucose concentrations up to 8 mmol/l. There is an excess of glucose entering the circulation compared with glucose uptake into the tissue. Glucose production is increased by hepatic glycogenolysis which is promoted by sympathetic adrenergic stimulation to the liver and increased circulating adrenaline concentrations. Glucagon, secreted from the A cells of the pancreas, also mediates glycogenolysis. In muscle, glycogenolysis results in increased production of lactate and pyruvate, which can be converted to glucose by gluconeogenesis in the liver. Gluconeogenesis is stimulated by the increased levels of adrenaline, glucagon and cortisol. Glycerol, released from fat during lipolysis, is also a substrate for gluconeogenesis. The actions of these counter-regulatory hormones are balanced by insulin. Glucose uptake into muscle and adipose tissue is stimulated by insulin, and in addition, insulin inhibits gluconeogenesis. Following injury plasma insulin concentrations are reduced with respect to the degree of hyperglycaemia. Glucose utilization is impaired, and this is thought to be caused by insensitivity of muscle and fat to insulin. This so-called insulin resistance is incompletely understood, but is some alteration of the insulin receptor on its effector mechanism.

Fat metabolism

Lipolysis of triglycerides to free fatty acids (FFAs) and glycerol is promoted by adrenaline and glucagon, potentiated by cortisol and inhibited by insulin. Following surgery plasma concentrations of glycerol are increased. FFAs are bound to albumin in the circulation. The oxidation of FFAs to acetyl-coA is enhanced by high glucagon and low insulin concentrations. Acetyl-coA units condense to form acetoacetyl-coA which is converted to acetoacetate in the liver, and subsequently to β-hydroxylase and acetone. These substances, called ketone bodies, can be metabolized as energy sources by tissues other than the liver.

Protein metabolism

Surgical trauma induces an alteration in protein metabolism which results in a net increase in urinary excretion of nitrogen. This so-called negative nitrogen balance reflects either a decrease in protein synthesis, increased protein break-down, or both. Sophisticated protein turnover studies are required to examine the precise balance of protein catabolism and synthesis. Following surgery, it is predominantly muscle but also visceral protein which is catabolized, and the amino acids mobilized in proteolysis are used as substrates for gluconeogenesis. In addition, new proteins are synthesized in the liver. These are the acute-phase proteins such as fibrinogen, CRP and ferritin. Synthesis of albumin and transferrin is decreased. The hormones adrenaline, cortisol and glucagon are involved in the mediation of proteolysis. The cytokines, particularly IL-1 and IL-6, are known to promote the formation of acute-phase proteins and have been implicated in the mediation of muscle breakdown to supply the amino acid requirements for new protein synthesis. The breakdown of muscle protein contributes to the weight loss which follows major surgical procedures, and in patients who are septic, or are already malnourished, protein catabolism may seriously impair postoperative recovery.

Recently, attention has focused on individual amino acids in an attempt to provide nutritional support of correct composition in a logical manner. Glutamine is an amino acid used by rapidly dividing cells of the gut mucosa and lymphocytes. It also acts as a precursor for the renal excretion of ammonia. Following surgery and other injury, the glutamine content of muscle and plasma glutamine concentrations decrease dramatically. Depletion of plasma glutamine may reduce the rate of lymphocyte proliferation and be associated with depression of immune function (Parry-Billings et al 1990). Glutamine has been shown to increase the rate of protein synthesis in vitro, hence recent studies have examined the effects of glutamine supplements in parenteral nutrition, in postoperative patients (Stehle et al 1989) and those with major catabolic illness (Ziegler et al 1990). Although the use of parenteral nutrition may improve nitrogen balance, there is little evidence of clinical benefit in patients following major surgery except for those who are severely malnourished (Veterans Group, 1991). Similarly, in postoperative patients, glutamine-supplemented intravenous nutrition was associated with improved nitrogen retention (Stehle et al 1989) but no evidence of improved outcome was presented.

EFFECT OF ANAESTHESIA ON THE ENDOCRINE RESPONSE TO SURGERY

Many groups have studied the effects of anaesthesia and analgesic techniques on the endocrine response to surgery. These investigations have included the examination of the effects of traditional and less conventional regimens such as xenon anaesthesia (Boomsma et al 1990) and acupuncture (Kho et al 1990). It should be noted that it may be difficult to make comparisons between studies as many variables may be uncontrolled or differ between investigations. Factors which may differ between studies include variations in intravenous fluid regimens, transfusions of homologous stored blood, extent of haemodilution, blood sampling intervals and the individual hormones and metabolites measured. The aim of these studies is usually to examine specific effects of individual agents and also to identify any beneficial consequences on postoperative morbidity and outcome associated with suppression of the hormonal and metabolic changes. Kehlet (1989) suggested that complete pain relief with appropriate analgesic techniques, when associated with a concomitant decrease in surgical stress response, may have important beneficial effects on postoperative morbidity. There is general agreement that it is beneficial to prevent the overt manifestations seen in the cardiovascular system as a result of the sympathetic nervous system response to anaesthetic and surgical stimulation, especially in patients with evidence of ischaemic heart disease. In such patients, vigorous attempts are often made to avoid potentially harmful tachycardia and hypertension. Other endocrine responses and the metabolic sequelae are less apparent, and the need to inhibit or prevent them may therefore seem questionable.

A recent study (Anand & Hickey 1992) has shown that neonates undergoing cardiac surgery given high doses of the opioid sufentanil showed less severe metabolic disturbance than a control group of neonates who received lighter anaesthesia with halothane and morphine. The study was small, and has been criticized, but suggested that in neonates requiring open heart surgery anaesthesia with sufentanil, continued into the postoperative period, may be associated with an improved outcome.

Opiates

It has long been known that opioids inhibit the hypothalamic–pituitary–adrenal axis. Therapeutic doses of morphine were shown to suppress ACTH secretion from the pituitary (McDonald et al 1959), while the adrenal cortex remained responsive to exogenous ACTH. Large doses of opioids were first employed in anaesthesia for cardiac surgery where it was felt that this technique conveyed superior haemodynamic stability than regimens using volatile agents. High-dose fentanyl — that is, doses of 50 µg/kg or greater — will inhibit cortisol and GH responses to pelvic surgery (Hall et al 1978). Larger doses (100 µg/kg) are required to prevent endocrine responses, including catecholamines, to upper abdominal surgery (Klingstedt et al 1987, Giesecke et al 1988). Such doses of opioids cause profound respiratory depression and are suitable only for patients in whom mechanical ventilation in the postoperative period is deemed necessary. In cardiac surgery, high-dose opioids suppress most of the hormonal responses until the onset of cardiopulmonary bypass, although different studies have not always given consistent results. Sufentanil, which is approximately 5–10 times more potent than fentanyl, does not suppress the rise in circulating catecholamines associated with the onset of cardiopulmonary bypass (Bovill et al 1983). Few studies of the effects of opioids on the endocrine responses to surgery are continued into the postoperative period. Of those investigations carried on after surgery ends, the inhibitory effect of intraoperative opioids on hormone secretion appears to be limited to the operative and immediate postoperative period (Walsh et al 1981). Bent et al (1984) demonstrated that an established hormonal response to pelvic surgery could not be 'turned off' by the addition of opioids after 1 hour. However, an investigation of the influence of pain relief with patient-controlled analgesia (PCA) on changes in circulating catecholamine, cortisol and glucose concentrations following cholecystectomy showed that in addition to reduced pain intensity scores, plasma cortisol values were significantly reduced postoperatively in patients who received PCA with fentanyl compared with those who received morphine subcutaneously on request (Moller et al 1988). These interesting findings require confirmation.

Anaesthetic induction agents

The imidazole drug etomidate suppresses adrenal cortical secretion by inhibition of the mitochondrial, cytochrome P450-dependent, 11β-hydroxylase step of the biosynthetic pathway. Following reports of increased mortality in critically ill patients sedated with etomidate, the drug is no longer licensed for long-term sedation. A single induction dose of etomidate will suppress the cortisol response to surgery and even decrease preoperative cortisol values, but this has not been associated with any adverse effects in healthy patients (Lacoumenta et al 1986). Both diazepam and midazolam may also compete with steroid mixed-function oxidases for cytochrome P450 and have been shown to inhibit cortisol production from isolated bovine adrenocortical cells in vitro. More importantly, midazolam, which has an imidazole ring in addition to its basic benzodiazepine structure, has been shown to reduce the adrenocortical response to peripheral and major upper abdominal surgery (Crozier et al 1987, Desborough et al 1991). However, unlike etomidate, the adrenal cortex responds to exogenous administration of ACTH following midazolam (Crozier et al 1987).

Volatile anaesthetics

The effects of volatile anaesthetics on the endocrine responses to surgery have been extensively studied. Oyama's group have examined the effects of a series of volatile agents used over the past 20 years, from ether to sevoflurane (Oyama et al 1989). In general terms, volatile agents have been shown to be less effective than narcotics in suppressing cortisol and other endocrine responses to surgery (Hall et al 1978). However, few studies compare equipotent doses of anaesthetic agents, and the possibility that the differences in endocrine endocrine responses arise as a result of different depths of anaesthesia cannot be excluded. Flezzani et al (1986) have shown that in patients who received approximately 50 µg/kg fentanyl for cardiac surgery, those who received 1% or 2% isoflurane added from a vaporizer during cardiopulmonary bypass had a decreased cortisol response compared with those who did not receive additional anaesthesia.

It may be difficult to differentiate the effects on the endocrine system of the anaesthetic agents themselves from the additional effects resulting from the surgical stimulus. Carli & Elia (1991) showed that a long period of anaesthesia without surgical stimulation was without effect on circulating concentrations of the metabolites glucose, lactate, glycerol and alanine. Values of glucose and lactate increased significantly only after the start of surgery.

Volatile anaesthetic agents may contribute to the hyperglycaemia of surgery. In vitro studies have demonstrated that halothane and enflurane inhibit glucose-induced insulin secretion directly from isolated rat islets of Langerhans (Ewart et al 1981). Results from a clinical study suggested that isoflurane may impair insulin secretion in response to infused glucose, although the doses of glucose used were excessive and non-physiological, and there was no comparison with a non-volatile anaesthetic technique (Diltoer & Camu 1988).

Local anaesthetic techniques

Epidural and spinal anaesthesia with local analgesics provide excellent pain relief and are extremely effective in preventing the endocrine and metabolic responses to surgery. For operations in the pelvis such as hysterectomy and prostatectomy, or surgery to the lower limbs, extensive regional blockade with local anaesthetic from dermatomal levels T^4 to S^5 will completely prevent the hormonal response (Engquist et al 1977). This extensive block prevents afferent neuronal input to the central nervous system and the hypothalamic–pituitary axis, and also the efferent neuronal pathways to the adrenal medulla, thus inhibiting both the pituitary and catecholamine responses to surgery.

For upper abdominal and thoracic procedures, regional analgesia is less effective in suppressing the endocrine responses to surgery, although studies have shown some inhibition of cortisol and catecholamine concentrations (Rutberg et al 1984). It is likely that the main reason for the lack of effect is incomplete afferent neuronal blockade. Similarly, a wide range of nerve blocks, such as paravertebral and intercostal, provide extrememly good postoperative analgesia but do not always inhibit the hormonal responses to surgery (Hall & Lacoumenta 1988). Where complete neuronal blockade can be readily achieved, for example retrobulbar block for cataract surgery, the cortisol and glycaemic responses to operation can be prevented (Barker et al 1990).

Spinal opioids

Epidural and intrathecal opioids provide excellent intraoperative and post-operative analgesia. However, these techniques have less impact on the endocrine responses than blockade with local anaesthetic agents, although the use of spinal opioids is often associated with a reduction in the glycaemic response to surgery in the postoperative period (Christensen et al 1982). Intraoperatively, the lack of sympathetic blocking properties of the opioids accounts for their inability to prevent the usual hyperglycaemia.

Specific hormonal blockade

Attempts have been made to inhibit the endocrine responses to surgery by a combination of techniques, including specific blockade of individual hormones. The GH response to surgery can be prevented using octreotide, a synthetic octapeptide analogue of somatostatin, but this has no beneficial effects on metabolism in the perioperative period (Desborough et al 1990). Octreotide also inhibits pancreatic endocrine secretion.

Combined regimens

Since individual anaesthetic or analgesic regimens may be associated with suppression of one aspect of the endocrine or acute-phase response to surgery, combinations of drugs have been used in an attempt to provide total analgesia and inhibition of the hormonal responses (Shulze et al 1988). The addition of the cyclo-oxygenase inhibitor, indomethacin, to neural blockade with epidural analgesia, reduced the febrile response to inguinal hernia repair compared with epidural or general anaesthetic alone (Shulze et al 1987).

In a further group of patients having similar surgery, H_1 and H_2 receptor and serotonin$_2$ antagonists indomethacin and tranexamic acid were added to neural blockade with epidural analgesia. The humoral blockade was without significant effect on the rise in temperature, change in leukocyte concentrations, or acute-phase protein measurements (Schulze et al 1988).

Regional blockade with epidural or spinal local anaesthesia is also without effect on circulating concentrations of IL-6 (Moore et al 1992). This would be expected since the cytokine is produced from activated macrophages following tissue injury. The effects of inhibition of the IL-6 response to surgery remain open to speculation, since this may be possible only with the advent of specific antibodies or cytokine receptor blockade.

It is apparent that exhaustive attempts have been made in an endeavour to inhibit endocrine responses to surgery. It is not possible from single, small studies to demonstrate whether this improves patient outcome following surgery. Scott & Kehlet (1988) reviewed a large number of studies in which a range of indices of postoperative morbidity was compared following surgery undertaken with either general or regional anaesthesia. The surgical procedures were of the lower limbs or the pelvic organs such as hip surgery, hysterectomy, prostatectomy or vascular surgery to the legs. Intraoperative blood loss and the incidence of thromboembolic complications were the only factors significantly reduced in patients receiving regional anaesthesia. It is not possible to state categorically that any improved postoperative outcome was caused by a diminution in the endocrine and metabolic responses to surgery, since these were not directly measured.

The majority of studies of this kind are performed on healthy patients, usually starved only overnight, in whom the benefits of inhibition of the endocrine responses to surgery may not be of overwhelming importance. However, a detailed understanding of the mechanisms involved in initiating and maintaining the responses and the techniques which modify them may have wide implications for the management of patients with critical illnesses and sepsis and also for diabetic patients undergoing surgery. In these groups of patients further derangements of metabolism may add to the potentially harmful effects of prolonged catabolic illness.

Very few investigations have addressed the effects of inhibiting the endocrine responses to surgery using regional analgesia in high-risk patients. Yeager et al (1987) studied 53 patients having major non-cardiac vascular surgery. The anaesthetic regimen was chosen by the clinician responsible for the patient. Twenty-eight individuals had intraoperative regional anaesthesia using epidural local anaesthetic which was continued into the postoperative period. The other patients received parenteral opioids. Although this study has been criticized for poor control, the results did suggest that epidural anaesthesia was associated with a reduction in postoperative complications, including major organ system failure such as cardiovascular system failure and chest infections. Consequently, length of hospital stay was reduced in this group of patients. The endocrine response to surgery, as demonstrated by urinary excretion of cortisol, was reduced in the patients who received epidural anaesthesia.

Tuman et al (1991) have investigated the effects of epidural anaesthesia and analgesia in patients with atherosclerotic disease having peripheral vascular reconstructive surgery to the lower limbs. This randomized, prospective study compared the effects of general anaesthesia or a combination of regional anaesthesia and general anaesthesia on coagulation status and postoperative outcome. Coagulability was assessed using thromboelastography. Hypercoagulability may be implicated in cardiovascular complications and thrombosis of peripheral vascular grafts. The authors of this study referred to evidence which suggests that epidural anaesthesia may have direct and indirect effects on coagulation, which reduce hypercoagulability after vascular surgery. The study showed that patients who received epidural and general anaesthesia were less coagulable than those receiving general anaesthesia alone and this was associated with fewer postoperative thrombotic episodes and a shorter stay in intensive care.

A recent review has called into question many aspects of the study of the effects of regional blockade with local anaesthetics on clinical outcome after surgery (Rigg 1991). This paper suggested methods of organizing and performing randomized controlled trials to address this issue. However, although regional anaesthesia may inhibit some of the hormonal and metabolic responses to surgical trauma, it is without effect on other parameters of the acute-phase response. Further work is necessary to elucidate the role of the cytokine response in determining outcome after surgery.

REFERENCES

Anand K J S, Hickey P R 1992 Halothane morphine compared with high-dose sufentanil for anaesthesia and postoperative analgesia in neonatal cardiac surgery. N Engl J Med 326: 1–9
Barker J, Robinson P N, Vafidis G C et al 1990 Local analgesia prevents the cortisol and glycaemic response to cataract surgery. Br J Anaesth 64: 442–445
Bent J M, Paterson J L, Mashiter K et al 1984 Effects of high-dose fentanyl anaesthesia on the established metabolic and endocrine response to surgery. Anaesthesia 39: 19–23
Boomsma F, Rupreht J, Man In 'T Veld, de Jong F H et al 1990 Haemodynamic and neurohumoral effects of xenon anaesthesia. Anaesthesia 45: 273–278
Bovill J G, Sebel P S, Fiolet et al 1983 The influence of sufentanil on endocrine and metabolic responses to cardiac surgery. Anaesth Analg 62: 391–397
Brandt M R, Skousted L, Kehlet H et al 1976 Rapid decrease in plasma triiodothyronine during surgery and epidural analgesia independent of afferent neurogenic stimuli and of cortisol. Lancet ii: 1333–1336
Bythell V E, Lacoumenta S, Breimer L H, Brooks S et al 1989 Effects on epidural anaesthesia on plasma calcitonin gene-related peptide. Acta Anaesthesiol Scand 33: 666–669

Carli F, Elia M 1991 The independent metabolic effects of enflurane anaesthesia and surgery. Acta Anaesthesiol Scand 35: 329–332

Christensen P, Brandt M R, Rem J, Kehlet H 1982 Influence of extradural morphine on the adrenocortical and hyperglycaemic response to surgery. Br J Anaesth 54: 23–27

Chwals W J, Bristrian B R 1991 Role of exogenous growth hormone and insulin-like growth factor I in malnutrition and acute metabolic stress: a hypothesis. Crit Care Med 19: 1317–1322

Crozier T A, Beck D, Schlaeger M et al 1987 Endocrinological changes following etomidate, midazolam or methohexital for minor surgery. Anesthesiology 66: 628–635

Cruickshank A M, Fraser W D, Burns H J G et al 1990 Response of serum interleukin-6 in patients undergoing elective surgery of varying severity. Clin Sci 79: 161–165

Cuthbertson D P 1932 Observations on the disturbance of metabolism produced by injury to the limbs. Q J Med 1: 233

Derbyshire D R, Smith G 1984 Sympathoadrenal responses to anaesthesia and surgery. Br J Anaesth 56: 725–739

Desborough J P, Hall G M, Hart G R et al 1990 Hormonal responses to cardiac surgery: effects of sufentanil, somatostatin and ganglion blockade. Br J Anaesth 64: 688–695

Desborough J P, Hall Gam, Hart G R, Burrin J M 1991 Midazolam modifies pancreatic and anterior pituitary hormone secretion during upper abdominal surgery. Br J Anaesth 67: 390–396

Diltoer M, Camu F 1988 Glucose homeostasis and insulin secretion during isoflurane anaesthesia in humans. Anesthesiology 68: 880–886

Dong Q, Hawker F, McWilliam D et al 1992 Circulating immunoreactive inhibin and testosterone levels in men with critical illness. Clin Endocrinol 36: 399–404

Engquist A, Brandt M R, Fernandes A, Kehlet H 1977 The blocking effect of epidural analgesia on the adreno-cortical and hyperglycaemic responses to surgery. Acta Anaesthesiol Scand 21: 330–335

Ewart R B L, Rusy B F, Bradford M W 1981 Effects of enflurane on release of insulin by pancreatic islets in vitro. Anesth Analg 60: 878–884

Flezzani P, Croughwell N D, McIntyre R W, Reves J G 1986 Isoflurane decreases the cortisol response to cardiopulmonary bypass. Anesth Analg 65: 1117–1122

Frayn K N 1985 Substrate turnover after injury. Br Med Bull 41: 232–239

Giesecke K, Hamberger B, Jarnberg P O et al 1988 High and low dose fentanyl anaesthesia: hormonal and metabolic responses during cholecystectomy. Br J Anaesth 61: 575–582

Hall G M, Lacoumenta S 1988 Local analgesic techniques for upper abdominal surgery — endocrine and metabolic effects. Br J Anaesth 61: 649–651

Hall G M, Young C, Holdcroft A et al 1978 Substrate mobilisation during surgery. A comparison between halothane and fentanyl anaesthesia. Anaesthesia 33: 924–930

Hall G M, Walsh E S, Paterson J L, Mashiter K 1983 Low-dose insulin infusion and substrate mobilisation during surgery. Br J Anaesth 55: 939–945

Hume D M, Egdahl R H 1959 The importance of the brain in the endocrine response to injury. Ann Surg 150: 697–712

Imura H, Fukata J I, Mori T 1991 Cytokines and endocrine function: an interaction between the immune and neuroendocrine systems. Clin Endocrinol 35: 107–115

Joris J, Cigarini I, Legrand M et al 1992 Metabolic and respiratory changes following cholecystectomy: laparotomy versus laparoscopy. Br J Anaesth 69: 341–345

Kehlet H 1989 Surgical stress: the role of pain and analgesia. Br J Anaesth 63: 189–195

Kho H G, van Egmond J, Zhwang C F et al 1990 The patterns of stress response in patients undergoing thyroid surgery under acupuncture in China. Acta Anaesthesiol Scand 34: 563–571

Klingstedt C, Giesecke K, Hamberger B et al 1987 High and low dose fentanyl anaesthesia circulatory and plasma catecholamine responses during cholecystectomy. Br J Anaesth 59: 184–188

Kono K, Philbin D M, Coggins C H 1981 Renal function and stress response during halothane or fentanyl anaesthesia. Anesth Analg 60: 552–556

Lacoumenta S, Paterson J, Myers M A, Hall G M 1986 Effects of cortisol suppression by etomidate on changes in circulating metabolites associated with pelvic surgery. Acta Anaesthesiol Scand 30: 101–104

McDonald R K, Evans F T, Weise V K et al 1959 Effect of morphine and nalorphine on plasma hydrocortisone levels in man. J Pharmacol Exp Ther 125: 241–247

Moller I W, Dinesen K, Sondergard S et al 1988 Effect of patient-controlled analgesia onplasma catecholamine, cortisol and glucose concentrations after cholecystectomy. Br J Anaesth 61: 160–164

Moore C, Desborough J, Burrin J, Hall G M 1992 IL-6 and the pituitary hormone response to surgery. J Endocrinol 132S: 207

Oyama T, Murakawa T, Matsuki A 1989 Endocrine evaluation of sevoflurane, a new inhalation anaesthetic agent. Acta Anaesthesiol Belg 40: 269–274

Parry-Billings M, Evans J, Calder P C, Newsholme E A 1990 Does glutamine contribute to immunosuppression after major burns? Lancet 336: 523–525

Philbin D M 1989 Antidiuretic hormone and surgery. Clin Anaesthesiol 3: 395–404

Rigg J R A 1991 Does regional block improve outcome after surgery? Anaesth Intensive Care 19: 404–411

Ross R J M, Miell J P, Buchanan C R 1991 Avoiding autocannabalism. Br Med J 303: 1147–1148

Rutberg H, Hakanson E, Anderberg L et al 1984 Effects of the extradural administration of morphine, or bupivacaine, on the endocrine response to upper abdominal surgery. Br J Anaesth 56: 233–238

Schulze S, Schierbeck J, Sparso B et al 1987 Influence of neural blockade and indomethacin on leucocyte, temperature and acute phase protein response to surgery. Acta Chir Scand 153: 255–259

Schulze S, Drenck N, Hjortso E, Kehlet H 1988 Influence of combined neural blockade, H_1 and H_2 receptor and serotonin$_2$ receptor blockade, indomethacin and tranexamic acid on leucocyte, temperature and acute-phase protein response to surgery. Acta Chir Scand 154: 329–333

Scott N B, Kehlet H 1988 Regional anaesthesia and surgical morbidity. Br J Surg 75: 299–304

Spangelo B L, Judd A M, Isakson P C, MacLeod R M 1989 Interleukin-6 stimulates anterior pituitary hormone release in vitro. Endocrinology 125: 575–577

Stehle P, Mertes N, Puchstein C et al 1989 Effect of parenteral glutamine peptide supplements on muscle glutamine loss and nitrogen balance after major surgery. Lancet i: 231–233

Thompson D, Milford-Ward A, Whicher J T 1992 The value of acute phase protein measurements in clinical practice. Ann Clin Biochem 29: 123–131

Tuman K J, McCarthy R J, March R J et al 1991 Effects of epidural anaesthesia and analgesia on coagulation and outcome after major vascular surgery. Anaesth Analg 73: 696–704

Vankelecom H, Carmeliet P, Van Damme J et al 1989 Production of interleukin-6 by folliculostellate cells of the anterior pituitary gland in a histiotypic cell aggregate culture system. Neuroendocrinology 49: 102–106

Veterans Affairs Total Parenteral Nutrition Cooperative Study Group 1991 Perioperative total parenteral nutrition in surgical patients. N Engl J Med 325: 525–532

Walsh E S, Paterson J L, O'Riordan J B et al 1981 Effect of high-dose fentanyl anaesthesia on the metabolic and endocrine response to cardiac surgery. Br J Anaesth 53: 21155–21164

Wang C, Chan V, Yeung R T 1978 Effects of surgical stress on pituitary testicular function. Clin Endocrinol 9: 255–266

Weissman C 1990 The metabolic response to stress: an overview and update. Anesthesiology 73: 308–327

Woolf P D, Hamill R W, McDonald J V et al 1985 Transient hypogonadotrophic hypogonadism caused by critical illness. J Clin Endocrinol Metab 60: 444–450

Yeager M P, Glass D D, Neff R K et al 1987 Epidural anaesthesia and analgesia in high-risk surgical patients. Anesthesiology 66: 729–736

Ziegler M G, Morrissey E C, Marshall L F 1990 Catecholamine and thyroid hormones in traumatic injury. Crit Care Med 18: 253–258

9. The management of burns

N. Parkhouse

Severe burn injury remains a major clinical problem despite a steady reduction in the incidence over the last few decades as result of active prevention and improved safety standards (Elberg et al 1987). The management of major burns necessarily involves collaboration between the burn surgeon and anaesthetist, ideally in the environment of a designated burns unit staffed by specially trained nurses and therapists. A large proportion of a contemporary burn practice in the UK is paediatric, children under the age of 5 accounting for 86% of the admissions to the Regional Burns Unit at Mount Vernon Hospital, Northwood in 1991, and paediatric input is therefore essential.

Improvements in an understanding of the pathophysiology and advances in the surgical management have resulted in some refinement of the management but the morbidity and mortality of a major burn injury have not changed substantially in most units since the introduction of fluid resuscitation therapy in the 1940s. Greater appreciation of the pathophysiology of the inhalational injury to the lung which accompanies many burns and a more interventional approach to its management have contributed to improved survival rates. There are wide variations in the choice of resuscitation fluid and the formula for fluid replacement in the early burn shock phase. Similarly there are variations in the methods of wound dressing and management. There is wide agreement as to the importance of supplementary nutrition in the early hypermetabolic phase of the burn injury which may be achieved in a variety of ways. These clinical aspects are well-summarized in comprehensive texts (Muir et al 1987) and in recent reviews (Deitch 1990).

There is a body of research into the pathophysiological response to burn injury in animal models and in human patients. The animal models allow standardization of the burn injury and generation of larger numbers for comparative studies but may be extrapolated to the human clinical situation only with caution. Human research into burn pathophysiology is dogged by multiple variables and difficulty in standardizing observation or experimental groups. While the volume of literature grows about a number of changes accompanying the burn injury, its impact on the clinical therapeutic management of the burned patient is yet to be fully realized. This reflects the complexity of the neurohumoral response to burn injury and its multiple effects on metabolism, immunity and organ function.

PATHOPHYSIOLOGY

Local changes

Tissue damage due to thermal injury is the result of direct heat damage and the secondary damage arising from inflammation. The severity of the direct damage reflects the temperature, mode of burn (scald, flash, flame, contact, electrical) and duration of exposure. The thermal damage extends from superficial to deep and the skin injury is classified according to depth into superficial partial-thickness damage, deep partial-thickness damage and full-thickness loss. Electrical injury has a different mechanism to pure thermal injury and causes both superficial and deep damage in the line of the path of least resistance taken by the current between the entry and exit wounds. This causes characteristic circumscribed full-thickness skin burns and necrosis of muscle and nerve due to Joule heating and electroporation. In the past routine electrocardiogram monitoring has been advised following electrical injury but in a recent analysis of 125 electrical burns, there were no cardiac complications (Haberal et al 1989).

Three zones of injury have been described (Jackson 1953): the zone of coagulation in which tissues are irreversibly coagulated; the zone of stasis, in which there is intense vasoconstriction adjacent to the coagulative necrosis, and the zone hyperaemia in which there is acute inflammatory vasodilatation. The hyperaemia is accompanied by an increase in capillary permeability which gives rise to local oedema. Hyperaemia is also characteristically visible surrounding the burn as an erythematous flare which may on occasion confuse assessment of the area of burn and may give rise to overestimation of the requirements for fluid therapy (Laing et al 1991).

The role of inflammatory mediators

In the stasis zone there is intense local vasoconstriction which may contribute to dermal ischaemia and a progressive necrosis which deepens the level of injury. Recent evidence has shown that burn blister fluid contains elevated levels of endothelin (Neild & Parkhouse 1992) and it is suggested that this potent vasoconstrictor may be released in response to endothelial trauma and may itself be responsible for the intense local vasoconstriction. An excess of endothelin in the circulation may also contribute to the increase in systemic vascular resistance and vasoconstriction of the splanchnic and renal circulations.

The vasodilatation and increased vascular permeability are presumed to have a neurogenic and a non-neurogenic component in common with any cutaneous response to injury. The initial phase is dependent on histamine and substance P while subsequent development and maintenance of inflammation are associated with a number of vasoactive amines including serotonin and bradykinin, prostaglandins and leukotrienes. Clinical pharmacological inhibition of these inflammatory mediators has been largely unsuccessful in modifying capillary permeability as judged by the formation of oedema. It seems likely that other factors contribute to the increased permeability such as direct endothelial cell damage, possibly mediated by xanthine oxidase or nitric oxide.

There is increasing evidence for lipid peroxidation in burned patients (Wooliscroft et al 1990) and this is presumed to occur in the injured tissue or in the stasis zone (Jackson 1953), where oxygen free radicals are generated (Kaufman et al 1989). Lipid peroxidation in burned patients may be prevented by superoxide dismutase (SOD — 500–1000 u/kg polyethylene glycol conjugated SOD) with a significant reduction in the plasma levels of conjugated dienes compared with untreated controls but the clinical relevance is uncertain since the levels of these lipid peroxidation products have not been shown to correlate with the burn mortality probability (Thomson et al 1990).

Evidence for the existence of a specific cutaneous burn toxin (CBT) has been generated steadily by its proponents since it was first isolated in 1959 as a dialysable toxin which was lethal to rodents (Sparkes et al 1990a). Sparkes et al used an enzyme-linked immunosorbent assay based on a sheep antihuman CBT immunoglobulin G (IgG) to show that CBT alters independently from lipid peroxide levels in plasma. Proposed effects include cardiotoxicity, hepatotoxicity and immunosuppression (Sparkes et al 1990b) but there is no widespread agreement as to its role and character, although its immunological specificity must raise the possibility of the therapeutic use of anti-CBT monoclonal antibody.

The endocrine response to burning includes the release of catecholamines and cortisol which are together responsible for the increased metabolic rate with accelerated nitrogen turnover and negative nitrogen balance, and hyperglycaemia with hyperinsulinaemia and insulin resistance. The reduction in plasma volume due to increased vascular permeability causes further release of catecholamines, vasopressin, aldosterone and activation of the renin angiotensin system. This results in decreased renal blood flow, vasoconstriction and sodium retention. It is possible that atrial natriuretic polypeptide plays a counter-regulatory part in this response, as shown by Wakabayashi (1990) in the rat.

RESUSCITATION

Despite the increase in understanding of the pathophysiology of burn injury and its systemic effects, there is currently no clinical useful pharmacological inhibitor of either the local or systemic response to the burn injury. The early clinical management is therefore concerned with resuscitation to treat the effects of the fluid shifts causing shock and to avoid the complications of secondary organ failure. Specifically, fluid therapy is directed at maintaining systemic blood pressure to preserve cerebral and renal blood flow and ventilatory support is used to treat the effects of inhalational injury or secondary respiratory distress. Table 9.1 summarizes the essential elements of the initial care of a burned patient. Miller et al (1992) describe a sophisticated algorithmic approach to the fluid resuscitation of cutaneous burns and Langford & Armstrong (1990) describe an algorithm for the management of smoke inhalation.

Fluid therapy

The initial consequence of a severe thermal injury is loss of fluid from the plasma into the extracellular space at the site of the burn. The electrolyte content of the exudate is the same as that of plasma and the protein content is a little less, being in the region of 80% initially and falling to 50%. The fall in plasma volume causes a compensatory sympathetic splanchnic vasocon-striction which contributes to the maintenance of a normal blood pressure. The rate of loss of fluid has been shown to increase with size of the area burned, which is conventionally expressed as a percentage of the body surface area. In larger burns, the splanchnic vasoconstriction results in renal and intestinal ischaemia and fails to prevent the hypotension. Formal fluid resuscitation is generally administered to adults with a burn of more than 15% body surface area and to children with greater than 10% burns. With burn areas less than this, absorption of an increased oral fluid intake is usually enough to compensate for the loss in plasma volume.

There are wide international variations in the fluid used for resuscitation and the way in which infusion is planned. Colloid-based regimes are widely used in the UK while crystalloid-based regimes are more common in continental Europe and in the USA. The volume of isotonic crystalloid solution is large compared to the corresponding volume of colloid required for resuscitation of an equivalent burn and crystalloid is reported to accentuate

Table 9.1 Initial assessment and treatment of a patient with major burns

---

Assessment
Examine for signs of inhalational injury
Assess cardiovascular status
Assess area of burn (use chart)
Assess depth of burn and need for escharotomies
Examine for other injuries

Treatment
Humidified oxygen 40% and intubation if indicated
Opioid analgesia
Begin fluid resuscitation according to the Mount Vernon formula (area of burn × weight in
    kg)/2-ml human plasma protein fraction to be given in the first 4 hours after injury
Insert nasogastric tube and commence enteral feeding (half strength)
Insert silicone Foley catheter to monitor urine output

---

the tissue oedema. Hypertonic saline may have advantages in lessening the oedema, possibly limiting burn-induced tissue injury.

The theoretical and practical advantages of resuscitation by transfusion of plasma are clearly set out by Muir et al (1987) and, although reconstituted human plasma protein fraction is now generally substituted for whole plasma, it remains the most consistent with our concept of burn shock as an oligaemic shock due to reduced plasma volume. Alternative colloid resuscitation fluids include the gelatins (Haemaccel, Gelofusine), dextrans (Dextran 40, 70 and 110) and starches (Hespan, Pentaspan). Haemaccel may interfere with the immune response by decreasing opsonin levels and with wound healing by lowering fibronectin levels. It has a considerable osmotic diuretic effect which may mask renal hypoperfusion. Anaphylaxis to the dextrans is commonly reported but this may be pre-empted by pretreatment with a hapten (Promit). Hespan 6% is very similar to 4.5% human albumin solution and could prove to be a cheap and efficacious alternative to plasma with an intravascular half-life of 18–30 hours. Pentaspan has a shorter plasma half-life but may have a specific action in reducing vascular permeability. It seems likely that the starches may have a useful role in the future.

Formulae have been devised for calculating the infusion volumes to help replace the loss as it occurs. The rate of loss of fluid is maximal in the first few hours postinjury and then declines over the next 24–48 hours. The infusion requirements are therefore greatest in the first few hours after the injury. The Mount Vernon formula has been in widespread use since first published in 1962 (see Muir et al 1987). The first 36-hour 'shock' phase may be usefully divided into six periods of increasing length, during each of which the fluid requirements are approximately the same. The volume required for the first 4 hours is (total percentage of burn × weight in kg)/2 = ml of fluid required. It should be emphasized that the first 4-hour shock period begins at the time of the injury. The progress of resuscitation is monitored and the volume requirements for the subsequent periods adjusted accordingly.

The first 4-hour period is followed by two more 4-hour periods, two 6-hour periods and a final 12-hour period during which the volume requirements are expected to be the same although in practice this is seldom the case. One reason for this is the current use of plasma protein fraction rather than dried whole plasma as used in the original studies. This has been suggested to increase the volume requirements by approximately 30% (Watson et al 1977). Murison et al (1991) compared the effectiveness of resuscitation using the two different formulae prospectively and showed no difference in morbidity or mortality between the two groups but found excessive urine output when the modified formula was used, suggesting overinfusion. There are no equivalent published data regarding the use of alternative plasma substitutes. A further reason for discrepancy between calculated and actual volumes is the presence of inhalational burn injury together with cutaneous burns. Hughes et al (1989) showed that normalization of physiological parameters using contemporary invasive monitoring techniques resulted in increased volume requirements of

75% for the first 24 hours and 110% for the second 24 hours respectively above the values predicted by the Mount Vernon formula.

The Odstock formula for calculating fluid requirements in the first 36 hours is based only on the blood volume calculated from the body weight of the patient; an amount of plasma equivalent to one blood volume is given regardless of the size of the burn (Griffiths & Laing 1981). One-third of the calculated volume is given in the first 8 hours, the second third over the next 12 hours and the remaining third over the subsequent 16 hours. This may result in overtransfusion of smaller burns and potential undertransfusion of larger burns compared to the Mount Vernon formula and readjustment in response to close clinical monitoring is recommended.

The calculations of plasma requirements based on burn area and body weight do not include the basal metabolic fluid requirements. These are provided either by oral water (60 ml hourly for an adult initially increasing to 100 ml/hour) or as an additional infusion of 5% dextrose. The oral route is preferred when it is not precluded by nausea and vomiting. Hourly gastric aspiration has been recommended in burns over 35% total area but interpretation of hourly aspirate volumes should take into account the volume of salivary and gastric secretions; aspiration of volumes approaching those given does not indicate a failure to absorb as absorption does not in any case occur in the stomach. It may indicate a relative impairment of gastric emptying but the aspiration of even equal volumes to those given implies that a proportion is passing into the duodenum and should not therefore be a sole indication to stop oral fluids or feeding (see section on nutrition below).

Resuscitation using isotonic crystalloid solutions requires much larger volumes and results in excessive enlargement of the extracellular space. The volume required in the first 24 hours is given by the Parkland formula as 4 ml/kg/% of total body surface area (TBSA) burned. Half of the total requirement is given over the first 8 hours and the remaining half over the next 16 hours. Crystalloid can be given according to the Mount Vernon scheme, in which case the volume for the first 4-hour period is given by weight in kg × percentage area, i.e. twice as much crystalloid as plasma. The massive oedema has led to the suggestion that hypertonic lactated saline (250 mmol of sodium per litre) should be used in an attempt to reduce osmotically the degree of fluid shift (Monafo et al 1973) and this was shown to reduce the oedema in the burned tissue. More recently Boeckx et al (1990) have shown that early administration of a high sodium load results in a considerable reduction in the overall volumes required to maintain renal perfusion and diminished oedema. In contrast, Gunn et al (1989) failed to show the expected benefits of hypertonic resuscitation in a prospective trial against isotonic lactated Ringer's solution. Horton et al (1990) showed that a combination of hypertonic saline and 6% Dextran 70 improved myocardial contractility. The concept of using a hypertonic load to reduce the degree of early fluid shift differs from that of replacement and deserves a critical clinical evaluation.

There is as yet no therapeutic manoeuvre to reverse the increase in vascular permeability which causes the loss of fluid from the circulation. Recent experimental research into the effects of large doses of vitamin C in a guinea pig burn model has shown a reduction in the water content of the burned skin, suggesting a reduction in the degree of increased capillary permeability; the volume of fluid required for resuscitation in the first 24 hours was correspondingly reduced (Matsuda et al 1992). The mechanism of this effect is not clear but may be related to the antioxidant effect of ascorbic acid. Further effects included maintenance of normal metabolism through an inhibitory effect on the production or release of cortisol and maintenance of normal body weight (Nelson et al 1992).

Inhalational injury

The presence of an inhalational component to a burn injury substantially increases the mortality rate over that expected from the extent of the cutaneous burn alone. An inhalational burn may be suspected when there is a smell of smoke, soot staining of the face, nares and oropharynx, and mucosal oedema. Fibreoptic bronchoscopy is valuable in confirming the diagnosis and for therapeutic suction and lavage under indirect vision. Treatment includes oxygen administration by mask, endotracheal intubation and mechanical ventilation with positive end expiratory pressure. The principles are well set out as an algorithm by Langford & Armstrong (1990). Hyperbaric oxygen may have a place in the treatment of severe carbon monoxide poisoning but transfer may jeopardize treatment of associated burn injury. Carboxyhaemoglobin measurement on admission may be a useful clinical diagnostic test with levels over 15% suggesting significant smoke inhalation.

Inhalation of fumes from certain plastics may cause cyanide poisoning which produces a cellular hypoxia due to reversible binding with mitochondrial enzymes. Blood cyanide concentration measurement is generally unhelpful in the acute situation but cyanide poisoning should be suspected when signs of hypoxia occur in conjunction with parameters, suggesting diminished oxygen consumption, i.e. normal arterial oxygen saturation, increased mixed venous oxygen saturation, decreased arteriovenous difference in oxygen content, metabolic acidosis, raised lactate and increased anion gap. Specific cyanide antidotes may be indicated when these features are present and cyanide poisoning is suspected. These fall into three groups: agents which convert haemoglobin to methaemoglobin (amyl nitrite, sodium nitrite 4-dimethylaminophenol), agents which facilitate endogenous metabolism of cyanide (sodium thiosulphate) and cyanide chelating agents (dicolbalt edetate). When amyl nitrite is used care should be taken to ensure that the oxygen-carrying capacity of the blood is not excessively reduced and that the sum of the percentages of methaemoglobin and carboxyhaemoglobin do not exceed 40%.The details of the management of cyanide poisoning are given in the algorithm of Langford & Armstrong.

Toxic shock syndrome

Toxic shock syndrome (TSS) has been recognized in recent times as a cause of life-threatening circulatory collapse complicating the early course of burns in children. The cause of the shock appears to be an enterotoxin produced by staphylococci. Eight different toxins may be produced including TSS toxin-1 (TSST-1) which is associated with the majority of menstrual cases of toxic shock. Cole & Shakespeare (1990) reported the staphylococcal phage types and toxins in 5 cases of probable TSS in burned patients and they emphasize the difficulty in diagnosis which can only be confirmed retrospectively. They propose a simplified set of criteria for the diagnosis of TSS in burned children in order to enable the initiation of treatment as early as possible. The criteria are:

1. Fever >39°C.
2. Rash.
3. Shock.
4. Diarrhoea and vomiting.
5. Irritability.
6. Lymphopenia.

They emphasize that there need not be active infection of the burn wound for toxin production and absorption to occur.

As a result of a current increase in awareness of the complication, possible TSS may be overdiagnosed at the present time. As the clinical course is characteristically precipitous, treatment is given as soon as the condition is suspected, consisting of transfusion of fresh frozen plasma and packed red cells. Antibiotics are given to decrease wound surface staphylococcal colony counts to prevent further toxin production. The polyvalent immunoglobulin in fresh frozen plasma and Sandoglobulin are presumed to neutralize toxin already in the circulation although prophylactic intravenous immunoglobulin does not alter the incidence of infection or the mortality rate in patients without the signs of TSS (Waymack et al 1989). Frame et al (1990) have identified a specific reduction in the IgG_2 subclass which responds to the administration of Sandoglobulin. It is possible that the recent apparent increase in incidence of TSS in burned children reflects the absence of gammaglobulin in the plasma fractions currently used for resuscitation.

WOUND MANAGEMENT AND SEPSIS

A detailed review of burn wound management is outside the scope of this chapter but the principles are detailed in Muir et al (1987) and more recent developments in Deitch (1990). The main aim of treatment is to prevent infection so as to allow superficial burns to heal and to prepare deeper burns for surgery.

The burn wound is sterile immediately after injury but despite aseptic precautions at the time of initial dressing and protective and source isolation in the environment of a burn unit, colonization of the wound commonly occurs within a few days of injury. It has been estimated that approximately 25% of patients with severe burns develop invasive infection after colonization of the wound with *Staphylococcus aureus*, coliforms and *Pseudomonas aeruginosa*. Topical antibacterial therapy of the burn wound has evolved in attempts to prevent or to slow colonization. Topical silver sulphadiazine cream is widely used in burn dressings and is particularly effective against coliforms. Silver sulphadiazine in combination with cerium nitrate has an improved antibacterial effect and transforms the burn into a leathery crust which remains dry and sterile.

General use of systemic antibiotics does not prevent colonization and selects for a more resistant bacterial flora. Flucloxacillin has been recommended for all burned children on admission in an attempt to prevent toxic shock (Frame et al 1990), though it remains of unproven benefit. Bacteraemia has been shown to occur at the time of burn wound manipulation (Sasaki et al 1979) and may cause septicaemia (Demling 1983) and it is rational to exhibit a short course of systemic antibiotics effective against the prevalent colonizing organisms at times of dressing change, debridement and skin grafting. The use of such prophylactic antibiotics to prevent invasive wound infection and septicaemia as a result of manipulation of the wound has never been studied in a prospective clinical trial. Zeigler et al (1988) identified an association between reduced intestinal permeability and systemic infection in burned patients and suggested that the effects of systemic infection may be compounded by absorption of bacteria or endotoxin from the gut. In order to pre-empt this, selective decontamination of the gut has been employed. Manson et al (1992) reported a retrospective study of 91 patients all treated with oral polymyxin and some additionally with co-trimoxazole and amphotericin B. The combination therapy decreased the incidence of wound infection with Enterobacteriaceae, eliminated *Proteus* species and diminished yeast colonization. Most importantly, no resistant strains were isolated and it was proposed that selective decontamination of the gut is an effective way of preventing wound colonization.

The timing of surgery depends on the depth of the injury. Clear-cut full-thickness burns may be excised on the day of injury if small and as soon as the state of resuscitation permits when large. Early excision of the damaged tissue removes the source of a number of toxic metabolites and the cutaneous burn toxin. There is no contraindication to the immediate excision of large areas of full-thickness burn and in certain cases it may be life-saving, as in the case of limb amputation in severe electrical burns (Haberal et al 1989).

When large areas are excised, skin cover may be achieved with mesh expansion of autograft. In very large burns alternative skin cover may be required. Fresh or banked cadaver allografts have been used to achieve temporary wound cover in patients with limited donor sites. Tissue culture techniques have been used to produce autologous or allogeneic epithelial grafts with cultured keratinocytes. The drawback is the lack of dermis and cultured keratinocytes alone have a limited place in practical therapy of the burn wound at present. In combination with allograft or synthetic dermal substitutes currently being developed, they appear likely to have a considerable place in the future.

NUTRITION

The hypercatabolic response to burn injury is responsible for the state of debility in which healing is retarded and immunity is compromised, exposing the patient to the risk of overwhelming sepsis. The negative nitrogen balance that follows all trauma is seen in its severest form following burn injury and commonly results in weight loss due mainly to loss of muscle mass. This may be superimposed on the requirements of growth in children; Childs et al (1990) found a maximum weight loss of 6–13% of the admission weight which was not regained at the time of discharge. Furthermore, children remained at a lower position on the weight percentiles up to 7 months following the burn. In the elderly, there may be pre-existing malnutrition and in the obese, selective protein and vitamin deficiency. Recognition of the impact of the hypercatabolic state on wound healing has led to attempts to minimize the response experimentally and clinically. Most recently, Breitenstein et al (1990) studied the effects of propranolol on the resting metabolic rate (RMR) in fasting burned patients. They demonstrated significant lowering of the RMR using either an intravenous infusion or oral propranolol but this was due solely to a decrease in lipid oxidation and not protein or carbohydrate oxidation. In a well-controlled study of the effects of human biosynthetic growth hormone (somatotropin) on the catabolic response, Belcher et al (1989) showed no improvement in nitrogen retention but a significant increase in insulin resistance. Breitenstein et al (1990) investigated the effect of beta-blockade on the resting metabolic rate using indirect calorimetry. The small reduction which they demonstrated was due to reduced lipid oxidation only, the propranolol having no effect on the metabolism of carbohydrate or protein. Large doses of vitamin C may normalize the hypermetabolic response in animals, possibly through an inhibitory effect on cortisol production or release. Currently no specific therapy has been shown to have a significant effect in reducing the hypermetabolism in humans and clinical efforts are directed toward adequate nutritional support to make good the losses.

The case for a coordinated team approach in the nutrition of the burned patient is well made by Henley (1989). Assessment of protein loss is generally by weight or body mass index (weight in kg divided by the square of the height) and although sequential weighing of adults with large burns may be difficult, an accurate measure may be regularly obtained. Serum protein measurements are routinely available and twice-weekly 24-hour urinalysis provides an indication of renal nitrogen loss, to which may be added 0.2 g for each per cent burn in the first 10 days postburn.

Replacement is with a high calorie to nitrogen ratio of between 120 : 1 and 150 : 1, with energy requirements met by equal provision of carbohydrate and lipid. Many formulae for determining energy requirements have been devised and Henley (1989) recommends a method in which the basal metabolic rate is calculated based on age weight and sex, and adjustments made for the extent of the burn, degree of activity and pre-existing abnormality, as described by Elia (1982). Similarly, the increased protein requirements are calculated to cater for the degree of hypermetabolism.

Administration may be through normal diet, oral supplementation, tubed enteral nutrition or parenteral nutrition. Saito et al (1987) drew attention to the effect of the route of nutrient administration on gut mucosal integrity after burn injury. Comparing immediate enteral feeding with parenteral feeding in a guinea pig model they showed that immediate postburn enteral nutrition was associated with maintenance of gut mucosal integrity while parenteral feeding was associated with gut mucosal atrophy. Luminal nutrients could have an effect on the maintenance of the integrity of the gut through their direct utilization by absorptive cells and by stimulating the systemic release of trophic hormones such as gastrin, cholecystokinin and secretin. It was suggested that preservation of mucosal integrity inhibited the passage of intestinal endotoxin and bacteria into the systemic circulation. Zeigler et al (1988) showed that reduced intestinal permeability in burned patients was associated with infection by measuring the absorption of lactulose which is normally efficiently excluded by the intestinal mucosa. Lactulose absorption was found to be increased threefold in burned patients with infections compared with non-infected burn patients but it was not clear from this study whether the increased permeability was the cause of infection or whether infection caused disruption of the gut barrier. Zeigler et al suggest that there may be an amplification loop whereby the effects of distant infection are compounded by the absorption of bacteria or endotoxin from the gut and they emphasize the importance of early enteral feeding in the maintenance and repair of the mucosal barrier.

Nasogastric fine-bore tube feeding is instituted as early as possible during the resuscitation phase using iso-osmolar feed. A low infusion rate is used initially and is then increased slowly to avoid diarrhoea. Under certain circumstances enteral feeding cannot be instituted or sustained, usually due to ileus. Parenteral feeding may then become necessary to avoid cachexia but enteral feeding should be resumed at the earliest opportunity.

ANALGESIA

The principles and special considerations for pain relief in burns are reviewed in detail by Kinsella & Booth (1991).

Opioid analgesics remain the mainstay of treatment in the acute management of major burns. During the shock-resuscitation phase, intravenous boluses are given rather than intramuscular or subcutaneous injections because of reduced blood flow and oedema which delay absorption. In severe burns, intravenous opioids may continue to be administered by intravenous bolus doses or by continuous infusion. Patient-controlled analgesia (PCA) is frequently appropriate and has been shown to be safe and suitable for children (Gaukroger et al 1991). On occasion, patients with extensive full-thickness burns have little pain because of the deep destruction of the nerve endings, in which case opioid analgesia should be used judiciously, especially during the palliative care of a non-survivable injury.

In the recovery phase the requirement for opioids may continue for some weeks depending on the severity of the burns and the need for dressing changes and physiotherapy. During this period, the severity of pain in the individual case reflects not only the depth and area of the burn but also the psychological response to the injury and fear of disfigurement and loss of livelihood. In most cases it is possible to reduce the dosage of opioids satisfactorily, increasing it as necessary prior to painful interventions. Enterally administered morphine sulphate has proved very useful and is replaced by buprenorphine or dihydrocodeine as requirements decrease.

Repeated major dressing changes may be performed using nitrous oxide in the form of Entonox in conjunction with the opioid analgesia, or using ketamine. Ketamine can be safely used repeatedly and can be given by either the intravenous or intramuscular route. This is particularly useful in children who may be less able to manage the Entonox. General anaesthesia is reserved for surgical procedures which generally involve debridement of burned tissue and skin grafting. Small areas of skin graft may be taken under local anaesthetic in the form of a subcutaneous field block or using topical eutectic mixture of local anaesthetics (EMLA), though this has a significant failure rate.

PHARMACODYNAMIC CHANGES

The pharmacokinetic parameters of many drugs may be influenced by the circulatory and metabolic changes which occur in response to burning and by secondary renal and hepatic dysfunction. As a result of this spectrum of interlinked changes, absorption, distribution, metabolism and elimination may all be variably increased or decreased at the different phases of the acute response and recovery. Certain generalizations may be made. Immediately after injury effective tissue perfusion is reduced and the rate of distribution and elimination of intravenous drugs is reduced. Splanchnic ischaemia lowers the concentration gradient across the gut which may reduce oral absorption, although changes in gastric acidity may accelerate dissolution of tablets. Drugs which are administered at the time of loss of fluid from plasma are distributed in the abnormally increased extracellular space from which they may be reabsorbed into the plasma as oedema resolves. The increased blood flow in the hypermetabolic phase results in a quicker onset of action of intravenous drugs and a shorter half-life because of increased elimination so that higher doses may be required. Oral drugs will be absorbed more rapidly because of the increased concentration gradient. Renal blood flow and glomerular filtration may be reduced in the acute phase of injury though this effect may be countered by effective resuscitation and both may become increased in the hypermetabolic phase.

Albumin is lost from the plasma during the shock phase and may reach low levels as a result of the catabolic phase. This reduces the protein binding of acidic and neutral drugs and increases their volume of distribution. Conversely, increased alpha$_1$ acid glycoprotein increases the protein binding of basic drugs.

Phase I hepatic metabolism is significantly depressed as a result of decreased enzyme activity and drugs principally metabolized by the liver have a prolonged half-life and may reach toxic levels when the usual therapeutic doses are used. Such drugs include lignocaine and pethidine. In contrast, phase II conjugation reactions are unimpaired so that the hepatic glucuronidation of drugs such as lorazepam and morphine are not altered by burn injury.

The implications of this pharmacodynamic flux are well-summarized by Bonate (1990) who draws attention to the difficulties in pharmacokinetic research in burned patients because of the heterogeneity of burned patients and the polypharmacy required for their treatment. He emphasizes the importance of therapeutic monitoring for adjusting drug dosage to suit the pharmacodynamics of the individual patient.

REFERENCES

Belcher H J C R, Mercer D, Judkins K C et al 1989 Biosynthetic human growth hormone in burned patients: a pilot study. Burns 15: 99–107

Boeckx W D, van Canneyt S, de Ridder D 1990 Practical guidelines for burnshock fluid therapy in the first 24 hours postburn. In: Boeckz W, Moserová J (eds) Progress in burn-injury treatment. Academic Publishing, Leuven

Bonate P L 1990 Pathophysiology and pharmacokinetics following burn injury. Clin Pharmacokinet 18: 118–130

Breitenstein E, Chiolero R L, Jequier E et al 1990 Effects of beta blockade on energy metabolism following burns. Burns 16: 259–264

Childs C, Hall T, Davenport P J et al 1990 Dietary intake and changes in body weight in burned children. Burns 16: 418–422

Cole R P, Shakespeare P G 1990 Toxic shock syndrome in scalded children. Burns 16: 221–224

Deitch E A 1990 The management of burns. N Engl J Med 323: 1249–1253

Demling R H 1983 Improved survival after massive burns. J Trauma 28: 179–184

Elberg J J, Schroder H A, Glent-Madsen L et al 1987 Burns: epidemiology and the effect of a prevention programme. Burns 13: 391–393

Elia M 1982 Effect of nitrogen and energy intake on the metabolism of normal, depleted and injured man. Clin Nutr 1: 173

Frame J D, Everitt A S, Gordon P W N, Hackett M E 1990 IgG subclass response to gamma globulin administration in burned children. Burns 16: 437–440

Gaukroger P B, Chapman M J, Davey R B 1991 Pain control in paediatric burns — the use of patient-controlled analgesia. Burns 17: 396–399

Griffiths R W, Laing J E 1981 A burn formula in clinical practice. Ann R Coll Surg Engl 63: 50–53

Gunn M L, Hansborough J F, Davis J W et al 1989 Prospective randomised trial of hypertonic sodium lactate versus lactated Ringers solution for burn shock resuscitation. J Trauma 29: 1261–1267

Haberal M, Oner Z, Gulay H et al 1989 Severe electrical injury. Burns 15: 60–63

Henley M 1989 Feed that burn. Burns 15: 351–361

Horton J W, White D J, Baxter C R 1990 Hypertonic saline dextran resuscitation of thermal injury. Ann Surg 211: 301–311

Hughes K R, Armstrong R F, Brough M D, Parkhouse N 1989 Fluid requirements of patients with burns and inhalation injuries in an intensive care unit. Intensive Care Medicine 14: 464–466

Jackson D M 1953 The diagnosis of the depth of burning. Br J Surg 40: 588

Kaufman T, Neuman R A, Weinberg A 1989 Is postburn dermal ischaemia enhanced by oxygen free radicals? Burns 15: 291–294

Kinsella J, Booth M G 1991 Pain relief in burns: James Laing Memorial Essay 1990. Burns 17: 391–395

Laing J H E, Morgan B D G, Sanders R 1991 Assessment of burn injury in the accident and emergency department: a review of 100 referrals to a regional burns unit. Ann R Coll Surg Engl 73: 329–331

Langford R M, Armstrong R F 1990 Algorithm for managing injury from smoke inhalation. Br Med J 299: 902–905

Manson W L, Klasen H J, Sauer E W et al 1992 Selective intestinal decontamination for prevention of wound colonization in severely burned patients: a retrospective analysis. Burns 18: 98–102

Matsuda T, Tanaka H, Shimazaki S et al 1992 High dose vitamin C therapy for extensive deep dermal burns. Burns 18: 127–131

Miller J G, Carruthers H R, Burd D A R 1992 An algorithmic approach to the management of cutaneous burns. Burns 18: 200–211

Monafo W C, Chuntrasokul V, Varian A Y 1973 Hypertonic sodium solutions in the treatment of burn shock. Am J Surg 126: 778–783

Muir I F K, Barclay T L, Settle J A D 1987 Burns and their treatment 3rd edn. Butterworths, London

Murison M S C, Laitung J K G, Pigott R W 1991 Effectiveness of burns resuscitation using two different formulae. Burns 17: 484–489

Neild G, Parkhouse N 1992 Unpublished data

Nelson J L, Alexander J W, Jacobs P A et al 1992 Metabolic and immune effects of enteral ascorbic acid after burn trauma. Burns 18: 92–97

Saito H, Tock O, Alexander J W et al 1987 The effect of route of nutrient administration on the nutritional state, catabolic hormone secretion and gut mucosal integrity after burn injury. J Parenter Enter Nutr 11: 1–7

Sasaki T M, Welch G W, Herndon D N 1979 Burn wound manipulation induced bacteraemia. J Trauma 19: 46–48

Sparkes B G, Monge G, Marshall S L et al 1990a Plasma levels of cutaneous burn toxin and lipid peroxides in thermal injury. Burns 16: 118–122

Sparkes B G, Gyorkos J W, Gorczynski R M et al 1990b Comparison of endotoxins and cutaneous burn toxin as immunosuppressants. Burns 16: 123–127

Thomson P D, Till G O, Wooliscroft J O et al 1990 Superoxide dismutase prevents lipid peroxidation in burned patients. Burns 16: 406–413

Wakabayashi G 1990 Atria natriuretic polypeptide after burn injury: blood levels and physiological role in rats. Burns 16: 169–175

Watson J S, Walker C C, Sanders R 1977 A comparison between dried plasma and plasma protein fraction in the resuscitation of burn patients. Burns 3: 108–111

Waymack J P, Jenkins M E, Alexander J W et al 1989 A prospective trial of prophylactic and intravenous immune globulin for the prevention of infections in severely burned patients. Burns 15: 71–76

Wooliscroft J O, Prasad J K, Thomson P et al 1990 Metabolic alterations in burn patients: detection of adenosine triphosphate degradation products and lipid peroxides. Burns 16: 92–96

Zeigler T R, Smith R J, O'Dwyer S T et al 1988 Increased intestinal permeability associated with infection in burn patients. Arch Surg 123: 1313–1319

10. Modern day-surgery

D. J. Wilkinson

Day-stay anaesthesia and surgery have been practised for many years. Nicoll in Glasgow wrote of his experiences in such a service in 1909 for paediatric surgery (Nicoll 1909) and Waters wrote of his 'Down-Town Anesthesia Clinic' some 5 years later (Waters 1919), while working in Sioux City, Iowa. These were isolated events in medical practice however and, although interesting historically, did little to influence day-to-day practice. There were other intermittent reports on the possibilities of day surgery over the years (Herzfeld 1938, Webb & Graves 1966), but it was not until the mid 1960s in the USA that the development of formal ambulatory surgery programmes became established.

In the UK there were many hospitals which initiated day wards and started to practise some form of day surgery around the same time. The concept was much slower to be accepted in this country however and has lagged a long way behind the US developments.

A TIME OF REPORTS

The redevelopment of the NHS over the last 5 years has provided new impetus to day surgery. Administrators have been looking for ways to improve efficiency in hospitals, which is their usual synonym for cost-saving exercises. An awareness that in the USA up to 60% of all surgery was being performed on a day-stay basis compared with about 18–20% in the UK provided a powerful incentive for research and report writing.

The Royal College of Surgeons of England's Commission on the provision of surgical services produced some guidelines for day case surgery (Royal College of Surgeons of England 1985) which reflected the deliberations of a multidisciplinary committee. The written report tried to provide a policy for day work, some definitions of what this type of work was, an idea of the accommodation and facilities required, and then some thoughts on patient selection, anaesthetic considerations and postoperative care. A list of possible surgical procedures was provided as well as some thoughts on economics and staffing levels. This document did a great deal to focus thinking on day-case work but it was still a distillation of UK practice and made outdated recommendations such as that no operative procedure should be longer than

30 min. The newer concepts of American and Australian development in this field were overlooked and so UK practice stagnated. Perhaps more importantly, those who began to increase their day-stay work did so under the provisions of this document and so inadequate facilities and limited practices resulted.

The Value for Money Unit of the NHS management executive produced a report later in the decade which became known as the Bevan report after the Chairman of the Committee (Bevan 1989). This document looked at all aspects of theatre work but suggested that:

The expanded use of Day Surgery, especially where dedicated facilities exist or can be provided, may be one way to increase overall theatre utilisation and throughput at least cost. A limiting factor here is often the lack of day beds or infrastructure geared to this form of treatment.

The report also highlights the lower cost of treating patients as day cases as opposed to inpatients. Hospital administration began to take notice of day surgery.

The Audit Commission then attempted to identify why this type of practice was not developing at the rate found in North America and why different district health authorities were performing at such variant rates (Audit Commission 1990). The Commission produced what they called a basket of 20 procedures which were particularly suited to day work and which could be used to compare district performance. They found that cases from this basket were treated in widely different manners from place to place and suggested that if district health authorities all performed these basket cases at reasonable levels then 186 000 extra patients would be treated at no extra cost, and that a further 300 000 additional patients could be catered for with ease. This would have immediate impact on waiting lists. The main reasons why these cases were not being performed were lack of audit, lack of specialized facilities, inappropriate and inefficient use of current facilities, poor management of existing day facilities, and lack of interest in this type of work by clinicians and administrators alike.

A second report by the Value for Money Unit evaluated day practice in much greater detail (National Health Service Management Executive 1991). Their conclusions echoed those of the Audit Commission, stressing the need for a major commitment by surgeons and anaesthetists to this type of work and the provision of dedicated facilities with adequate ancillary support. These three reports received widespread publicity and hospital administrators and clinicians all started to take notice.

ENTHUSIASM FOR DAY SURGERY

Many of the recommendations made by all these reports had been published in the past by a wide variety of health care personnel from the UK, but their innovative ideas had been overlooked (Ogg 1985, Kallar & Whitwam 1988). A series of books were published at this time relating to day care in the UK

(Bradshaw & Davenport 1989, Healy 1990, Klepper et al 1991), and the British Association of Day Surgery was inaugurated. This society rapidly expanded, attracting membership from all disciplines related to the specialty — surgical, anaesthetic, nursing and clerical.

The first European Congress on Ambulatory Surgery was held in Brussels in March of 1991 and delegates from all over Europe were joined by practitioners from North America. It was soon apparent that there was a wide gulf between most of the rest of Europe and the UK, with the UK well ahead in terms of facilities and practice, but there was still a huge gap between UK and North American practice.

In the UK there is now a widespread building programme by hospitals both in the public and private sectors, joining this new enthusiasm for day work. Unfortunately many have failed to appreciate the needs of day surgery as exemplified in North American and Australian practice. New centres have been built and opened which are totally out of date and which will not meet the needs of present or future patients. This is often a result of trying to include too many other facilities, or of adding a day centre on to existing structures which are not suited to the concept.

LATEST REPORTS

The Royal College of Surgeons of England has now published an updated version of its 1985 report (Royal College of Surgeons of England 1992), which is a marked step forward from the original but does not embrace what I believe to be modern practice. There is an acceptance of mixed medical and surgical facilities in the report, so that endoscopy, oncology and surgery are all potentially housed in the one unit. This does not provide the correct ambience for surgical day work. Surgical day cases are patients who are essentially well — they are not ill — they have different requirements to medical patients who are often quite unwell. There are statements such as 'The elderly and the infirm will ordinarily be excluded . . . ', this is again outdated practice; it is often the elderly who benefit the most from day stay as they do not then become disoriented by overnight stay in hospital. 'Even if accompanied, patients should not go home by public transport": why ever not? If they are walking around, eating, drinking and comfortable and have a sensible escort, what is the problem? Patients go home from the wards by public transport and they are often a great deal less well than patients after day-case surgery. The report is a useful step forward but on the whole does not go far enough and is too conservative and didactic in its views.

The Audit Commission also produced another of its NHS occasional papers in March 1992 in conjunction with the Royal College of Surgeons' report, entitled *All in a Day's Work* (Audit Commission 1992). This report shows a potential 214 000 patients who could be treated as day cases and this is based on more accurate data-collecting systems than had been available in the 1990 report. It highlights the importance of purchasers and providers working together to provide the right facilities and standards of care for these day cases and then providing adequate audit of that work.

THE 'NEW AGE' OF DAY SURGERY

Day surgery must now move further into the 20th century in the UK with the development of special centres which can be either free-standing or associated with existing hospitals. One such centre has recently opened at St Bartholomew's Hospital, London. This centre has been built within the shell of a listed building and therefore suffers from the constraints that English Heritage and planning authorities apply; nevertheless it has set new standards in design, facilities, and operational policy for a UK day centre. Its design and working practice will be reviewed.

Planning team

A group of interested personnel within the hospital designed and oversaw the whole project from start to finish. All design was performed in-house by the District Works Department with input from all members of the committee. The pivotal event in the planning of this centre was a trip to Boston, Massachussetts which assessed five day facilities in that city. The plans that had been made up to that point were abandoned and a totally new design made. Weekly meetings by the planning committee then sorted the myriad problems as they arose in the construction phase. This same group provided the initial operational policy of the centre as well as planning staffing levels and instigating the timetable and designing the booklets and information sheets that have proved to be so innovative and successful in the centre.

Design

The original floor space of about 810 m^2 was made up of an operating theatre and three Nightingale wards on the ground floor of the East Wing of the hospital (Fig. 10.1). There was a central access point to the wing which led to a lift area and stairwell which services the rest of the wing, which includes an orthopaedic theatre in the basement, and facilities for psychiatric patients on the first floor and for oncology on the second and third floors. These facilities had been recently refurbished and access had to remain from the ground floor via the staircases and lifts. On the ground floor area there were a variety of slopes and steps between the wards and theatre. Plans of the area were available but their accuracy was suspect and details of services such as water and electrical lines were sketchy.

The basic design of the new centre is a reception area, two theatres, a recovery room and a secondary recovery or step-down unit (Fig. 10.2). The patients rotate through these areas in a circular pattern without retracing their steps. The reception area has a large desk area and secure storage room for

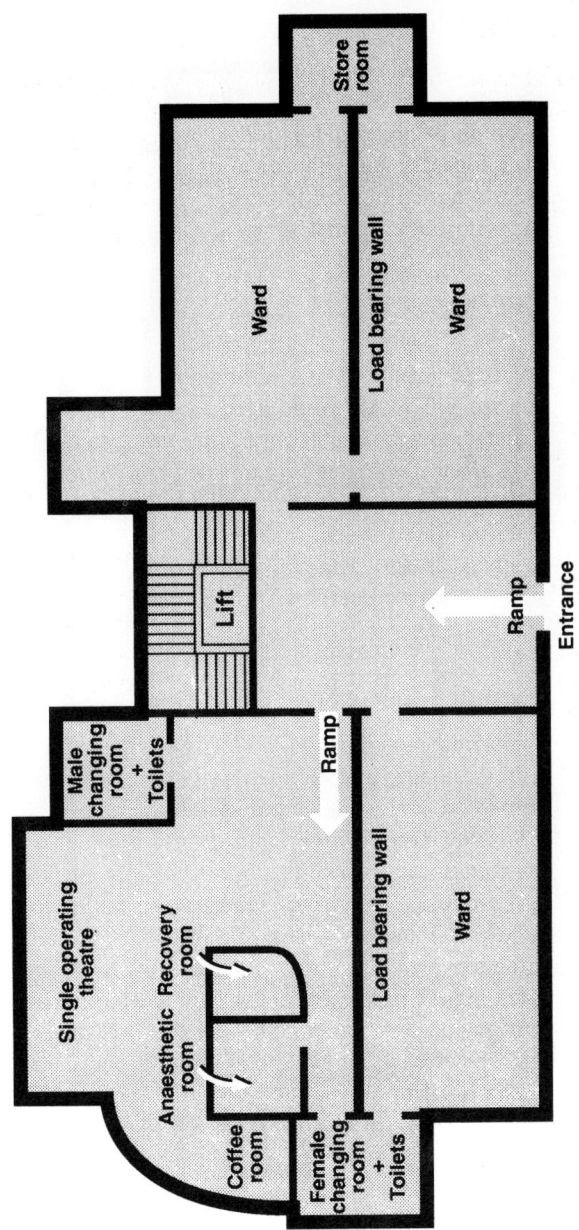

Fig. 10.1   Original plan of East Wing site, St Bartholomew's Hospital.

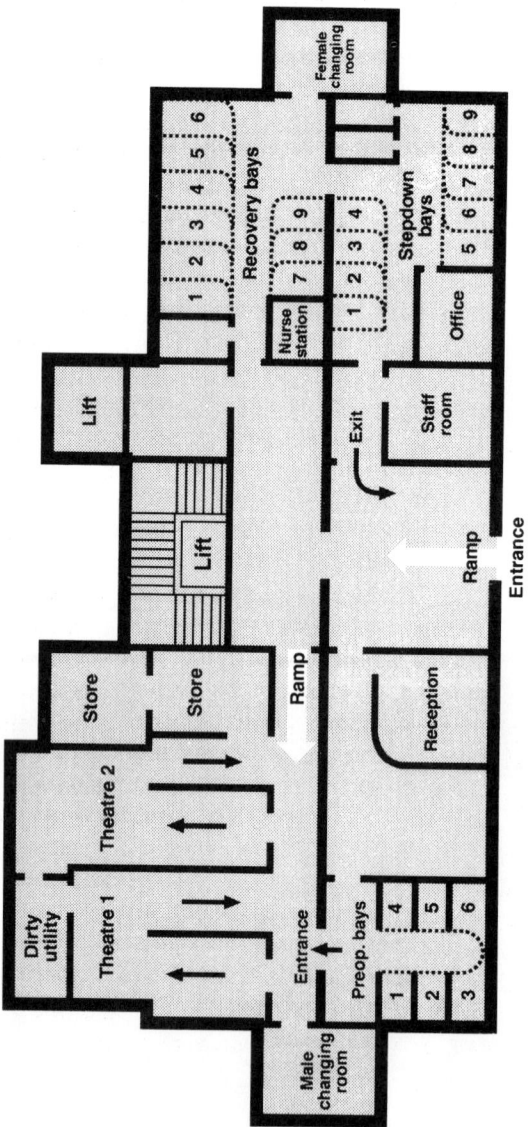

Fig. 10.2 Day Surgery Centre, East Wing, St Bartholomew's Hospital.

notes and files. The room is non-clinical in nature and has been likened to a hotel reception area with its diffuse lighting, pleasant soft furnishings, potted plants and so forth. The preoperative area next to the reception is divided into six cubicles, each of which contains a comfortable chair and a table, and ensures complete privacy for any patient. There is a patient toilet in this area also.

The theatre zone is subdivided into two fully self-contained theatres both with separate anaesthetic rooms. There is a shared dirty utility room with all facilities and a very large communal storage area. Additional storage facilities are incorporated in the two theatres and anaesthetic rooms in the form of fitted cupboards and drawers. The male changing room with toilet and shower facilities is also in this zone. The scrub-up area for theatres is in the patient exit corridor adjacent to each theatre and it is in this area that trolleys are laid up. Both theatres are built to the standard required for the use of X-ray imaging, and the larger of the theatres has full laser usage provision. This is a high-technology area appropriately coloured and finished, although without antistatic properties.

The recovery zone is on the other side of the central lift and stair area, and also contains the linen store, a nursing desk area, and the female changing rooms, again with toilets and showers. Individual trolleys, of which there are eight in this area, can be separated by curtains from each other in what is otherwise an open-plan area. Each patient area has full monitoring facilities, suction, piped oxygen, and lighting.

The step-down zone has nine reclining chairs in an open-plan formation which can be turned into individual private cubicles with curtains. There are patient toilets, a beverage bar, a nursing desk area, a secure patient clothes store, a linen room, a drug dispensary, and an office additionally in this zone. There is also a paediatric cot area here. This zone adjoins the central lift and stair access to which the patients pass on their way out of the building (Fig. 10.1). There is an adjacent staff room here with all facilities.

The theatre area is air-conditioned and the other patient areas are supplied with large ceiling fans. There is a television and video in both the reception and step-down unit and all areas have piped music which can be individualized to each main zone. All areas have communications via intercoms which can be public or private, as well as the usual alert and cardiac arrest call buttons. Telephone facilities for the staff are available in all areas and for the patients in all of the step-down bays. Computer links with the rest of the hospital are available in reception and recovery zones.

Patient flow

Outpatients

Patients are referred to outpatients by their general practitioners. The referring doctor or the surgeon, or nowadays, interestingly, due to all the publicity attending this type of work, the patient, may suggest the procedure be performed under day-stay conditions. If all parties agree to this approach, a special booklet is completed there and then, and the patient takes this to the day centre and books in. The booklet contains sections which display the results of clerking and examining the patient; these are simple tick questionnaires which can be completed by the patient alone or with some nursing help (Fig. 10.3). The junior doctor of the surgical team checks this questionnaire in outpatients and performs a simple physical examination of the patient. Consent forms are signed and any laboratory investigations needed are performed.

One of the most important aspects of this assessment is the height : weight ratio. Short obese patients provide too great a challenge for monitoring, airway and vascular access as well as inhalational agent consumption. It may be that total intravenous or regional anaesthesia for these patients may limit some of these problems, but they are not all obtunded. While the Royal College of Surgeons report centres on calculations of obesity based on the body mass index (unclothed weight (kg) divided by the height (m^2) should be less than 30), this is too complex a calculation for the average nurse, surgeon or anaesthetist to perform in outpatients. I have developed a simple height weight nomogram graph (Fig. 10.4) in which the height and weight are plotted so that if the patient falls above the line he or she is fit for day surgery and if below the line, he or she is not. This has proved very effective, although numerous revisions of the graph have been made as our experience grows. It is interesting to note that the US centres make no such limitations and will take on 150–200 kg adults with equanimity!

This may be completed by a Houseman or by Nursing Staff

FOR GENERAL ANAESTHESIA/REGIONAL BLOCK PATIENTS ONLY				DO YOU HAVE; OR HAVE EVER HAD:			
	Yes	No	Don't Know When		Yes	No	Don't Know When
Chest pain	☐	☐	☐ ☐	Kidney Disease	☐	☐	☐ ☐
Palpitations	☐	☐	☐ ☐	Liver Disease	☐	☐	☐ ☐
Shortness of breath	☐	☐	☐ ☐	Deep Vein Thrombosis	☐	☐	☐ ☐
Oedema	☐	☐	☐ ☐	Fits	☐	☐	☐ ☐
High Blood Pressure	☐	☐	☐ ☐	Cough Regularly	☐	☐	☐ ☐
Heart Attack	☐	☐	☐ ☐	Smoker	☐	☐	☐ ☐
Rheumatic Fever	☐	☐	☐ ☐	Asthma	☐	☐	☐ ☐
TB	☐	☐	☐ ☐	Bronchitis	☐	☐	☐ ☐
Diabetes	☐	☐	☐ ☐				

cont.

Fig. 10.3   Part of outpatient clerking form for Day Surgery Centre, St Bartholomew's Hospital

This may be completed by nursing staff

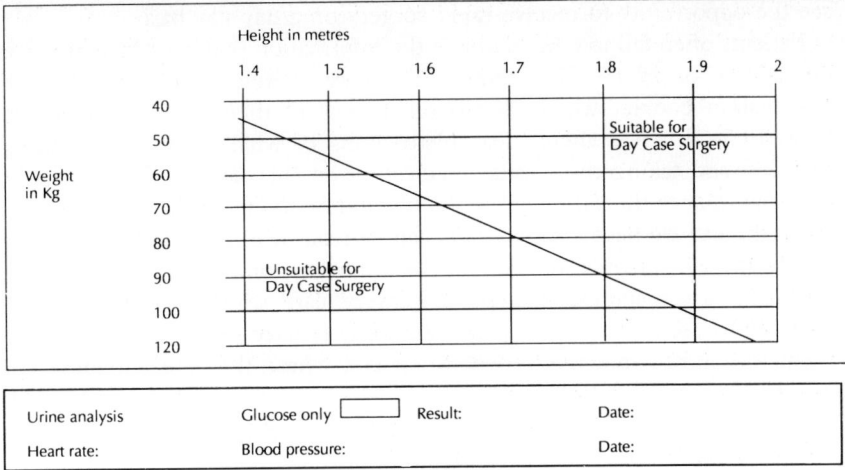

Fig. 10.4 Height/weight nomogram for Day Surgery Centre, St Bartholomew's Hospital.

Laboratory investigations are minimal. Sickle cell tests are performed where indicated; haemoglobin levels for menstruating women are checked, but nothing else is routine. Urine testing may be performed as part of outpatient assessment but is not repeated in the day centre. It is the concept of patient wellness rather than illness that must be remembered at all times (Michel & Myrick 1990). Admission for day surgery is not a time to provide medical screening for patients; that must be performed elsewhere.

Booking in

When patients have completed this outpatient work-up they walk to the day centre, bringing their booklet with them, and book in for their surgery. The operating lists are made up by the reception clerical and nursing staff who are well aware of the time it takes to perform a specific operation. The patient is offered the next available time on their surgeon's operating list. They are given a date and time to attend together with some general advice about their future time in hospital. They are shown round the centre and meet as many of the nursing staff as they can so that there are a few familiar faces on the day of surgery.

The reception staff check that all aspects of the booklet relating to the surgery have been completed and if this has not been the case the patient is directed back to outpatients for this to take place or alternatively a member of the surgical team is invited to the day centre to complete the process.

Potential problems of a social or medical nature can often be determined at this time and suitable advice and assistance sought. This may be from the anaesthetic department or Social Services or from community nursing. It must be remembered that patients are often economical with the truth if they see the opportunity to receive rapid surgery on a day-stay basis.

Patients often fail to take in any of the information they are given either in outpatients or in the day centre. They are therefore provided with an information booklet which details all aspects of their time in the centre (Fig. 10.5). It gives them clear instructions of what to do about eating, drinking and taking their usual medication on the day of their surgery. It explains what to do if they fall ill beforehand or simply do not wish to come in on the day we have chosen. This can be read by all the members of their family and can provide very useful basic information. The last page of this booklet is a self-addressed, prepaid stamped card which is completed and returned to the centre by the patients once they have returned home. It asks them to confirm that they know when and where they are attending and

The Day Surgery Centre

Please attend the Centre at ————————————————— **(time)**

Date/Day ——————————————————————————

Name of Consultant ————————————————————————

INTRODUCTION

This is a purpose built multi-speciality centre with its own operating suite and modern equipment designed to serve patients who require an operation or procedure which does not necessitate staying in hospital overnight. It is run by experienced staff who are enthusiastic about your care in the Day Surgery Centre and who have been specially trained for this work.

We realise that however routine a procedure is to us, it is not routine to you, the patient. Do ask any member of staff questions if you are concerned about any aspect of your admission and care.

Our aim is to provide you with efficient personalised care, and to enable you to return home soon after surgery to recuperate in familiar home surroundings. As you are coming in from home and not staying in hospital, it is VERY IMPORTANT to understand and comply with all information in this booklet.

BEFORE COMING TO THE CENTRE

Food and Drink

If you are to have a general anaesthetic or a local anaesthetic, the following instructions **MUST BE OBSERVED UNLESS** you have had instructions to the contrary from your own Consultant in Out-patients.

Fig. 10.5 Page 1 of the patient information booklet for Day Surgery Centre, St Bartholomew's Hospital.

for what purpose, and that they have read and understood the booklet and have arranged for someone to collect them and stay with them overnight (Fig. 10.6). The patients then go home with their instruction booklet. The reception staff then contact the patient's general practitioner by letter to inform him or her that one of their patients has been booked into the centre for a specific procedure and to ask if there is any medical or social reason of which the practitioner is aware that might be a constraint to this process.

Preoperative week

In the week prior to an admission the reception staff ensure that all is ready for the forthcoming surgery. They check that the patient has confirmed attendance and if not, they contact him or her either directly by telephone or indirectly via their general practitioner or through the community nursing service. They check that the patient's notes are available, that all tests requested are complete, that all X-rays are available and that the surgical instrumentation to perform the procedure is available. The planned list is reviewed by the surgical team and approval obtained for the content and order. The essence is to prevent there being any failure to attend on the patient's part and then any cancellation for anaesthetic or surgical reasons. Any patient may cancel an appointment at any time for any reason, by simply telephoning the centre, and the reception staff can then offer them a new date and also offer other patients an earlier operation.

CONFIRMATION SLIP

Your name: _____

I am able to report to the Day Surgery Centre on (date)_____

_____

at (appointment time)_____

Under
(Dr/Surgeon/Professor) _____

I have read and understood the instructions outlined in the booklet and I confirm that I am able/unable to arrange for someone to collect me and that someone will remain with me overnight.

Name _____

Date _____

Contact telephone number (if possible) _____

Fig. 10.6 Patient confirmation slip for Day Surgery Centre, St Bartholomew's Hospital.

Day of surgery

Patients arrive in the centre at a time appropriate to their planned surgery. They move through into the preoperative bay area where they are assessed by nursing and medical staff. They change into appropriate garments for the intended surgery. There is no place for the removal of teeth, hearing aids and underclothes from the patient having a lesion removed under local anaes- thetic on the arm, for example. Each patient is different and therefore requires suitable preparation; the preservation of dignity and control is of paramount importance. Relatives can accompany patients at this stage or may leave, taking with them a paging device. This device has a range of some 25 miles, allowing relatives complete freedom to pursue their normal daily events and yet allowing the day centre to call them back at any stage. They do not need to phone to check at any time; if and when the bleep sounds, they return to the centre.

Simple physiological measurements on each patient are made at this time — blood pressure, pulse etc. — and the time of last eating, state of dentition and current state of health are ascertained. The anaesthetist can see and examine the patient in privacy at this point and the surgeon can review the procedure and mark the area for surgery.

Premedication is optional. Perhaps the only really useful therapy at this time is the use of eutectic mixture of local anaesthetics (EMLA) cream, which should be available for adults as well as children. Short-acting benzodiaz- epines are popular in many units but while some claim significant anxiolysis without discharge delay postoperatively and others prefer to accept some degree of apprehension rather than polypharmacy for day work, it is up to individuals to make up their own minds and develop their own safe practices. Many premedicants can be titrated intravenously once the patient is either in theatre or the anaesthetic room, but each centre must develop the practice in the manner which suits their caseload and staffing structures. As in all aspects of anaesthetic care there are not absolute right and wrong ways of doing any procedure. The basic *raison d'être* has to be to tailor the practice to the needs of the individual patient.

Into theatre

The patient, who is well and walked into the centre and who will walk out again at the end of the day, can walk through into the anaesthetic room where he or she positions him- or herself on a trolley. Full monitoring is then applied before any further treatment is started. This includes an electrocar- diogram, a pulse oximeter and a non-invasive blood pressure monitor. Local anaesthesia or general anaesthesia is then instituted according to the needs of the surgeon and patient. If general anaesthesia is utilized then analysis of respired gases is essential, as is the use of disconnection alarms and exhaled tidal volume measurement for patients undergoing intermittent positive pressure ventilation. Peripheral nerve stimulators and temperature monitoring facilities must be available in addition.

Again there are no absolute methods of practice which are correct. Each anaesthetist must develop techniques which permit patients to undergo their surgical procedure with the minimum of stress and the maximum of comfort. Analgesia is paramount and must be long-lasting. Morbidity such as nausea and vomiting must be minimized.

The ideal technique for day surgery probably will involve a blending of local anaesthesia with a varying degree of unconsciousness for all patients. Some will happily remain wide awake during local blockade and surgery while others will wish to be totally unconscious. The use of short-acting opioids such as fentanyl and alfentanil usually, but not always, carries the price of some degree of postoperative nausea, especially on ambulation. Non-steroidal anti-inflammatory (NSAIDs) are becoming more and more popular, utilizing a variety of routes of administration, and these drugs can certainly provide dramatically effective analgesia for quite major surgery and are synergistic with the opioids. Upper and lower gastrointestinal bleeding can follow their regular use by these routes and parenteral forms have considerable side-effects, many of which are still being evaluated. These drugs certainly have a place in day surgery but are not an universal panacea.

Many recent studies seek to compare opioids with NSAIDS for day-stay work but these drugs should be used together. The patient can have a short-acting opioid at induction both to facilitate the induction and to provide the initial operative analgesia; a NSAID can then be given either rectally (usually diclofenac) or intramuscularly (particularly if intramuscular ketoralac is available), which will provide the later analgesia; then, wherever possible, a long-acting local anaesthetic should be used prior to the start of surgery, to produce profound intra- and postoperative analgesia and to decrease the requirement for postoperative analgesic medication.

There may be a place for the routine administration of a muscarinic blocking agent if opioids are used in conjunction with propofol. These latter two agents frequently produce profound bradycardia which may be augmented by vagal reflexes if NSAID suppositories are then utilized. The complete absence of surgical stimulation found with the judicious use of local anaesthesia may then enhance this slow pulse. Intravenous glycopyrolate in a low dosage of 0.1 mg on induction will usually mask these effects without producing an unwanted tachycardia.

Some practitioners like to use prophylactic antiemetics for all patients. Routine intravenous metoclopramide on induction does carry the potential risk of postoperative oculogyric problems but does not appear to be a major problem. The use of propofol certainly seems to minimize nausea, as does the use of NSAID and local anaesthetics in preference to opioids. Ephedrine has been used extensively in the USA for its antiemetic properties and warrants greater investigation. In addition the forthcoming launch of ondansetron may prove very valuable in this field if similar results are obtained in anaesthesia as have been demonstrated in chemotherapy treatment.

Sedation can be provided by the shorter-acting benzodiazepines such as midazolam, which may or may not require reversal with flumazenil, or from the standard intravenous induction agents methohexitone, propofol, etomidate and possibly soon the newly reformulated althesin. These sedatives can be used as single doses, which may then be augmented by inhalational agents, or alternatively they can be given as continuous infusions. The inhalational agents can be utilized according to each practitioner's own preference. The emergence times from these agents play little part in the final recovery of patients and their use and mode of administration should be according to local preferences. Closed-circuit anaesthesia may be appropriate on cost grounds for the most recently introduced agents.

Once either the local or the general anaesthesia is complete patients are moved into the operating theatre. They are here transferred on to a high-quality operating table for their surgery; this table can be adjusted and positioned in a myriad of ways to suit the surgeon. There is minimal effort involved in transfer of such patients from trolley to table and then back again with the use of roller devices or Pat-slides. The use of a trolley as an operating table limits the potential procedures that may be carried out both now and in the future. Full monitoring as described in the anaesthetic room is maintained and augmented where appropriate throughout surgery. Once the surgical procedure is complete the patient is transferred to recovery.

Recovery

In this area all patients must be cared for by specifically trained nurses on a one-to-one basis until they are fully conscious. Full monitoring is maintained as before and once awake patients are questioned on their level of comfort. Pain and sedation scores are charted. Once patients can sit in comfort they are encouraged to do so. As soon as they feel able to walk they are escorted to a secondary recovery or step-down area to complete their recovery. In this zone they can rest in reclining chairs until they wish to dress themselves and increase their mobilization. Here they can eat and drink once more, utilize the toilet facilities, and be visited by a member of the surgical team who can give the patient further information. Relatives and friends can join the patient at any stage of the recovery process at the discretion of the medical and nursing staff.

Discharge

The majority of patients attending for day surgery can be discharged by the nursing staff who are able to follow simple discharge criteria protocols (Fig. 10.7). Any patient can be 'flagged' to be discharged by the anaesthetist at any stage in their stay in the centre. The patients receive all appropriate medication which is dispensed by the centre. These usually comprise

Registered General Nurse please confirm that the Patient:

PRIOR TO DISCHARGE	YES	NO
1. has stable B.P. and pulse - results	☐	☐
2. can swallow and cough	☐	☐
3. can walk without feeling faint	☐	☐
4. has minimal nausea and is not being sick	☐	☐
5. can breathe comfortably and looks a normal colour	☐	☐
6. is wide awake and knows what is going on	☐	☐
7. has passed urine	☐	☐
8. has had something to eat or drink	☐	☐
9. has had the operation site checked	☐	☐
10. has their post-operative instructions	☐	☐
11. has their post-operative medications	☐	☐
12. has their doctors letter	☐	☐
13. knows when to come back to outpatients	☐	☐
14. has someone to take them home	☐	☐
15. has someone to stay with them tonight	☐	☐
16. has their audit check questionaire	☐	☐

I confirm that these discharge criteria have been met and the patient can go home at...
and I believe that this patient will/will not benefit from a visit from the community care nurses and this has/has not been arranged (delete as required)

Signed..(Day Ward Nurse)

Fig. 10.7 Discharge criteria for Day Surgery Centre, St Bartholomew's Hospital.

analgesics, often in two formulations, a small number of tablets for severe to moderate pain (say DF118) and a larger number of less potent drugs (such as mefenamic acid or paracetamol).

Patients are also given detailed sheets of instructions which outline the 'do's' and 'don'ts' of their immediate and late postoperative management (Fig. 10.8). Patients are then allowed to go home with an escort, provided assurance has been given that they have someone to care for them that night.

The general practitioners involved are informed for their patient's discharge by letter at present but we are currently evolving a method of either faxing a full discharge summary to their practice before the patient has left the centre or, for those without a fax, telephoning the practice and leaving a message that the patient is about to be discharged. We hope in this way to minimize any potential gap in the patient's care and allow both the hospital and community to have proper input into that care.

Postoperative care

Until patients next attend for outpatient review by the surgeon they are cared for by their own practitioners, the community nursing services and, more

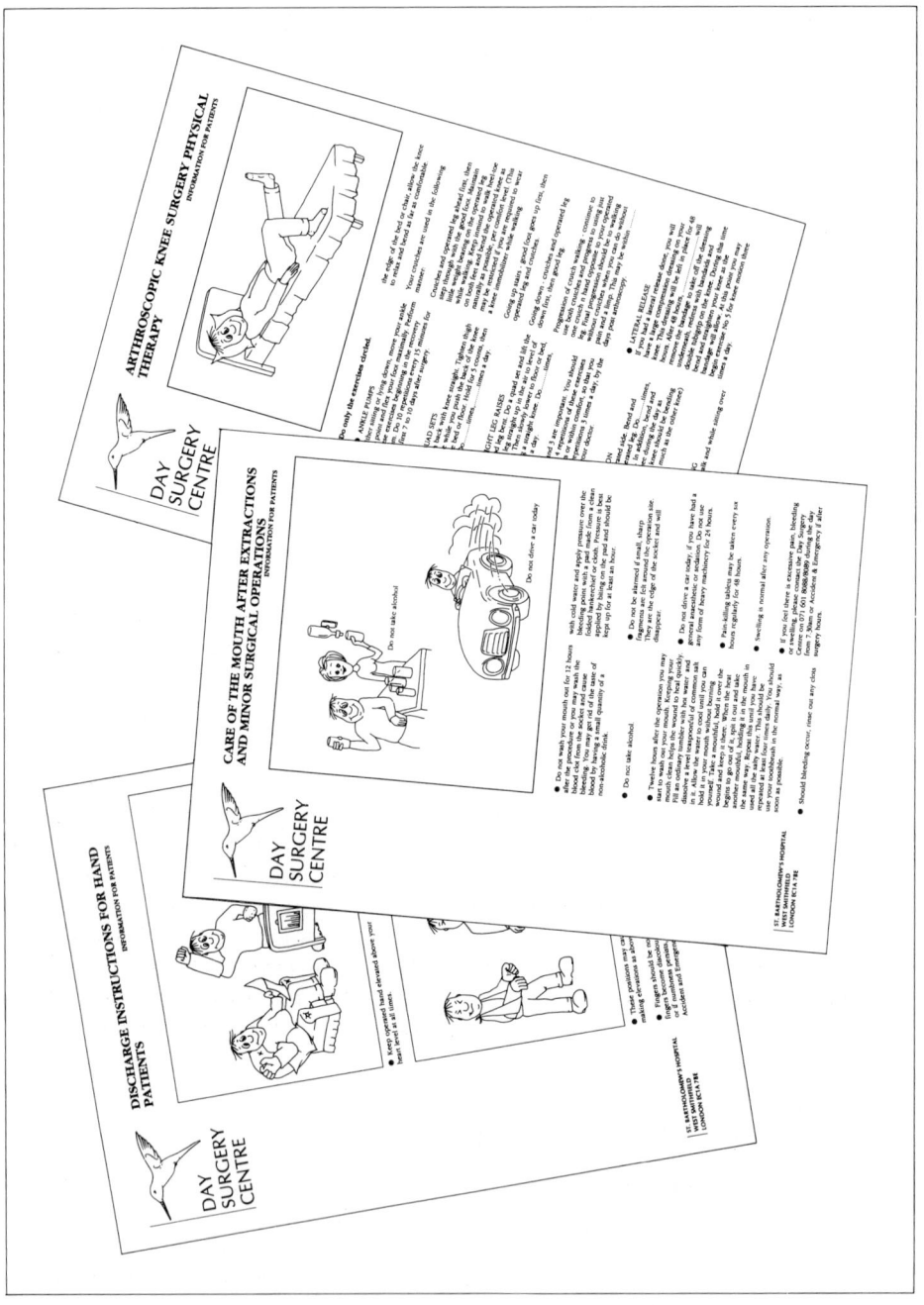

Fig. 10.8   Patient information sheets from Day Surgery Centre, St Bartholomew's Hospital.

usually, their immediate family. We believe that our centre can still augment that care and so we provide a follow-up service postoperatively. This currently involves a telephone questionnaire of the patient on the day after discharge from the centre which permits audit of our work and a chance for the patient, or relative, to clarify any problems that they foresee (Fig. 10.9). Further detailed audit of our work is carried out by postal questionnaires which are based on those designed by the Audit Commission (Audit Commission 1991).

MANAGEMENT

Day-to-day management of the centre is provided by a medical director (an anaesthetist) and a clinical nurse manager. They report to a management committee which comprises a senior member of the hospital management team, a senior surgeon, the senior audit manager, the senior community nursing officer, a financial advisor, and the director, service manager and senior nurse of the anaesthetic directorate. Additional members are co-opted to any meeting as appropriate. This group reports through the clinical policy group to the general manager of the hospital.

SPECIAL FEATURES OF THIS CENTRE

The patients flow in a circular fashion through the various areas in the centre without back- or cross-tracking. There is a special ambience created in the centre by the attitude of the staff and the non-clinical appearance of the various rooms. Staff are selected not only for their clinical skills but because of their ability to relate to patients. This has been termed the 'people-people' concept, only employing people who really like being with and caring for other people, and this concept is vitally important. The centre is self-sufficient in personnel and equipment within the umbrella of a large hospital. Staff are flexible in their working practices — there are no longer theatre or ward staff — staff can and do work wherever there is a need. Detailed information, both verbal and written, is given to all patients at all parts of their hospital stay. Patients are encouraged to participate in, and comment on, their care at all stages. Close communication is preserved between the centre and the medical and nursing facilities of the community. Audit of practice, both medical and nursing, is made and evaluated.

NOT THE PERFECT DAY CENTRE

This day surgery centre is reported here as an illustration of what can be achieved in the NHS by careful planning. It is not the universal panacea for all day centres. It is by no means the ideal such centre. There is inadequate space (because of being a central and listed site) for many other features such as showers for patients, lay-up areas in theatres, plant space for full air-conditioning, more storage space, teaching and lecture rooms etc. Each

TELEPHONE QUESTIONNAIRE ON POSTOPERATIVE DAY

	Yes	No
Time/Date of call..		
1. Do you feel well?	☐	☐
2. Did you feel well whilst travelling home?	☐	☐
3. Have you had any bad pain since the operation?	☐	☐
Details:		
4. Did you need to take your pain relieving tablets?	☐	☐
How many? How many left?		
5. Did they work ? i.e. is the pain better?	☐	☐
6. Have you felt sick since you have been home?	☐	☐
Details:		
7. Have you been sick?	☐	☐
Details:		
8. Can you do what you would normally undertake whilst at home?	☐	☐
Specify:		
9. Are you able to go to work/school?	☐	☐
10. Have you had any problems passing urine since you came home?	☐	☐
Specify:		
11. Have you arranged for your GP to recieve your discharge letter?	☐	☐
12. Do you need to see your GP?	☐	☐
Why:		
13. Do you need to see your community nurse?	☐	☐
Why:		
14. When is your next medical appointment?	Please check page 6	
15. Have you any questions about anything?	☐	☐
Details:		
16. Have you any suggestions about how we could improve anything about your time in the Day Surgery Centre?		
Details:		

Questionaire completed by... Date..

Seen by Nursing Manager.. Date..

Medical Director... Date..

Fig. 10.9 Postoperative telephone questionnaire from Day Surgery Centre, St Bartholomew's Hospital.

centre will incorporate those features that it believes to be the most important and which will be appropriate for the patients for whom they will be caring in their practice.

THE FUTURE

Day-stay surgery will increase more and more in the future. All aspects will undergo change and development. Surgeons will increase the complexity and duration of their day-stay practice as newer techniques such as 'key-hole surgery' expand the possible procedures which can be attempted. Anaesthetists will continue to improve postoperative morbidity, utilizing newer and hopefully less toxic agents. Epidural and subarachnoid anaesthesia will expand in frequency and scope in this country as it has in the USA. Hotel facilities will be built close to hospitals to extend the possibilities of day care. Community and domiciliary nursing will extend its remit in these fields to cater for their patients' needs, much in the way as can be seen with US surgeons performing day-stay thyroidectomy, hysterectomy and cholecystectomy at present.

Few of the features of design, managment and care provided by our centre are necessarily unique. It is instead the blending of what we consider to be the best of American and UK practice which gives this day surgery centre its special place in current UK medicine. It is to be anticipated that many more new centres will evolve over the coming decades and they will incorporate aspects from this centre in their designs, much as we have utilized others to produce our plans. Day surgery is not a static process but one which is constantly evolving in new directions. All involved in this type of work must be prepared to adopt a flexible approach and constantly to re-evaluate their practice in the light of new developments.

REFERENCES

Audit Commission 1990 A shorter cut to better services. Day surgery in England and Wales. HMSO, London
Audit Commission 1991 Measuring quality: the patient's view of day surgery. HMSO, London
Audit Commission 1992 All in a day's work: an audit of day surgery in England and Wales. HMSO, London
Bevan P G 1989 The management and utilisation of operating departments. NHS Management Executive Value for Money Unit. HMSO, London
Bradshaw E G, Davenport H T (ed) 1989 Day care; surgery, anaesthesia and management. Edward Arnold, London
Healy T E J (ed) 1990 Anaesthesia for day case surgery. Bailliere's clinical anaesthesiology, vol 4. Bailliere Tindall, London
Herzfeld G 1938 Hernia in infancy. Am J Surg 39: 422
Kallar S K, Whitwam J G (ed) 1988 Outpatient anaesthesia. Proceedings of an International Symposium at Antwerp, Belgium, 9 June 1988. Medicom, Bussum, The Netherlands
Klepper I D, Sanders L D, Rosen M (eds) 1991 Ambulatory anaesthesia and sedation: impairment and recovery. Blackwell Scientific Publications, Oxford

Michel L L, Myrick C 1990 Current and future trends in ambulatory surgery and their impact on nursing practice. J Post Anesth Nursing 5: 347–349

National Health Service Management Executive, Value for Money Unit 1991 Day surgery: making it happen. HMSO, London

Nicoll J H 1909 The surgery of infancy. Br Med J 2: 753–755

Ogg T W 1985 Aspects of day surgery and anaesthesia. Anaesthesia Rounds no 18. ICI, Macclesfield, Cheshire

Royal College of Surgeons of England 1985 Guidelines for day case surgery. Royal College of Surgeons of England, London

Royal College of Surgeons of England 1992 Guidelines for day case surgery. Royal College of Surgeons of England, London

Waters R M 1919 The down-town anesthesia clinic. Am J Surg 33 (suppl): 71–73

Webb E, Graves H 1966 Anesthesia for the ambulant patient. J B Lippencott, Philadelphia

11. The laryngeal mask airway — a review

J. Brimacombe   N. Shorney

The laryngeal mask airway (LMA) is undoubtedly the most significant advance in airway management since the endotracheal tube (ETT) and has succeeded where many other attempts at alternative airways have failed. Invented by Brain in 1981, it was released on the UK in 1988 following extensive testing and modification. The advantages of having a non-invasive airway which avoided the hazards of intubation while affording greater security than a facemask soon became apparent.

Over the last 4 years the LMA literature has greatly increased, helping to define the LMA's uses, its merits and demerits. A survey from 1983 to 1991 reveals a total of 183 publications on the LMA and over 70% of these papers have been in British journals, notably *Anaesthesia*, with 52% of world publications. The international popularity of the LMA is increasing markedly and, as judged by sales and publications, is having a considerable impact in Australia, Europe, South-east Asia, Canada and Japan (Fig. 11.1). Release of the LMA in the USA was delayed until 1992.

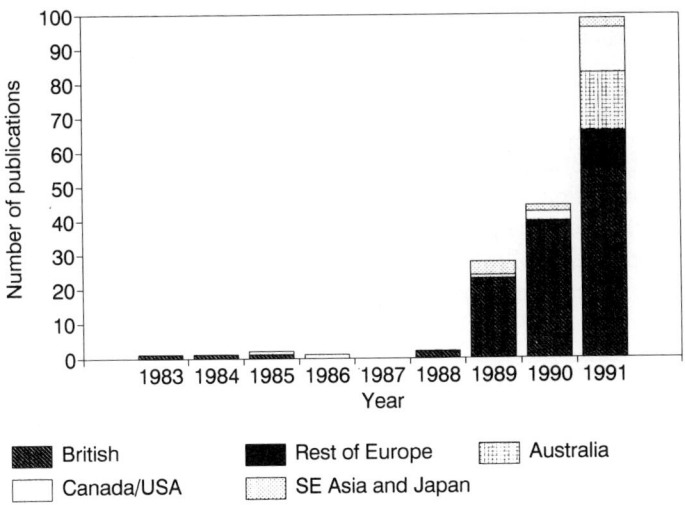

Fig. 11.1 The rise of the laryngeal mask airway (LMA) as judged by the number of publications describing its use.

183

An account of the early history of the LMA has been published by Brain (White 1991) and details of its usage can be found in the comprehensive Intavent instruction manual. The LMA literature has been reviewed by Leach & Alexander (White 1991), since when publication numbers have doubled. This chapter sets out to review the world literature on the LMA to June 1992.

ANATOMY UPDATE

The LMA was designed following anatomical studies of the cadaveric adult pharynx. When perfectly positioned, it lies with the tip resting against the upper oesophageal sphincter, the sides facing the pyriform fossae, with the upper surface behind the base of the tongue and the epiglottis pointing upwards. Fibreoptic and radiological studies have revealed that the actual position of the LMA is much more variable, but the functional result remains excellent.

Epiglottic downfolding is common and frequently blamed for poor functioning of the LMA. It has been demonstrated fibreoptically that 60% of patients have a posteriorly displaced epiglottis and 6% had a visible oesophagus. These findings have been confirmed in both anaesthetized and awake patients. The discrepancy between anatomical positioning and function is more marked in children. Rowbottom et al (1991) showed that, despite a clinically patent airway in 98%, perfect fibreoptic positioning occurred in only 49%. Brain's explanation for this is that the fibreoptic laryngoscope only offers a two-dimensional view when, in reality, gas is moving freely through the lateral spaces on either side of the mask aperture bars and therefore function is maintained.

Radiological, magnetic resonance and computed tomography studies confirm that the position of the LMA is variable and that severe malpositioning can occur in the presence of a clear airway.

Secondary to airway function, the anatomical feature of most interest is the degree of isolation the LMA provides from the gastrointestinal tract and oropharynx. In addition to demonstrating the oesophagus in visible communication with the larynx, a study using dye swallowed preinduction demonstrated regurgitation in 5 of 15 patients with the LMA, compared with none of 15 with the facemask, suggesting that the presence of the LMA may affect lower oesophageal sphincter tone (Barker et al 1991). Isolation from the oropharynx appears more reliable; the inflated cuff acts as an airtight throat pack. John et al (1991) placed dye in the upper airway of 64 patients and found no leakage.

PHYSIOLOGY UPDATE

Cardiovascular system

The LMA has minimal effect on the cardiovascular system. Comparative studies have shown that, at insertion, it produces a mild stress response compared to standard intubation and is haemodynamically comparable to insertion of a Guedel airway. This has led some authors to suggest that the LMA may be preferable to intubation in patients at risk from a marked stress response, such as those with hypertension, coronary or cerebrovascular disease. Where intubation is necessary in such high-risk cases, it may be worth considering intubation through the LMA; however, studies about the stress response to intubation through the LMA have not yet been published.

Respiratory system

The non-invasiveness of the LMA also applies to the respiratory system where it forms a highly physiological communication with the larynx. During spontaneous ventilation glottic opening and closing occur, airflow is unimpeded, the ciliary tree still functions and coughing is possible during light anaesthesia.

Intermittent positive pressure ventilation (IPPV)

Ventilation through the LMA is easily achieved in up to 98% of patients, but leaks occur between 10 and 30 cm H_2O, making the LMA unsuitable for high airway pressure ventilation, though a benefit of this is that normal patients are protected against barotrauma. During straining higher airway pressures may be achieved because the constricting pharyngeal muscles produce a tighter seal. Also there is no change in leak pressure when the head is moved. Gastric dilatation is an obvious hazard where pressures exceed upper oesophageal sphincter pressure and is a particular concern in children, although it can also occur in adults.

Gastrointestinal system

Insertion of the LMA frequently provokes a swallowing reflex, causing transient glottic closure that can be mistaken for laryngospasm and at light levels of anaesthesia or in awake patients, recurrent swallowing can occur, leading to gastric dilatation. Of greater concern is a small study by Rabey et al (1992), who, using a slow pull-through technique, suggested that lower oesophageal sphincter pressure may be reduced after insertion of the LMA. The clinical implications of this await further studies.

Intraocular pressure and bacteraemia

A study on the effects of the LMA on intraocular pressure showed that there was little increase in pressure compared with endotracheal intubation. The risk of bacteraemia occurring on insertion of the LMA is similar to that during oral intubation and is less than most reported series of nasal intubation.

INSERTION TECHNIQUES AND INDUCTION AGENTS

Insertion techniques

The standard insertion technique for the LMA has evolved through many different stages. Brain's first prototype was inserted facing backwards and then rotated through 180° (1983). Later prototypes used an introducer designed to prevent epiglottic downfolding. This was phased out in favour of a refined insertion technique and the final design was a compromise between the most efficient seal with the glottis and ease of insertion. A wide variety of alternative techniques have been described, which are perhaps best used only where the standard insertion technique fails (Table 11.1).

Successful insertion may not always be rewarded with a clear airway. Correct functional placement can be verified by observation of the reservoir bag, gentle IPPV, capnography, fibreoptic laryngoscopy and use of the oesophageal detector device. Optimal stability for the LMA can be achieved by bending the tube downward over the chin and connecting it to the anaesthetic hosing below the chin. There have been no reports of problems when inserting modifications of the LMA, but it would be surprising if insertion rates were similar to the standard model. Finally, when inserting the LMA in awake patients, asking the patient to swallow may be helpful.

Induction agents

When used for spontaneous ventilation the LMA is best inserted either immediately postinduction or when anaesthesia is deepened with a volatile

Table 11.1 Alternative insertion techniques

Technique	Notes
Back to front	Especially in children (size 2)
Partial removal and reinsertion	
Repositioning head	
Anterior traction of glottis	
Introducer	Now abandoned due to potential trauma
Laryngoscope	Controversial
Superior laryngeal nerve block	
Anteriorly deflated rim	Controversial
Partially inflated cuff	Success rate of 97%
Fully inflated cuff	
Extra mouth opening	
'Jaw jerk'	
'Twisting'	In children
Finger on postpharyngeal wall	In tonsillar hypertrophy
Anterior traction of tongue	In tonsillar hypertrophy
Lateral approach	In children

agent. It is widely believed that propofol is the induction agent of choice with the LMA because it provides more upper airway relaxation than thiopentone. However the evidence for this is limited and the outcome is dependent on the induction dose chosen and the use of additional agents. A comparative study of thiopentone 5 mg/kg, methohexitone 1.1 mg/kg and propofol 1.9 mg/kg in 50 patients found that propofol was the induction agent of choice, but no data were presented (Miranda & Reddy 1990). It has been noted, however, that thiopentone with or without opioid provided adequate conditions for insertion. Brown et al (1991) compared propofol 2.5 mg/kg and thiopentone 4 mg/kg for postinduction LMA insertion and found that propofol provided slightly better conditions; however, the use of additional agent resulted in no significant difference, suggesting that a higher-dose thiopentone might be comparable to propofol as an induction agent. Brain suggests that the induction agent of choice for insertion in children is deep volatile anaesthesia, but this is not proven.

INSERTION RATES AND LEARNING

Insertion rates

Most published studies on the LMA have quoted first-time insertion rates and their relationship to experience: 72–99% of LMAs are inserted at the first attempt, 8–14% at the second and 1–4% at the third. The time taken to insert is less widely reported, but is quoted at between 7 and 20 seconds. Anaesthetists of all grades achieve good results with minimal prior experience. Approximately 98% of cases achieve a satisfactory result within three attempts. Most first-time failures are attributed to inadequate depth of anaesthetic and poor technique; however, as with intubation, a small percentage will present as impossible.

Although Brain suggests that paediatric application demands more experience and skill, the published series do not substantiate this, first-time rates being quoted as 89% and 89.5%. However, although there are few data available, it is thought that infants under 6 months may be more difficult.

Learning

Brain considers that the learning curve is long for perfect insertion even though adequacy is rapidly acquired. It is intrinsically logical that experience should lead to more successful use of the LMA, but the high insertion rates in novices make this difficult to demonstrate. A study of 200 children, however, showed that the number of problems encountered did relate to experience (Mason & Bingham 1990) and a further study of 200 adults concluded that success rates were better after 15 insertions, but not related to the grade of anaesthetist (McCrirrick et al 1991). Additional evidence for a learning curve is provided in a study of 687 cases where more problems were encountered in the first 6 months than the second 6 months (White 1991).

Whilst the LMA is technically easy to insert at all levels of experience, knowledge about when it is appropriate to attempt insertion and recognition of insertion failure is less easily acquired. Some authors have cautioned that this apparent ease of insertion will lead to inappropriate use by junior anaesthesists for failed obstetric intubation and that the more demanding and basic skill of holding a mask and airway will be lost to trainees.

PRIMARY CARE AND RESUSCITATION

The use of the LMA for emergency medicine was first described by Brain in 1984, but there has been hesitancy in its adoption due to the risk of aspiration and problems with high airway pressure ventilation. Several reports illustrate the value of the LMA on the failed intubation trolley and it clearly has a place in the hospital setting where intubation is difficult or impossible. The unresolved controversy is its use in prehospital care. Brain believes that the LMA's primary advantage in an emergency is its speed and simplicity of insertion. Hypoxia can be rapidly corrected, thereby removing a major stimulus to regurgitation — a view shared by others.

Davies et al (1990) compared intubation with the LMA in paramedics and concluded that the LMA was inserted more rapidly, more frequently and was easier to learn, but emphasized that the ETT remains first choice in the emergency situation. Hassan et al (1990) criticize this paper. Davies et al suggested that the end-point for any trial of resuscitation should be successful ventilation, not successful insertion and establishment of spontaneous respiration. Hassan and colleagues remarked that anaesthesia does not simulate the field situation where it may be more difficult to insert an LMA.

Whilst these reservations are indeed valid, the LMA is preferable to obstruction and its hypoxic sequelae and the ability to insert an LMA where access is limited or laryngoscopy contraindicated suggests it should have a role in emergency medicine.

REFLUX AND ASPIRATION

At its inception it was hoped that the unique shape of the LMA would isolate the gastrointestinal from the respiratory tract. Brodrick et al's (1989) early series specifically mentioned no evidence of aspiration amongst 100 patients; however, Brain (White 1991) noted a case occurring in 1987 and it soon became apparent that the airway was not reliably protected.

The risk of aspiration is widely perceived as the single most limiting feature of the LMA and the majority of publications worldwide make mention of it, even without direct evidence. McCrirrick et al (1991) reported a series of 200 patients; Miranda & Reddy (1990) published a series in which patients were ventilated in a variety of postures, and Mason & Bingham (1990) report its use in 200 children, all without evidence of aspiration. Experience by Leach & Alexander (White 1991) with over 7000 cases leads them to suggest that the incidence of aspiration is very low indeed. In contrast, Wilkinson et al (1990) reported 8 cases of regurgitation from a series of 546, 2 of whom aspirated. No fatalities have been reported from pulmonary aspiration syndrome associated with the LMA. Brain has reported 4 cases of regurgitation in which no attempt was made to remove the LMA and all patients rapidly recovered; management included Trendelenburg tilt, 100% oxygen, deepening anaesthesia, suction and dexamethasone.

Of prime concern are cases of aspiration in fasted patients. Griffin & Hatcher (1990) reported aspiration pneumonia during the recovery phase after elective cholecystectomy which required intensive care unit management. In their discussion the authors draw attention to the factors making the LMA unsuitable for abdominal surgery: possible incompetence of the oesophageal sphincter; increased intragastric pressure from IPPV; and the possibility that the LMA preferentially directs regurgitated gastric contents into the trachea. There was considerable criticism of this case, condemning the use of the LMA for cholecystectomy. Brain comments that the LMA should never be removed, or the cuff deflated, until the patient is completely awake and the reflexes have returned. It is well-known that many routinely prepared patients have stomach contents that place them at risk of acid aspiration and this is more likely in patients having upper abdominal surgery.

Physiologically, vomiting differs from simple regurgitation as the glottis is closed and aspiration is less likely. Wilkinson et al (1990) have reported cases of vomiting at the end of the procedure with vomitus being noted in the anaesthetic breathing system, and they support Koehli's (1991) concern that the mask preferentially directs vomitus into the trachea. Brain contests this view. He believes that because the LMA obliterates the pharyngeal reservoir there is less fluid available to be aspirated at any one moment, and indeed fluid will often travel up the LMA tube on expiration – a valuable early sign.

A prototype of the LMA included a dorsal groove allowing the passage of regurgitated fluid, or a nasogastric tube. Brain alternatively suggested passing a lubricated ETT behind the partly deflated cuff of the LMA into the oesophagus to allow gastric drainage. It was thought that a nasogastric tube might also permit the escape of gases blown into the stomach during IPPV, but a comparative study with tracheal intubation concluded that this was not worthwhile. It is also a widely held view that a nasogastric tube is not only ineffective at emptying the stomach, but also increases the risk of aspiration by compromising the lower oesophageal sphincter.

The risk of aspiration with the LMA may not be greater than with the facemask; however, a short series by Rabey et al (1992) suggests the physical presence of the LMA may decrease oesophageal barrier pressure and this view is supported by Barker et al's (1991) studies with dye. The use of the LMA for laparoscopy has been discussed by Brimacombe & Shorney (1992a). They suggested that although the LMA offers some possible advantages, there has been no work to substantiate its use in laparoscopy and that caution is needed until such information is available. Careful selection of cases will help to preserve the reputation of the LMA: the LMA should be considered as an alternative to the facemask and never an alternative to the ETT. Wilkinson et al (1990) urge constant vigilance as, in the inexperienced user, the relative ease of maintaining an airway gives a false sense of security. The reputation of the LMA may rest on the publication of a large controlled series to determine if its physical properties increase the risk of aspiration.

OBSTETRICS

Any attempted diversion from the accepted techniques of anaesthesia for caesarean section tends to provoke polarized discussion and the role of the LMA is no exception. The earliest reference to its use in caesarean section was from Chadwick & Vohra in 1989 and, like all subsequent reports, it was used in a case of failed intubation. Tunstall (1989), in an editorial on failed intubation, sees some future for the LMA in the updated drill. De Mello (1991) has reported its routine and successful inclusion in a failed intubation kit. The LMA may have a role in obstetric anaesthesia where elective tracheostomy is the only alternative. However, there has been a report of inadequate oxygenation with an LMA after failed intubation for caesarean section.

The opponents to its use in obstetrics are primarily concerned about aspiration, whereas its proponents concentrate on the maintenance of maternal oxygenation and concurrent use of cricoid pressure. Brimacombe (1991) has shown that cricoid pressure does not prejudice ease of insertion of the mask; however, an early communication of a blind, controlled study has challenged this view and further studies are clearly needed. There have been several reports of insertion with the patient in the left lateral, head-down position with cricoid pressure applied and most authors recommend main-tainence of spontaneous ventilation in this position.

The key to any successful failed intubation drill (FID) is oxygenation without aspiration. The value of the LMA in FID, however, is controversial. Clearly if there is failure to intubate and to oxygenate then insertion of the LMA is a valid alternative.

A worst case scenario was imagined by Freeman et al (1990): they emphasized that unskilled use of the LMA is of no value in failed intubation. However, most deaths from failed intubation were from tracheal tube misplacement, not aspiration (DHSS 1991: Confidential Enquiry into Maternal Deaths in England and Wales, 1985–1987), and the appropriate use of the LMA may well have alleviated the situation.

Whether the LMA should be used to aid intubation during FID or how safe it is to proceed with an LMA and cricoid pressure is uncertain.

MANAGEMENT OF AIRWAY PROBLEMS

A key role for the LMA is in maintaining the airway where intubation has failed or facemask anaesthesia is impossible. Three cases of difficult intubation, managed with the LMA, were described by Brain in 1985 and since then its use in this area has been widely reported. Brain has suggested on anatomical grounds that there may be an inverse relationship between difficult intubation and ease of insertion of the LMA, but Frerk (1991) has emphasized that this has not been substantiated.

The use of an LMA as an aid to intubation has been reviewed by Silk (White 1991). The angle the tube enters the bowl was partly designed to allow blind tracheal intubation, which was first reported by Brain in 1984. In 1989 Chadd et al passed a gum elastic bougie (GEB) down the LMA of 2 anaesthetized patients and railroaded an ETT after removal of the LMA. Allison & McCrory (1990) then refined this and directed the bougie into the trachea under fibreoptic guidance. They reported 100% success rate for correct placement of the GEB when guided directly and 84% when passed blind. Blind passage of a bougie down the LMA was used to perform a difficult awake intubation by McCrirrick & Pracilio (1991) and this technique has been updated using a hollow bougie-like introducer. Health & Allagain (1991) found that 90% of patients could be intubated blindly with a 6 mm cuffed tube through an LMA. This success rate was reduced to 56% by the application of cricoid pressure, which has the effect of tipping the laryngeal inlet anteriorly, thus making the angle of approach more difficult (Brimacombe 1991). Heath & Allagain's paper has been criticized by Frerk (1991) who argued that since this research was performed on normal patients, it didn't necessarily apply to patients who would be difficult to intubate. Rowbottom et al (1991) have advised caution with blind intubation techniques in children where fibreoptic positioning is more variable, but this technique has been used successfully with a success rate similar to adults.

A number of other aids and modifications have been described to help intubation through the LMA. A modified split LMA can act as a guide for the fibreoptic scope so that direct railroading of a large ETT can be performed. A rectal tube railroaded over the fibreoptic scope can act as a bougie whilst allowing oxygenation. Also a nasogastric tube plus oesophageal detector device has been used to confirm tracheal placement. Finally a prototype large-bore LMA is being developed which will allow the passage of a size 8 ETT.

EAR, NOSE AND THROAT/HEAD AND NECK SURGERY

The LMA has gained a place in anaesthesia for ear, nose and throat (ENT) and head and neck surgery, both electively and where distorted anatomy makes tracheal intubation difficult. In 1989, Alexander & Leach reported its use for ENT procedures. The benefits of the LMA are recognized as the avoidance of intubation, a clear intraoperative airway and a quiet recovery period with an absence of coughing and stridor. Although airway and surgical access are usually adequate, some restrictions can occur, most notably tube compression by a tonsillar gag. The satisfactory use of a flexometallic modification has been described to overcome this problem.

John et al (1991) showed that the LMA cuff forms an adequate seal across the pharynx to protect the airway from blood and secretions. They injected methylene blue into the pharynx of 64 adults breathing spontaneously and no evidence of dye in the larynx was seen in any case. Some authors however have found blood clots on the underside of the LMA following oropharyngeal procedures, which suggests a pack is advisable when practical.

Johnston et al (1990) in a series of 48 children for otological procedures concluded that the LMA was a safe and effective technique, providing a better airway than a mask during head-turning and for long procedures.

Insertion difficulty may be encountered in patients with tonsillar hypertrophy and the following manoeuvres have been suggested to overcome this: an antisialagogue, adequate head extension, a lateral approach, a guiding finger on the posterior pharyngeal wall, anterior traction of the tongue and the use of a laryngoscope.

DENTAL AND FACIOMAXILLARY SURGERY

The LMA has achieved wide acceptance for minor oral surgery. Young (White 1991) in a recent review outlined the advantages of the LMA over the nasal mask for oral surgery:

1. ease of airway maintenance;
2. the insertion of a pharyngeal, rather than an oral pack;
3. a smooth wake-up for the patient with continuous airway protection from debris after the removal of the pack.

Bailie et al (1991) compared the use of the LMA with the nasal mask in 50 children. The LMA group had fewer hypoxic episodes and there was no significant difference with regard to access or ease of surgery. Noble & Wooller (1991) have reported the use of the LMA in dental chair anaesthesia. They found it an excellent alternative to the nasal mask with an easier airway and better protection of the pharynx from debris.

There is some concern over restricted surgical access, but for minor procedures, this is not a significant problem. However, the LMA may require positional adjustment during the procedure, making a hands-on technique preferable. Respiratory obstruction can still occur, most notably when the mandible is depressed, but this is usually only a transient occurrence. Most studies suggest that although surgical time is slightly prolonged, anaesthetic time is shortened and no overall time loss occurs. Where airway maintenance is difficult with a nasal mask, or the passage of a nasotracheal tube is undesirable, as in day surgery units, the LMA offers an excellent alternative for minor cases, but for the more difficult case where perfect oral access is required, the nasal ETT should still be preferred to the oral LMA.

In case of faciomaxillary surgery where intubation may be difficult, the LMA is a useful alternative and it has been successfully used in a case of bilateral mandibular fractures.

RECOVERY

Brain recommends that the LMA should be left in situ until the full recovery of pharyngeal reflexes, when it should be removed with the cuff inflated. Patients will often determine this end-point by removing the mask themselves. Some reports, however, suggest the patients are more at risk of complications during recovery with the LMA in situ. Wilkinson et al (1990) report a case of laryngeal stridor during recovery where it was considered that the LMA held secretions on to the larynx. Others have reported cases where the patient has vomited during emergence in the supine position. Koehli (1991), while reporting a case of aspiration with the LMA, raises two points of practice with regards to position: firstly, that due to the secure airway and the fear of dislodging it, patients tend to be transferred to recovery in the supine position and, secondly, that since gastric contents are prevented from escaping via the pharynx, one key advantage of the lateral position is negated. He argues that since the LMA preferentially directs gastric contents into the trachea – a point disputed by Brain – it may be better to remove the LMA while the patient is still deeply anaesthetized and transfer the patients in the lateral position. Brain points out that high intraabdominal pressure generated by moving the partially anaesthetized patient may provoke regurgitation – a problem that is avoided if the patient is transferred whilst still deeply anaesthetized.

Kumar (1990) reported the use of the LMA for inadequate reversal and suggested its appropriateness in the partially reversed, semiawake patient in respiratory distress, thus avoiding further drugs and reintubation.

PAEDIATRICS

The earliest report of the LMA's use in children was in 1988 when prototypes were successfully used for juvenile chronic arthritis. In 1989, Beveridge reported its use in an unintubatable case of Pierre Robin syndrome requiring cleft-palate surgery.

The paediatric LMAs are scaled-down versions of the adult model and therefore difficulties in its use in children might be expected. In fact the incidence of clinical problems is similar to adults, despite more variable fibreoptic placement. In an early series Mason & Bingham (1990) reported a clear airway in 178 out of 200 cases and recommended using an antisiala-gogue. Similar success has been reported for dental outpatients.

Infants and neonates

In their series of 200 children, Fawcett et al (1991) included 9 children younger than 6 months and they found airway patency was clear in only 6 cases. No problems were associated with gentle hand ventilation, although Brain does not recommend this in children due to the risk of gastric distention. There have been limited reports of its usage in neonates: Denny et al (1990) have recorded the resuscitation of a 2.75 kg Pierre Robin girl at birth, but its role in this area remains ill-defined.

A particular application in children is for remote and repeat anaesthesia where intubation may be avoided. Several authors have reported its successful use in children undergoing repeat anaesthesia for radiotherapy. Considerable vigilance must be maintained during such procedures. A size 2 LMA was noted incidentally to kink on the computed tomography scan and there has been a report of pharyngeal wall trauma after 14 anaesthetics for cranial irradiation. It might be wise to inspect the pharynx regularly to avoid problems.

PROLONGED USE, INTENSIVE CARE AND CORONARY ARTERY BYPASS GRAFTING

Prolonged use

No series about the prolonged use of the LMA have been published, but procedures lasting from 6 to 7 hours, using both spontaneous ventilation and IPPV, have been incidentally reported and no technique-related problems have been noted. Intubation and ventilation have always been the favoured technique for very long procedures, but it has been pointed out that there is no evidence that prolonged anaesthesia with the LMA is contraindicated and the advantages it offers may lead to an alteration of basic teaching in certain circumstances. Possible problems to consider, however, are pharyngeal trauma, respiratory fatigue and an increased risk of aspiration, particularly where IPPV is used. Brimacombe & Shorney (1992b) reported an 8-hour procedure in which a patient spontaneously ventilated through an LMA as part of a balanced regional anaesthetic. They found no changes in respiratory function or evidence of fatigue using an extensometer and no macroscopic pharyngeal trauma. They suggest such techniques are valid, but recommend rigorous monitoring of respiratory function whenever they are applied. Using indirect stroboscopic laryngoscopy, it has been shown that the incidence of pharyngeal erythema and wave irregularity was 27.3% and 9.1% respectively, 18–24 hours postoperatively, following routine use in singers. It has also been shown that the size 4 LMA exerts a substantial pressure on the pharyngeal mucosa which decreases with time. The clinical implications of these latter findings are unclear.

Intensive care

The role of the LMA in intensive care is also unclear and is probably limited to areas such as weaning or the short-term delivery of continuous positive airway pressure. Its use in the intensive care unit has only been reported once, in an alcohol-intoxicated patient, who was too deeply anaethetized to maintain an airway and yet too lightly anaestheized to tolerate an ETT. Theoretical advantages for the LMA are that it may be better tolerated than an ETT and could allow more normal cardiorespiratory physiology to be maintained during spontaneous ventilation. However, it is more difficult to secure, does not reliably protect the lungs and high airway pressures cannot be achieved. In addition information about the effects of prolonged insertion on the pharynx and patient tolerance is lacking.

Coronary artery bypass grafting (CABG)

The LMA was resorted to for a CABG procedure by White et al in 1991 when intubation was impossible. They removed the LMA shortly after the end of the operation. Foster & Clowes (1991), however, in a similar case, chose to perform a tracheostomy rather than using an LMA in the intensive care unit, but such management has been questioned. Although it seems doubtful that the LMA has a use in elective CABG, the haemodynamic stability it offers at induction may provide it with a role in certain subgroups.

USE IN AWAKE PATIENTS, LARYNGOSCOPY AND BRONCHOSCOPY

Awake

Insertion of the LMA under anaethesia is considerably less stimulating than endotracheal intubation and this has led to an interest in its insertion in awake patients. Brain (White 1991) was probably the first person to self-insert the LMA under local anaesthesia, but others have also reported performing this impressive feat. McCrirrick & Pracilio (1991) were the first to report its use in an awake patient, in whom they used it as an aid to intubation. Subsequently Brimacombe (1992) reported its use in an awake patient with stridor.

Laryngoscopy

The dynamic view of the larynx afforded by the LMA has led to its use in thyroid surgery for the prevention of recurrent laryngeal nerve injury;

however, others have urged caution when used in this area since sudden loss of the airway can occur and rapid correction of problems may be difficult. It has also had some limited use in microlaryngeal surgery where it may become more popular when a larger-bore LMA is available.

Bronchoscopy

The LMA and the flexible bronchoscope can assist not only in the diagnosis of laryngeal and bronchial pathology, but also in its subsequent management. Bronchoscopy can be performed down the LMA in both awake and anaesthetized patients and its use has also been reported in children. The advantages of the LMA for these procedures are listed in Table 11.2. Brimacombe et al (1992) have studied the use of the LMA for awake diagnostic bronchoscopy in 50 patients. They state that it may have a role where respiratory function is critical, but recommend training in insertion under anaesthesia before adopting this technique in awake patients. Insertion rates and fibreoptic positioning were the same as for general anaesthesia. They encountered some minor problems such as recurrent swallowing (18%), but these were easily overcome with adequate sedation and topical anaesthesia.

EQUIPMENT AND MODIFICATIONS

Modifications

Brain has remarked that many specialized forms of the LMA should be possible. Two modifications for ENT/dental anaesthesia have already been described where a proportion of the tube is replaced with armoured tubing. Brain (White 1991) has described the development of an LMA that can be used nasally and a large-bore LMA which will accommodate a size 8 ETT.

Accessory equipment

As well as modifications to the LMA, many items of accessory equipment have been described to aid in its use (Table 11.3). The introducer, originally

Table 11.2 Advantages of the laryngeal mask airway for bronchoscopy

Easy to insert
Permits close respiratory monitoring
Can be performed in awake and anaesthetized patients
Facilitates administration of anaesthesia
Facilitates administration of 100% oxygen
Facilitates administration of continuous positive airway pressure intermittent positive pressure ventilation
Large internal diameter enables use of larger instruments
Avoids intubation
Easy intubation with bronchoscope
Allows laryngoscopy

designed to aid insertion and prevent epiglottic trapping, is no longer recommended because of the potential for trauma. A combination of two Portex swivel connecters has been suggested to provide flexible connections to the anaesthetic breathing system. A bite guard and holder have been described. Supplementary oxygen for recovery can be given using a Venturi T-piece system, a modified Brain circuit, a Portex thermovent T, or an open-ended T-piece.

COMPLICATIONS

Although problems associated with the LMA are uncommon and for the most part easily overcome, a number of major and minor complications have been described, many of which can be attributed to inappropriate use (Table 11.4). Major complications include aspiration, which is rare but potentially lethal, and has been discussed elsewhere in this chapter. Airway obstruction is also lethal where it goes unrecognized and may be due to gross malpositioning, epiglottic downfolding or forward displacement of the postcricoid area. Other causes of obstruction are cuff overinflation, increased cuff volume due to warming and nitrous oxide, kinking of the tube due to a taut pilot tube and the presence of a foreign body. The manufacturer now advocates checking for foreign bodies routinely before use of the LMA. Other complications include: coughing, laryngospasm, excessive salivation, retching, vomiting, biting, breath holding, recurrent swallowing and pharyngeal bleeding. Postoperatively hoarseness, dry mouth, dysphagia and sore throat have been reported. The incidence of sore throat is between 4 and 12%, but this is usually mild. The incidence may be higher following head-turning, although this has been contested.

Table 11.3 Modifications and accessory equipment to the laryngeal mask airway (LMA)

Modification or accessory	Notes
All armoured tube	For ENT
Partially armoured tube	For ENT
Nasal LMA	Under development
Split LMA	Aid to intubation
Rectal tube	Aid to intubation
Large-bore LMA	Aid to intubation and microlaryngoscopy (under development)
Reinforced size 2	Prevent kinking
Introducer	Now obsolete
Bite guard	
LMA holder	
Two swivel connectors	Link to circuit
T-piece	Supplementary oxygen
Modified Brain circuit	Supplementary oxygen
Portex thermovent-T	Supplementary oxygen
Open-ended T-piece	Supplementary oxygen

Table 11.4 Complications associated with the laryngeal mask airway

Complication	Notes
Airway obstruction	Partial and complete
Aspiration	Rare—2/546–0/7000
Biting	Common on emergence
Breath holding	Uncommon in adults
Coughing	Inadequate anaesthetic
Dry mouth	Uncommon
Dysphagia	Uncommon
Epiglottic trapping	
Excessive salivation	
Gastric dilatation	Mostly from intermittent positive pressure ventilation
Hoarseness	Uncommon
Laryngospasm	1–3% often misdiagnosed
Recurrent swallowing	In awake or light anaesthesia
Retching	
Sore Throat	4–12%—mild
Stridor	Rare
Trauma	Tonsils, pharynx, uvula, epiglottis
Vomiting	

Transient reflex glottic closure on induction can often be misdiagnosed as laryngospasm. It may occur if anaesthetic depth is insufficient and no doubt the tip of LMA can occasionally rest against the laryngeal inlet (White 1991). The reported incidence of laryngospasm is 1–3% and has been noted at both induction and education. Interestingly, the LMA has also been used in the treatment of laryngospasm.

Trauma can also occur to the uvula and the tonsils. Posterior pharyngeal wall trauma has been reported after repeat anaesthesia with the LMA. Epiglottic trapping in the mask aperture bars has also been reported. Stridor has been noted on removal of the LMA in 2 patitents with Chronic obstructive airways disease (COAD).

Mechanical problems with the LMA

The mean life expectancy of an LMA is approximately 200 uses. There are few reports of unexpected mechanical problems; however, kinking with a size 2 has been reported, since when the tubes have been strengthened by the manufacturer. The separation of a 2-month-old LMA into two pieces on removal from a patient has been reported; this was attributed to severe heat ageing by the manufacturer, who noted no other similar occurrences in over 200 000 uses worldwide.

MISCELLANEOUS

Respiratory disease

There has, been some opposition to the use of the LMA in patients with respiratory problems, but Brain emphasizes the need for adequate anaesthetic depth, not abandonment of the LMA; this leaves the ciliary tree intact and permits a smooth emergence. Indeed there are anecdotal reports that the LMA may be better than the ETT with regard to lung function in patients with respiratory impairment (White 1991, Brimacombe & Shorney 1992b), but this has not been substantiated.

Obesity

In an instruction manual, Brain (1991) suggests that the LMA is suitable for patients who are moderately obese, provided care is taken to ensure adequate anaesthetic depth for both insertion and maintenance and that measures are taken to ensure the stomach is empty in all cases. A size 4 LMA is probably suitable for both sexes, but the LMA is not recommended for severe or morbid obesity. There have been no studies about the use of the LMA in obesity.

Stridor

The use of the LMA in the assessment and management of stridor has been described by McNamee et al (1991) and Brimacombe (1992). The LMA allows adequate oxygenation whilst the obstruction is assessed fibreoptically; it can be inserted under either local or general anaesthesia, and it can act as a guide to intubation enabling the airway to be secured for other management strategies. Its use for elective surgery in a child with tracheal stenosis has been reported where minimal interference with airflow and lack of further tracheal damage is essential.

Others

The LMA may be the airway of choice for a great variety of procedures where a secure, non-invasive airway is required. Its use has been described for repeat computed tomography radiotherapy, nuclear magnetic resonance, facial burns, foramen ovale electroencephalograms, laser treatment for portwine stains and eye surgery. Finally it has been shown that the LMA results in minimal theatre pollution during spontaneous ventilation.

CONCLUSIONS

It is over a decade since Brain invented the laryngeal mask airway. Following a rather subdued introduction into anaesthetic practice the LMA has become very successful worldwide. Many of its applications have already been explored, but considerable work remains to consolidate these findings and allow more precise delineation of the role of the LMA in specific areas such as resuscitation, obstetrics and intensive care.

It remains to be seen if this remarkably practical invention can evolve into an ultimate LMA — offering the advantages of a clear non-invasive airway and protection from aspiration.

REFERENCES

Alexander C A, Leach A B 1989 The laryngeal mask — experience of its use in a district general hospital. Today's Anaesthetist 4: 200–205

Allison A, McCrory J 1990 Tracheal placement of a gum elastic bougie using the laryngeal mask airway. Anaesthesia 45: 419–420

Bailie R, Barnett M B, Fraser J F 1991 The Brain laryngeal mask — a comparative study with the nasal mask in paediatric dental outpatient. Anaesthesia 46: 358–360

Barker P, Murphy P, Langton J A, Rowbotham D 1991 Regurgitation of gastric contents during general anaesthesia using the laryngeal mask airway. Br J Anaesth 65: 660P

Beveridge M E 1989 Laryngeal mask repair of cleft palate. Anaesthesia 44: 653–657

Brain A I J 1983 The laryngeal mask — a new concept in airway management. Br J Anaesth 55: 801

Brain A I J 1984 The laryngeal mask airway — a possible new solution to airway problems in the emergency situation. Arch Emergency Med 1: 229–232

Brain A I J 1985 Three cases of difficult intubation overcome by the laryngeal mask airway. Anaesthesia 40: 353–355

Brain A I J 1991 The Intravent laryngeal mask instruction manual (2nd ed.). Intravent

Brimacombe J 1991 Cricoid pressure and the laryngeal mask airway. Anaesthesia 46: 986–987

Brimacombe J 1992 The laryngeal mask airway — use in the management of stridor. Anaesth Intensive Care 20: 117–118

Brimacombe J, Shorney N 1992a Laparoscopy and the laryngeal mask airway? Anaesth Intensive Care 20: 245

Brimacombe J, Shorney N 1992b The use of the laryngeal mask airway for prolonged anaesthesia. Can J Anaesth (in press)

Brimacombe J, Newell S, Swainston R, Thompson J 1992 A possible new technique for awake diagnostic bronchoscopy. Med J Aust 156: 876–877

Brodrick P M, Webster N R, Nunn J F 1989 The laryngeal mask airway — a study of 100 patients during spontaneous ventilation. Anaesthesia 44: 238–241

Brown G W, Patel N, Ellis F R 1991 Comparison of propofol and thiopentone for laryngeal mask insertion. Anaesthesia 46: 771–772

Chadd G D, Ackers J W L, Bailey P M 1989 Difficult intubation and the laryngeal mask airway. Anaesthesia 44: 1015

Chadwick L S, Vohra A 1989 Anaesthesia for emergency caesarean section using the Brain laryngeal mask airway. Anaesthesia 44: 261–262

Davies P R F, Tighe S Q M, Greenslade G L, Evans G H 1990 Laryngeal mask airway insertion and tracheal tube insertion by unskilled personnel. Lancet 336: 977–979

de Mello W F 1991 Management of failed endotracheal intubation at caesarean section. Anaesth Intensive Care 19: 303–304

Denny N M, Desilva K D, Webber P A 1990 Laryngeal mask airway for emergency tracheostomy in a neonate. Anaesthesia 45: 895

DHSS 1991 Report on confidential enquiries into maternal deaths in England and Wales 1985–1987. HMSO, London

Fawcett W J, Ravilia A, Radford P 1991 The laryngeal mask airway in children. Can J Anaesth 38: 685–686

Foster S J, Clowes N W B 1991 Laryngeal mask airway for coronary artery bypass grafting. Anaesthesia 46: 701

Freeman R, Baxendale B, McClune S, Moore J A 1990 Laryngeal mask airway for Caesarean section. Anaesthesia 45: 1094–1095

Frerk C M 1991 Intubation through the laryngeal mask. Anaesthesia 46: 985–986

Griffin R M, Hatcher I S 1990 Aspiration pneumonia and the laryngeal mask airway. Anaesthesia 45: 1039–1040

Hassan T B, Mowbray M J, Gevirtz C 1990 The laryngeal mask airway Lancet 336: 1329–1330

Heath M L, Allagain J 1991 Intubation through the laryngeal mask. Anaesthesia 46: 545–548

John R E, Hill S, Hughes T J 1991 Airway protection by the laryngeal mask. Anaesthesia 46: 366–367

Johnston D F, Wrigley S R, Robb P J, Jones H E 1990 The laryngeal mask airway in paediatric anaesthesia. Anaesthesia 45: 924–927

Koehli N 1991 Aspiration and the laryngeal mask airway. Anaesthesia 46: 419

Kumar C M 1990 Laryngeal mask airway for inadequate reversal. Anaesthesia 45: 792

McCrirrick A, Pracilio J A 1991 Awake intubation: a new technique. Anaesthesia 46: 661–663

McCrirrick A, Ramage D T O, Pracilio J A, Hickman J A 1991 Experience with the laryngeal mask airway in two hundred patients. Anaesth Intensive Care 19: 256–260

McNamee C J, Meyns B, Pagliero K M 1991 Flexible bronchoscopy via the laryngeal mask: a new technique. Thorax 46: 141–142

Mason D G, Bingham R M 1990 The laryngeal mask airway in children. Anaesthesia 45: 661–663

Miranda A F, Reddy V G 1990 Controlled ventilation with Brain laryngeal mask. Med J Malaysia 45: 65–69

Noble H, Wooller D J 1991 Laryngeal masks and chair dental anaesthesia. Anaesthesia 46: 591

Rabey P G, Murphy P J, Langton J A et al 1992 The effect of the laryngeal mask airway on the lower oesophageal sphincter during anaesthesia. Br J Anaesth — Abstracts 68: 440P

Rowbottom S J, Simpson D L, Grubb D 1991 The laryngeal mask airway in children — a fibreoptic assessment of posioning. Anaesthesia 46: 489–491

Tunstall M E 1989 Failed intubation in the parturient. Can J Anaesth 36: 611–613

White A, Sinclair M, Pillai R 1991 Laryngeal mask airway for coronary artery bypass grafting. Anaesthesia 46: 234

White D C (ed) 1991 The laryngeal mask airway. Eur J Anaesth 4: (suppl) 1–59

Wilkinson P, Cyna A M, Macleod D M et al, 1990 The laryngeal mask: cautionary tales. Anaesthesia 45: 167–168

12. Control of gas flow into anaesthetic apparatus

D. C. White

In the very earliest anaesthetic apparatus such as Morton's ether inhaler and its various successors air was the only gas employed other than anaesthetic vapour. When nitrous oxide came into widespread use it was chiefly for very brief dental procedures and was administered unmixed with other gases. Nitrous oxide compressed into metal cylinders became available in London in 1868 (Duncum 1947) and was administered via various forms of the 'two-way stopcock' which in many cases allowed the anaesthetist to admit variable amounts of air as well as nitrous oxide. Nevertheless, to judge from the articles written at that time, it was not customary to administer anything other than 100% nitrous oxide or air.

The extensive researches of Paul Bert showed the value of combining variable amounts of oxygen with nitrous oxide and focused attention on the importance of the proportioning of anaesthetic gas mixtures. Frederic Hewitt started to study the use of nitrous oxide/oxygen mixtures in 1886 and in a paper (Hewitt 1894) he describes the last of a series of 13 machines for nitrous oxide/oxygen anaesthesia. This apparatus, shown in Figure 12.1, has separate oxygen and nitrous oxide cylinders both controlled by a foot key (two nitrous oxide and one oxygen) connected by a coaxial tube to a double bag. The bag has a central partition. Keeping the two halves of the bag equally distended helped to ensure equal pressures at the mixing stopcock. This stopcock (Fig. 12.1B) had wide bore entrance and exit ports and a mixing control which could admit air to the mixing chamber, or alternatively, nitrous oxide to which could be added a controllable amount of oxygen. The further the control lever was turned the greater the number of small holes that were exposed, thus admitting more oxygen to the mixing chamber. Not shown in Figure 12.1 are the check valves in the gas inlet ports which, together with the overflow valve mounted on the outlet port from the stopcock, prevent rebreathing and make this the first in the line of intermittent flow machines which have been so widely used for dental anaesthesia.

Following Alfred Coleman's paper to the Society of Anaesthetists in 1898 the use of the nasal route for the administration of nitrous oxide became widespread for dental anaesthesia. This technique necessitated the gas coming from the machine at above atmospheric pressure, which 'was found to disturb excessively the proportion of oxygen in the mixture' (Thomas 1975). This

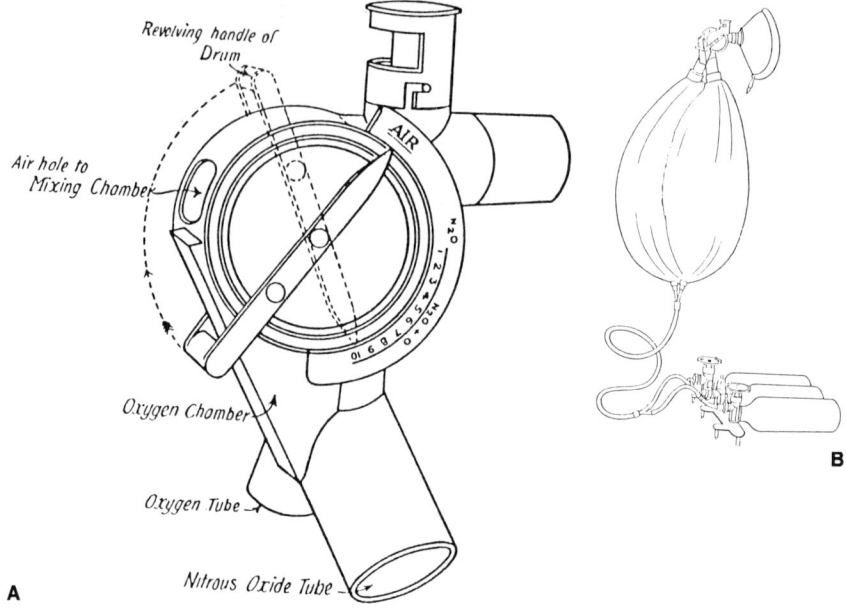

Fig. 12.1 **A** Hewitt's nitrous oxide/oxygen apparatus (1894). **B** mixture regulating stopcock.

was due, at least in part, to the difficulty of equalizing pressures at the gas inlet ports. This problem was not solved until Goodman Levy modified the apparatus by putting the oxygen bag inside the nitrous oxide bag.

The next development in the control of gas mixtures was perhaps the most important one of all. It was the introduction of a flow meter incorporated in an apparatus for nitrous oxide–oxygen–ether anaesthesia by Cotton and Boothby (1912). The use of the Rotameter in anaesthesia probably preceded this event (see below). The water sight-feed flow meter or 'bubble bottle' was a relatively crude device which nevertheless gave a quantitative indication of the passage of gas. Figure 12.2 shows such a meter for three gases. The gas flows down the perforated tubes; the higher the gas flow the more holes it can be seen to escape from. The escaping gas is led away from the top of the bottle. Such meters require individual calibration for each gas but as with all gas flow meters this can be quite easily done with a stop watch and a gas volume measuring device such as a spirometer. These meters were usually made (in the UK) with 6 holes corresponding to flows of 2, 4, 6, 8, 10 and 12 litres. Tests on a meter of this sort showed it to be remarkably accurate and therefore adequate for many, if not all, clinical purposes (Ward 1985).

Water sight-feed meters are not suitable for high gas flows because of foaming of the water; the meter shown has a nitrous oxide bypass fitted for use when a high flow of this gas is needed. In some cases water sight-feed meters were heated in order to warm the inspired gases. A further refinement was to place the perforated tube at an angle in the bottle so that the chain of bubbles

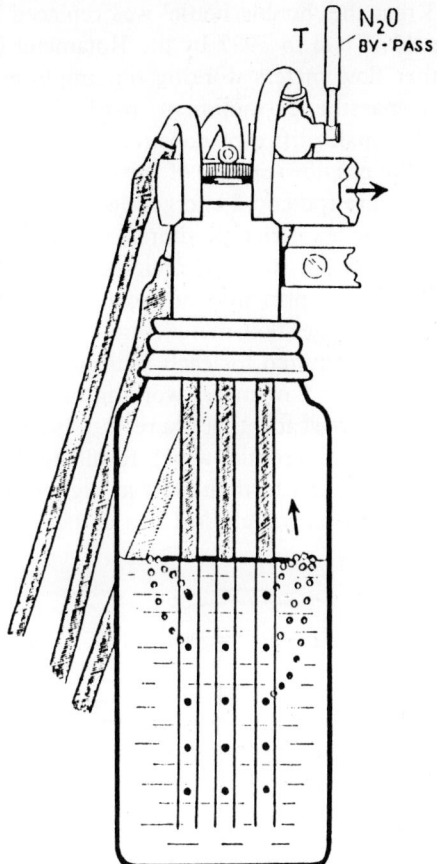

Fig. 12.2 Water sight-feed meter bottle for three gases.

emerging from each individual hole could be seen more easily. A meter incorporating this principle is seen in Figure 12.7. The flow of gas to these meters was at first controlled by needle valves attached directly to the gas cylinders. Reducing valves were available in connection with gas lighting and heating, welding, etc as early as the 1820s, but do not seem to have been applied to anaesthetic equipment until the beginning of the twentieth century. Jay Heidbrink is credited with their introduction in 1912 (Thomas 1975). The original Gwathmey apparatus (1912) did not have reducing valves but the first Boyle's machine (1917) did. Precision in the adjustment of flow meters was unlikely before reducing valves became available.

The introduction of the water sight-feed meter was a major step in the evolution of the modern anaesthetic machine because for the first time the (fairly) accurate proportioning of gas mixtures became possible.

In the UK the water sight-feed meter continued in use for many years. In the chronological series of Boyle's machine in the Charles King collection it was not until 1933 that the 'bubble bottle' was replaced by the Coxeter dry bobbin meter (Fig. 12.3) and in 1937 by the Rotameter (see below).

A number of other flow meters working on simple principles have been sucessfully used in anaesthetic equipment, particularly in the USA. If an obstruction such as a small orifice or constriction is placed in a gas stream then the velocity of the gas downstream of the obstruction (kinetic energy) is increased and the pressure (potential energy) decreased. Measurement of the pressure drop across the constriction therefore gives a measure of flow. Measurement of the pressure drop is straightforward (Figure. 12.4A, B). Figure 12.4B illustrates the principle of the water depression flow meter which was used in the Foregger flow meter (Fig. 12.5A, B). In this flow meter a separate constriction is required for each indicator tube.

The use of an orifice in a flow meter working on the principle described above suffers from the drawback that there is a square root relationship between flow and pressure differential which results in the graduations being close together at low flows and further apart at higher flows. This is clearly the least satisfactory situation for clinical use and is a consequence of the

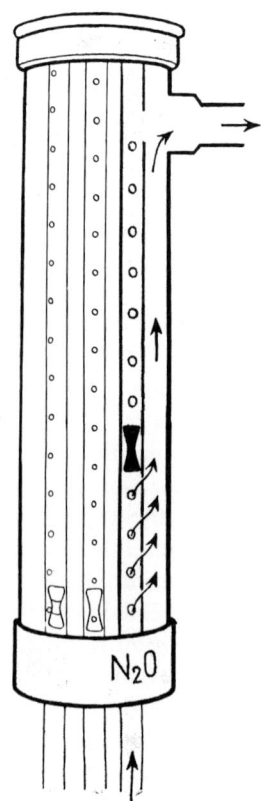

Fig. 12.3 Coxeter dry bobbin meter.

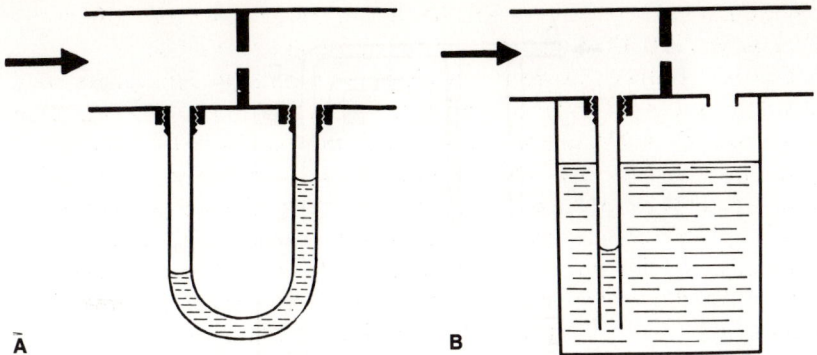

Fig. 12.4 **A** Orifice with U tube. **B** Water depression meter.

flow through the orifice being turbulent in nature. If a capillary tube is substituted for the orifice then flow through it is laminar (up to a certain level) and the calibration becomes more nearly linear. Figure 12.6 illustrates a water depression meter using two capillaries and having two ranges (Pask 1940). Meters of this sort which make use of capillaries are governed by Poiseuille's Law so that the calibration is affected by very small changes in capillary diameter. Figure 12.7 illustrates an unusual flow meter using a water sight-feed meter for oxygen and a water depression tube for nitrous oxide. It was fitted to Magill's endotracheal apparatus of 1927 (Charles King collection).

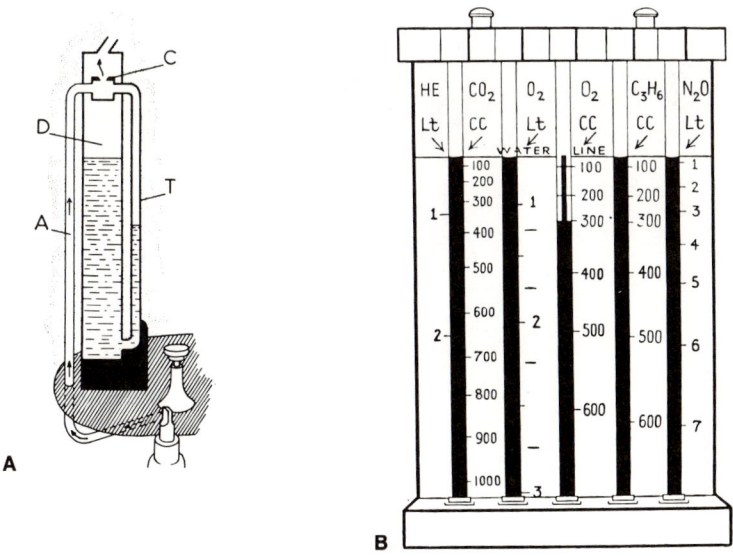

Fig. 12.5 Foregger flow meters: **A** Cross section of block (A = gas from control valve, C = orifice, D = mixing chamber, T = gauge tube. **B** front view.

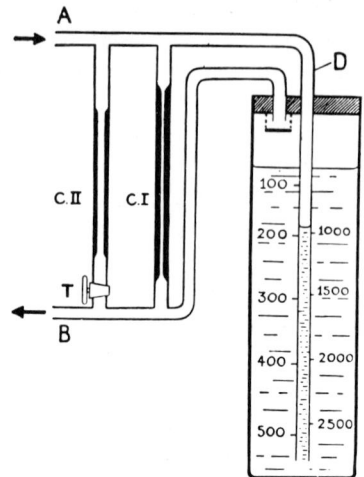

Fig. 12.6 Pask's low flow water depression meter (1940).

The pressure drop across both orifices and capillaries is high and one way of reducing this is to use a laminar flow element (LFE) instead of an orifice. An LFE is a bundle of capillary tubes through which the gas flow is linear even though the flow upstream may be turbulent. Because the pressure drop across the LFE is low it is desirable to use a more sensitive differential pressure transducer than a water-filled U tube.

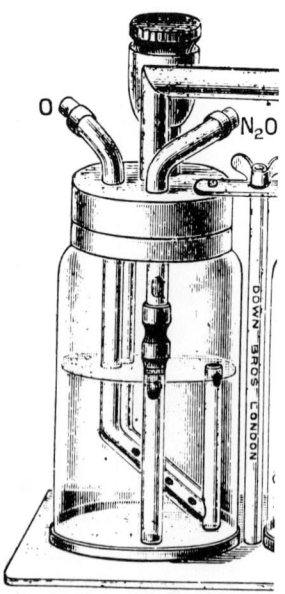

Fig. 12.7 Combined water sight-feed (O_2) and water depression (N_2O) meter (1927).

The flow meters described above, together with similar meters employing Venturi tubes, nozzles, etc. are together classified as variable pressure fixed orifice devices. They contrast with constant pressure–variable area devices in which the pressure drop is kept constant by varying the area of the obstruction to the gas flow. In meters of this type a bobbin or other occluding object lies within a tapered tube up which the gas passes. The bobbin is forced up the tube by the gas which passses around the bobbin. The 'orifice' is therefore the space around the bobbin, between it and the wall of the tapered flow tube. The pressure drop is generated by the weight of the bobbin. An example of a variable area flow meter was the Connell meter (Figure. 12.8) in which the tapered low tube was mounted in an inclined manner and the 'float' consisted of a pair of ballbearings. This gave a more stable reading than a single ball. The reading was taken at the point of contact between the two balls. Another variable area flow meter was the Heidbrink meter illustrated in Figure 12.9. As can be seen from the scales of both the Connell and Heidbrink meters a complex taper was employed in both so that they were capable of reading both low and high flows.

The Rotameter, the patent for which was applied for in 1908, is a variable area meter distinguished by the presence of small channels or vanes placed obliquely round the rim of the bobbin so that when it is pushed up by the gas stream the bobbin rotates. In other variable area meters the bobbin or ball can give a false reading if it sticks in the flow tube (usually from dirt or static charges in the tube). This rotation gives visual evidence of the passage of gas and it is this assurance which is the feature chiefly responsible for the

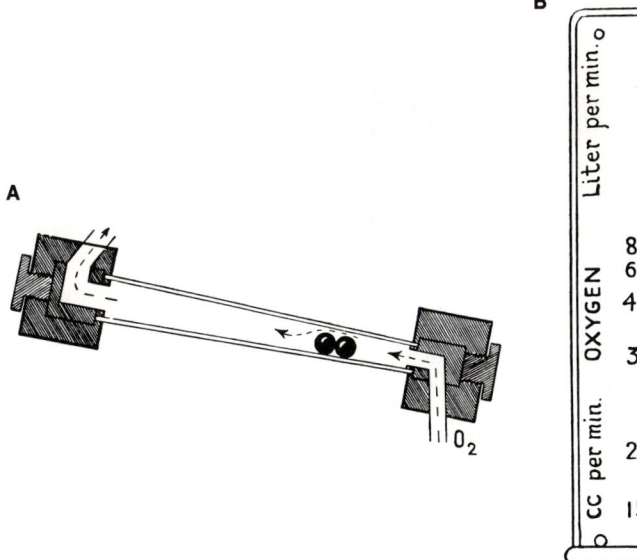

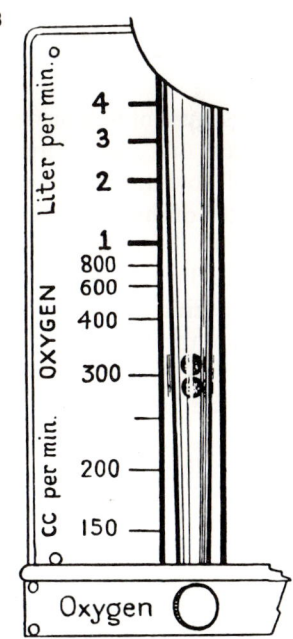

Fig. 12.8   A & B Connell inclined plane meter.

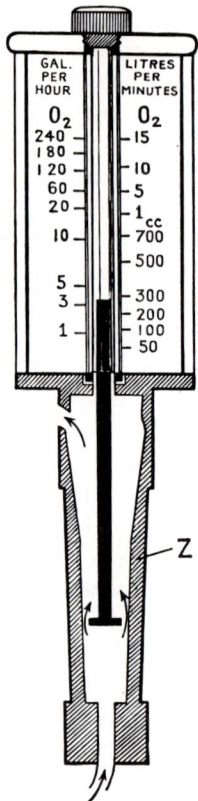

Fig. 12.9   Heidbrink meter.

universal use of Rotameters in modern anaesthetic equipment. So universal is their use that many current anaesthetic textbooks do not refer to any other type of flow meter. Figure 12.10 is a useful illustration showing clearly the principle of the Rotameter. Figure 12.10A shows the bobbin within the flow tube with the vanes around the rim of the bobbin. Figure 12.10B shows the pressure drop across the bobbin when the top of the bobbin (from which the scale reading is made) indicates 3. Figure 12.10C shows that when the gas flow rate through the tube has nearly trebled (to 8) the pressure drop across the bobbin remains the same. Since the tube is tapered, the higher up the tube the bobbin lies the greater is the space between the bobbin and the tube wall permitting gas to pass.

When the bobbin is near the bottom of the tube the constriction through which the gas passes resembles a tube rather than an orifice. This is because its length (the depth of the rim of the bobbin) is greater than its diameter. The space between the rim of the bobbin and the flow tube wall is actually an annulus so it is more accurate to refer to the area of this annulus as if it was a circle rather than an annulus.

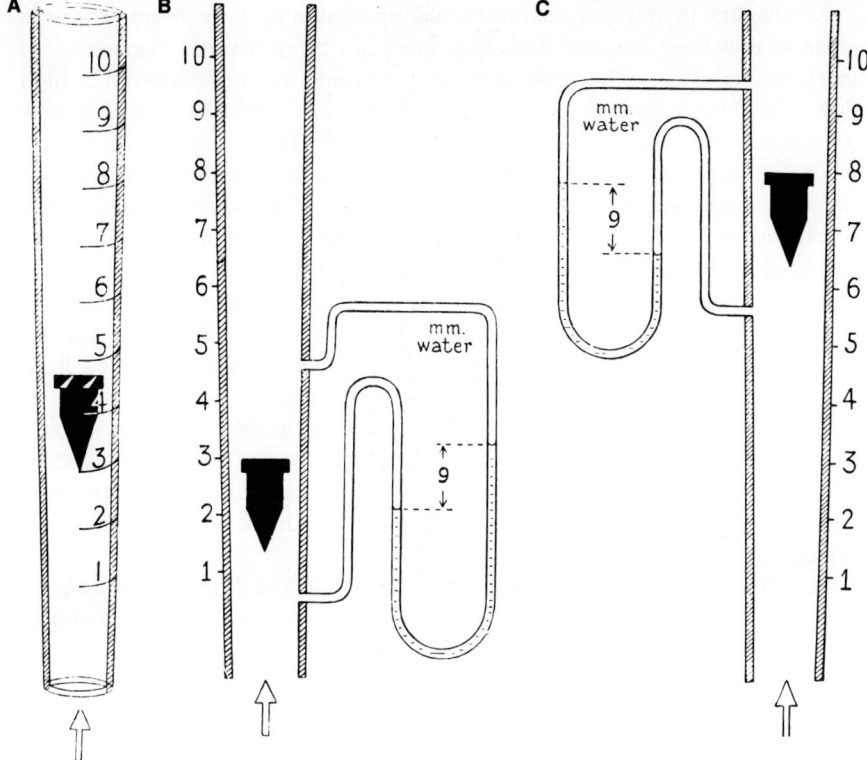

Fig. 12.10 A, B & C Rotameter (see text). Reproduced with permission from Macintosh RR, Muslin W W, Epstein H G 1963 Physics for the anaesthetist 3rd edition. Blackwell Scientific Publications, Oxford.

When the bobbin is near the top of the tube the length of the constriction (bobbin rim depth) is unchanged but the diameter of the constriction has become greater than its length, i.e. it resembles an orifice rather than tube.

The reason for this close scrutiny of the shape of constriction around the Rotameter bobbin is that if the constriction is an orifice and the pressure drop across it is kept constant then the flow rate of gas through it is related to the density of the gas:

$$\frac{1}{\sqrt[2]{\text{density.}}}$$

If the constriction is tubular the relationship is more complex but viscosity is the factor chiefly determining flow rate. If the flow tube is of uniform taper there is a gradual transition from a tubular constriction at the bottom of the tube to an orificial one at the top. This is a complicating factor in calibrating Rotameters which is best performed empirically by timed collection of measured volumes or timed ascent of soap films (Barr 1934). Once calibrated, Rotameters are accurate instruments provided the flow tube is vertically mounted and is kept clean.

Rotameters in modern anaesthetic equipment may have more than one taper so that both low and high flow rates can be measured. Many modern machines have a low flow tube mounted alongside, but in series with, a high flow tube. This is done to give a long, more accurately readable low-flow scale (0–1 l) together with a similar long scale for high flows (e.g. 1–10 l).

The earliest flow meters were controlled from the cylinders and this was the case with the earlier models of the Coxeter dry bobbin flow meter illustrated in Fig. 12.3. A later model of this flow meter had needle valves mounted at the base of each tube and this became standard practice. There is an alternative position for the needle valve controlling flow through the flow tube. If the valve is mounted downstream of the flow tube then it controls the flow through the meter and the tube is largely protected from pressure fluctuations due to changes in resistance down stream (e.g. a minute-volume divider type of ventilator such as the Manley). The bobbin remains steady during the ventilator cycle. A flow meter having this feature is termed 'pressure compensated'. Since it is operating at a higher pressure than a normal flow meter the flow tube requires calibrating at the operating pressure.

Because of its now universal use the history of the Rotameter has been studied (Forreger 1952). It is of interest that it was patented by Karl Kuppers in Germany in 1909 and that two were used in a nitrous oxide–oxygen machine demonstrated by Dr Maximillian Neu of Heidelberg in 1910 and 1911. The 'Rota machine' was reported in at least two other German papers but there were major drawbacks: firstly, no provision was made for using ether; secondly, nitrous oxide had to be imported from Britain or the USA; and thirdly the machine was almost twice the price of other machines. For these reasons the use of Rotameters in anaesthetic machines did not develop after 1913 except for a brief period of revival in connection with the use of acetylene as an anaesthetic agent in Germany in 1923–1925. Neu had appreciated that Rotameters made it possible to make gas mixtures of known composition accurately. The 1923 acetylene apparatus of Gauss and Wieland used a mixing tap to control the composition of the acetylene–oxygen mixture. The single Rotameter measured only the total gas flow to the patient.

The early use of Rotameters in Germany was not known to workers in Britain and the USA. The Cotton and Boothby bubble bottle is therefore the beginning of a continuous line of development of flow meters on anaesthetic machines. Rotameters were used industrially in Britain as long ago as before the First World War and were used by the manufacturers of medical gases after the war (Rendell-Baker 1963). All these Rotameters were very large; the ones used by Dr Neu appear to be about a metre long. There is evidence that Dr W J McCaskie of Birmingham (Macintosh 1952), Magill (1941) and Charles King (Trost 1942) considered the use of Rotameters in anaesthesia, and indeed Magill's endotracheal apparatus of 1932 (in the Charles King collection) has bobbin-type flow meters but the bobbins do not rotate. These are presumably the flow meters made by Siebe-Gorman referred to by Magill in his letter of 1941.

The credit for the introduction of Rotameters into modern anaesthesia must therefore go to Richard Salt of the Anaesthetic Department, Oxford who was given a month's study leave to study flow meters and visited the Rotawerke in Germany (Macintosh 1942). This visit resulted in the introduction of Rotameters on the 1937 Boyle's machine.

Rotameters have now achieved universal use in anaesthesia machines; they are well suited to manual use (but not automatic control — see below), have a high degree of accuracy if properly maintained [±2% is claimed by the manufacturers but this figure requires interpretation (Hodge 1979)] and give visual evidence of the flow of gas. Problems reported include loss of accuracy due to the flow tube not being vertical, dirt in the tube and build up of static electricity from the rotation of the bobbin (Clutton-Brock 1972, Hagelsten & Larsen 1965). Problems due to static build-up inside the flow tube have now been largely overcome. Inaccuracy in calibration is not usually of great clinical importance except at very low flow rates, eg during closed or low flow anaesthesia. Even new O_2 flow meters have been found to have deviations of up to 70% flows less than 1 l/min (Waaben et al 1978).

The future development of anaesthetic machines will involve the automatic control of the composition of anaesthetic gas mixtures and the increasing use of servo-mechanisms for various purposes. For example an oxygen sensor may be used to monitor the oxygen concentration in the gas mixture inspired from the machine, and via a computer (or hard-wired system) control a valve which admits oxygen to maintain a pre-set concentration. A similar mechanism can of course regulate the concentration of other gases in the anaesthetic machine. The anaesthetic concentration in the system can be controlled by, for example, the end-expired anaesthetic concentration or, better still, by a signal giving a measure of anaesthetic depth. All the preceding types of control have been used experimentally and, with the exception of the last named, have been successfully used experimentally.

All these mechanisms involve, in addition to a sensor, a mechanized valve of some sort to control gas flow and in most cases a gas flow meter to measure and record the gas flow required to bring about and maintain the pre-set level.

Volatile anaesthetic agents can be treated in this manner, for instance the Oxford vaporizer Type II passed ether vapour, from a heated pressure vessel through a Rotameter. The new agent desflurane, having a boiling point close to ambient temperature, can be similarly treated and this assists accurate gas mixture proportioning.

Unfortunately the conventional Rotameter–needle valve device does not easily lend itself to electronic control. The needle valve can be driven by a servomotor and the position of the bobbin can be optically sensed by a row of light sources (LEDs) mounted on one side of the flow tube and a row of photo-cells mounted on the side. This is a measurement system of low resolution and the highly non-linear scale of, e.g. a triple taper flow meter, presents considerable problems.

For these reasons a constant area–variable pressure type of flow meter of the kind already described is more suitable for these electronic control applications. Clearly an electronic differential pressure transducer must be used rather than a water manometer. The orifice type of meter is not the best for electronic control purposes, not just because of the square root relationship between pressure and flow already mentioned. For this relationship to be maintained accurately fully turbulent flow must be present at the orifice at all measured flow rates and this is not easy to guarantee. Because of this a capillary tube is usually used in the constriction. Such a device is the 'linear resistance laminar flow meter' described by Calkins et al (1982). In this instrument the differential pressure across a standard distance in the laminar flow path is linearly proportional to flow rate. An accuracy of better than 1% of full scale is claimed for this flow meter when used within a defined range of flow rates.

The remaining flow meters to be described which are suitable for electronic control systems can be classified as thermal transfer devices. In the hot wire flow meter (or anemometer) a resistance wire is heated by the passage of electric current and because it is mounted in the gas flow it is cooled by the gas. A servocircuit provides and records the current required to maintain a constant temperature which is a measure of gas flow rate. Linearization of this device is not easy.

A number of other thermal transfer devices have been described, one having considerable use in electronically controlled gas flow equipment is the stream temperature rise thermal flow meter. The principle of operation of these devices is shown in Figure 12.11. In this flow meter the whole of the gas stream is heated by a constant heat source, H, and the rise of the stream temperature thus produced is sensed by the difference between the temperatures T_1 and T_2. Devices of this sort measure the mass of gas passing. They are mass flow meters and as such have the considerable advantage that no corrections are required for temperature or pressure.

The equations governing the behaviour of most of the flow meters so far described are complex but the equation characterizing stream temperature

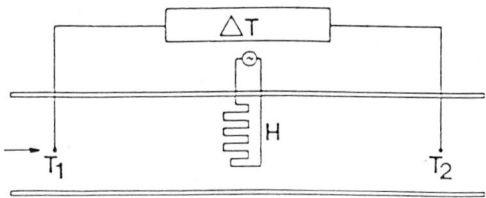

Fig. 12.11   The Thomas flow meter (Reproduced with permission from Baker W C & Pouchot J F 1983.)

rise flow meters is relatively simple:

$$M = \frac{H}{C_p \triangle t}$$

where M = massflow, H = heat input, C_p = specific heat of gas,
t = temperature change.

Calibration can be transferred from one gas to another by a correction based
on specific heat.

The device shown in Figure 12.11 requires a large amount of heat to heat
the entire gas stream, and this may be undesirable. More commonly the
arrangement shown in Figure 12.11 is applied to a small tube in which the
flow is laminar and bypasses a laminar flow element through which the main
gas stream flows. The measuring bypasss takes a known proportion of the total
flow. A refinement of the circuitry measures the heating current required to
maintain a constant thermal gradient in the face of changing flow rates. This
gives greater accuracy than a fixed heat output and allows observation of
changes in gradient. These devices are usually used in association with a
variable solenoid valve controlled by the flow meter, the whole assembly
constituting a mass flow controller.

Mass flow sensors using thermistors are used in the gas mixer of the
Engstrom ELSA anaesthetic machine (Davey et al 1992). An anaesthetic
machine in which the oxygen and nitrous oxide are servo-controlled using
mass flow controllers has been described (Humphry & White 1990).

The electrical flow meters so far described are used in conjunction with
continuously variable electrically controlled valves (taps).

An alternative which particularly lends itself to computer control is the
digital flow controller which combines the functions of needle valve and flow
meter. There are two ways in which these valves can be employed. In one
(Boaden & Hutton 1986) an array of solenoid-controlled binary (i.e. on–off)
valves is used. Eight valves are attached individually to eight pre-set fixed
orifice needle valves. These are critical flow valves (also called sonic or
choked flow). The needle valve's orifice is designed to operate with a pressure
drop of half the upstream pressure and provided this ratio is not reduced the
velocity of flow through the valve nozzle exceeds the speed of sound and the
flow rate through the valve is almost independent of downstream pressure
fluctuations. In the design referred to the smallest valve is preset to permit a
flow of 50 ml/min, the next smallest valve to 100 ml/min and so on upwards,
each valve having a flow rate twice that of the one below it in the series. The
maximum flow rate from the whole array is therefore 12 750 ml/min and any
flow rate between full flow and zero is obtainable in steps of 50 ml. This
device works well in practice. A computer-controlled gas mixer (Figure 12.12)
has been constructed using three digital flow controllers (Boaden et al 1988)
which has been used successfully in feedback control of end-tidal CO_2 in
anaesthetized, ventilated patients.

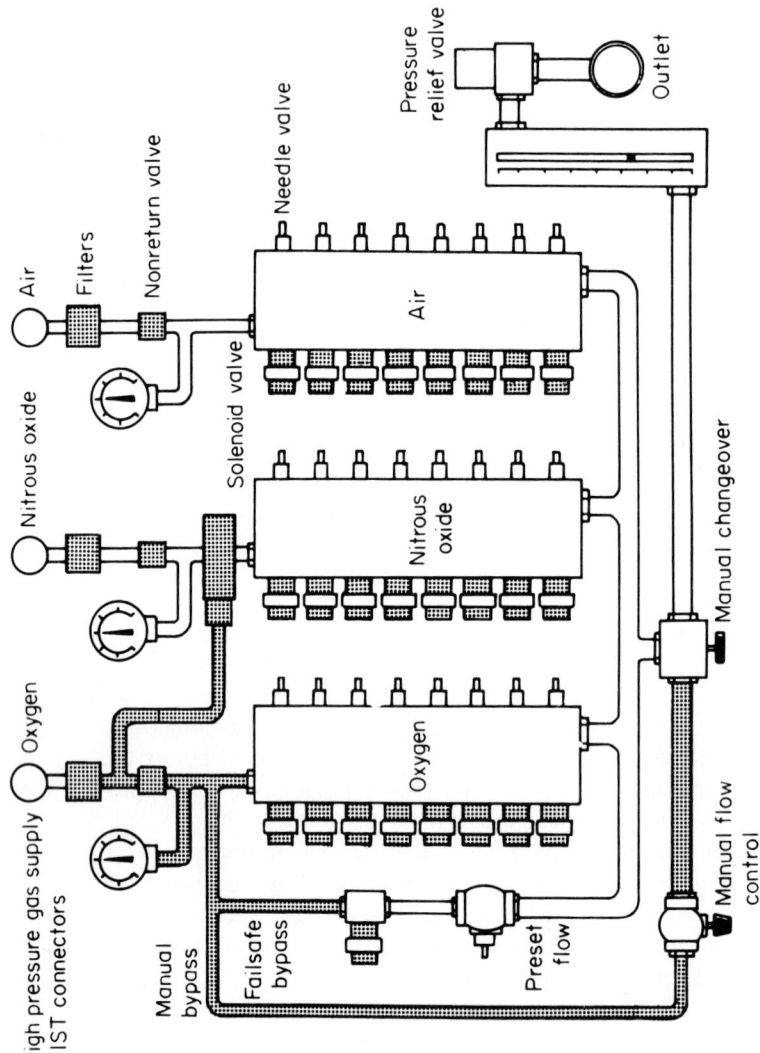

Fig. 12.12 A digital anaesthetic gas mixer (Reproduced with permission from Boaden et al 1989.)

An alternative method of using solenoid valves has been described by Palayiwa et al (1986) in which valves in the gas supply line are pulsed so that they open and close rapidly. The mark-space ratio (ratio of 'on' to 'off' time) can be electronically controlled so that control of the flow rate per minute through the valve is obtained.

Devices of this sort can be used not only to control gas mixtures but also to control vaporizers and to construct ventilators.

This review of gas flow into anaesthetic apparatus is far from comprehensive. A variety of other types of flow meter, particularly fluidic and ultrasonic have considerable potential for use in anaesthetic machines of the future.

REFERENCES

Baker W C, Pouchot J F 1983 The measurement of gas flow. J Air Pollution Control Assoc 33 :156–161
Barr G 1934 Two designs of flowmeter and a method of calibration. J Scientific Instruments 11: 21–324
Boaden R W, Hutton P 1986 The digital control of anaesthetic gas flow. Anesthesia 41: 413–418
Boaden R W, Hutton P, Monk C 1989 A computer controlled anaesthetic gas mixer. Anesthesia 44: 665–669
Calkins J M, Saunders R J, Waterson C K 1982 In: Brown B R (ed) Gas and vapour delivery in future anesthesia delivery systems. Philadelphia: FA Davis
Clutton-Brock J 1972 Static electricity and Rotameters. Br J Anaesth 44: 86–90
Cotton F J, Boothby WM 1912 Nitrous oxide–oxygen–ether anesthesia. Surg, Gynecol, Obstet 15: 281–289
Davey A, Moyle J T B, Ward C S 1992 An electronically controlled anaesthetic machine. In: Ward's anaesthetic equipment, 3rd Edn. London: WB Saunders
Duncum B 1947 The development of inhalation anaesthesia. Oxford: Oxford University Press
Foregger R 1952 Early use of Rotameter in anaesthesia. Br J Anaesth 24: 187–195
Hagelsten J O, Larsen O S 1965 Inaccuracy of anaesthetic flowmeters caused by static electricity. Br J Anaesth 37: 637–641
Hewitt F W 1984 Further observations on the use of oxygen with nitrous oxide. J Br Dent Assocn 19 380–387
Hodge E A 1979 Accuracy of anaesthetic gas flowmeters. Br J Anaesth 51: 907
Humphrey S J E, White D C 1991 A servo-controlled anaesthetic machine. Br J Anaesth 66: 400–401
King A C 1946 The evolution of anaesthetic apparatus. Br Med Bull 4(2): 12–139
Macintosh R R 1942 Letter. Lancet i: 27
Magill I W 1941 Letter. Lancet ii: 776
Palayiwa E, Hahn C E W, Sugg B R, Lindsay-Scott D, Tyrrell P J 1986 A microprocessor-controlled gas mixing device. Anesthesia 58: 1041–1047
Pask E A 1940 A double range flowmeter. Lancet ii: 680–681
Rendell-Baker L 1963 History of thoracic anaesthesia. In: Mushin W W (ed) Thoracic anaesthesia. Oxford: Blackwell Scientific
Thomas K B 1975 The development of anaesthetic apparatus. Oxford: Blackwell Scientific
Trost A H 1942 Letter. Lancet i: 92
Waaben J, Stokke D B, Brinlow M M 1978 Accuracy of gas flowmeter determined by the bubble method. Br J Anaesth 50: 1251–1256
Ward C S 1985 Anaesthetic equipment, 2nd Edn. London: Bailliére Tindall

13. Update

ABDOMINAL ANAESTHESIA

This was considered in Review 9 and only recent references to the subject are included. Inhalation of gastric contents is still a major cause of postoperative morbidity. Opioids are known to delay gastric emptying and it has been suggested that calcium channel blockers are also implicated. However, Yavorski et al (1991) were unable to show that verapamil or diltiazem significantly delayed gastric emptying in normal subjects.

Gastrointestinal bleeding may also be a risk factor not only for inhalation of gastric contents but also in patients who are being nursed in intensive care units. Ranitidine has been advocated to inhibit gastric acid secretion but Brunner & Chang (1990) found that omeprazole was more effective in inhibiting gastric acid secretion, reducing the need for invasive therapy in the treatment of bleeding peptic ulceration. Sucralfate, a complex salt or sucrose sulphate and aluminium hydroxide, inhibits pepsin A and also protects the mucosa via prostaglandin stimulus of mucus and bicarbonate secretion. It is effective in preventing stress ulcers in patients who have been ventilated and it is said to lead to a reduction in nosocomial pneumonia (McCarthy 1991).

Pre- and postoperative nutrition

In a prospective randomized trial in patients with gastric or colorectal cancer, 10 days' preoperative nutrition in severe depleted patients reduced the incidence of major postoperative complications (Meijerink et al 1992). Following an intestinal anastomosis many surgeons rely on a 'nil by mouth' regime until there is a return of bowel sounds or the passing of flatus. However, prolongation of this technique may lead to absorption of intestinal toxins as the bowel is a reservoir of micro-organisms (Maynard & Bihari 1991). This also applies to burns in which early feeding is advocated to minimize the absorption of intestinal pathogens. It is also noted that it is only the stomach and large intestine which do not function in the immediate postoperative period and Maynard & Bihari (1991) advocate feeding by nasojejunal tube or jejunostomy.

Blood transfusion

It has been suggested that blood transfusion impairs the antitumour immune response and that blood transfusion may be responsible for the spread of metastases or early recurrence. Francis (1991) found that at present it was impossible to conclude that there was a definite association between blood transfusion and tumour growth. In patients with metastatic carcinoma there may be haemostatic abnormalities including:

1. increased platelet aggregation;
2. abnormal activation of the coagulation cascade;
3. release of plasminogen activator;
4. decreased synthesis of anticoagulation proteins in the liver (Nand & Messmsore 1990).

During surgery, including those for carcinoma, the fibrinolytic response was variable, with some patients showing an increase of tissue plasminogen activator especially during clamping of the bowel (Johnson et al 1990). Curiously aspirin, which has anticoagulant properties, is said to reduce the risk of developing colorectal cancer (Baron & Greenberg 1991). It has also been suggested that blood transfusion is beneficial in the prevention of recurrent attacks of Crohn's disease but this has not been confirmed by Scott et al (1991).

Intravenous therapy

During major surgical procedures Hartmann's solution is often infused to replace the normal daily requirements. Many intravenous solutions are acidic and the pH of Hartmann is approximately 6.8. Postoperatively there is a tendency to prescribe dextrose saline in view of the fact that it is unlikely to produce sodium overload. However, Kruegener et al (1991) argued against the use of the solution despite its popularity (because of ease of administration) as it does not necessarily consider the patient's needs. They are also more likely to develop hyponatraemia. The ease with which it is possible to measure serum and urinary electrolytes as well as osmolality makes it possible to administer the appropriate fluid.

Fluid replacement in the critically ill is still subject to debate and despite theoretical reasons for the use of albumin, its value appears to be limited and treatment by synthetic colloid appears to be just as effective (Stockwell et al 1992a). Although the serum albumin concentration was less in those patients given colloid, there was no significant difference in the incidence of pulmonary oedema or renal failure (Stockwell et al 1992b).

Posture

It has been claimed that the prone jack-knife position is detrimental to cardiac output. However, Hatada et al (1991) confirmed that turning the patient from the supine to the prone position resulted in a significant fall in cardiac index, but if the patient were also in the head-down position the cardiac index increased and returned to the control value. In the jack-knife position there was slowing of the heart rate but an increase in mean arterial pressure.

Hypoxaemia

Catley et al (1985) and Rosenberg et al (1992) have drawn attention to the pronounced period of oxygen desaturation following major abdominal or orthopaedic surgery. [In fact desaturation also occurred during the insertion of cement into the femur during total hip replacement and Al Shaikh (1991) recommended during this phase that the inspired oxygen concentration should be increased to at least 50%.] Rosenberg et al (1989) reported oxygen desaturation and variations of heart rate following major abdominal surgery and this appeared to be related to preoperative tachycardia (Rosenberg et al 1990). Reeder et al (1991) described 3 patients, 2 of whom developed myocardial ischaemia during the 48 hours following surgery, even though their arterial oxygen saturation was greater than 90%. After this period, nocturnal hypoxaemia developed, increasing the severity and duration of the myocardial ischaemia. Tachycardia was also a feature in these patients and it appears that this, in combination with decreased oxygen saturation, may result in an increase in postoperative myocardial infarction. Reeder et al (1992) found that the oxygen saturation could be maintained greater than 90% during the *early* postoperative period, but in 50% of patients undergoing abdominal vascular surgery, it fell to less than 85% in the *late* postoperative period. In fact some patients were still hypoxaemic until the 5th postoperative night and there may be a place for continuing supplementary oxygen saturation during the whole of the first postoperative week. Incidentally, nocturnal hypoxaemia may also be present on the 4th postoperative night following thoracotomy (Entwistle et al 1991). Rather disappointingly, inhalation of 30% oxygen by face mask improved oxygen saturation but did not decrease the episodes of sudden oxygen desaturation (Rosenberg et al 1992).

Sphincter of Oddi

Nifedipine relaxes smooth muscle and it has been shown that it is effective in relieving spasm of the sphincter of Oddi in patients in whom there is an elevated basal pressure and the sphincter of Oddi phasic contractions of the predominantly antegrade type (Khuroo et al 1992).

Transurethral prostatectomy

Hahn (1992) noted the serum sodium decreased by 5 mmol/l in some patients and in others it was greater than this. Although this corresponded to the absorption of 1 litre of 2.2% glycine solution, only mild metabolic acidosis developed (Leading article 1991). Absorption of glycine used for irrigating the bladder during transurethral prostatectomy can lead to transurethral resection syndrome, the features of which include loss of consciousness, hypotension, hyponatraemia, renal failure, low arterial Po_2, a normal pH or metabolic acidosis. Apart from the absorption of electrolyte-free fluid and glycine there is also a dilution of protein (Hahn 1991).

REFERENCES

Al-Shaikh B 1991 Effect of inspired oxygen concentration on the incidence of desaturation in patients undergoing total hip replacement. Br J Anaesth 66: 580–582

Baron J A, Greenberg E R 1991 Could aspirin really prevent colon cancer? N Engl J Med 325: 1644–1645

Brunner G, Chang J 1990 Intravenous therapy with high doses of ranitidine and omeprazole in critically ill patients with bleeding peptic ulcerations of the upper intestinal tract; an open randomized controlled trial. Digestion 45: 217–225

Catley D M, Thorton C, Jordan C et al 1985 Pronounced episodic oxygen desaturation in the postoperative period; its association with ventilatory pattern and analgesic regimen. Anesthesiology 63: 20–28

Entwistle M D, Roe P G, Sapsford D J et al 1991 Patterns of oxygenation after thoracotomy. Br J Anaesth 67: 704–711

Francis D M A 1991 Relationship between blood transfusion and tumour behaviour. Br J Sur 78: 1420–1428

Hahn R G 1991 The transurethral resection syndrome. Acta Anaesthesiol Scand 35: 557–567

Hahn R G 1992 Acid–base status following glycine absorption in transurethral surgery. Eur J Anaesthesiol 9: 1–5

Hatada T, Kusunoki M, Sakiyama T et al 1991 Hemodynamics in the prone jack knife position during surgery. Am J Surg 162: 55–58

Johnson E J, Harisman H, Hampton K K et al 1990 Fibrinolysis during major abdominal surgery. Fibrinolysis 4: 147–151

Khuroo M S, Al Zargar S, Yattoo G N 1992 Efficacy of nifedipine therapy in patients with sphincter of Oddi dysfunction: a prospective, double-blind, randomized, placebo-controlled, cross over trial. Br J Clin Pharmacol 33: 477–485

Kruegener G H, Kerin M J, MacFie J 1991 Postoperative fluid therapy — put not thy faith in dextrose saline: discussion paper. J R Soc Med 84: 611–612

Leading article 1991 Monitoring TURP. Lancet 338: 606–607

McCarthy D M 1991 Sucralfate. N Engl J Med 325: 1017–1205

Maynard N D, Bihari D J 1991 Postoperative feeding. Br Med J 303: 1007–1008

Meijerink W J H J, Von Meyenfeldt M F, Rouflart M M J, Soeters P B 1992 Efficacy of perioperative nutritional support. Lancet 340: 187–188

Reeder M K, Muir A D, Foex P et al 1991 Postoperative myocardial ischaemia: temporal association with nocturnal hypoxaemia. Br J Anaesth 67: 626–631

Reeder M K, Goldman M D, Loh L et al 1992 Postoperative hypoxaemia after major abdominal vascular surgery. Br J Anaesth 68: 23–26

Rosenberg J, Dirkes W E, Kahlet H 1989 Episodic arterial oxygen desaturation and heart rate variations following major abdominal surgery. Br J Anaesth 63: 651–654

Rosenberg J, Rasmussen V, Von Jessn F et al 1990 Late postoperative episodic and constant hypoxaemia and associated ECG abnormalities. Br J Anaesth 65: 684–691

Rosenberg J, Pedersen M H, Gebuhr P, Kehlet H 1992 Effect of oxygen therapy on late postoperative episodic and constant hypoxaemia. Br J Anaesth 68: 18–22

Scott A D N, Ritchie J K, Phillips R K S 1991 Blood transfusion and recurrent Crohn's disease. Br J Surg 78: 455–458

Stockwell M A, Soni N, Riley B 1992a Colloid solutions in the critically ill. A randomised comparison of albumin and polygeline. 1. Outcome and duration of stay in the intensive care unit. Anaesthesia 47: 3–6

Stockwell M A, Scott A, Day A et al 1992b Colloid solutions in the critically ill. A
    randomised comparison of albumin and polygeline. 2. Serum albumin concentration and
    incidence of pulmonary oedema and acute renal failure. Anaesthesia 47: 7–9
Yavorski R T, Hallgren S E, Blue P W 1991 Effects of verapamil and diltiazem on gastric
    emptying in normal subjects. Dig Dis Sci 36: 1274–1276

MUSCLE RELAXANTS

Studies of muscle relaxants usually involve the abductor pollicis muscle and recording the tension developed following indirect stimulation. It is agreed that the small muscles of the hand may not necessarily reflect activity elsewhere, such as the diaphragm or the laryngeal muscles. This has been confirmed by Isono et al (1992) who found that in animals the geniohyoid was more sensitive to vecuronium than the diaphragm, an effect accentuated by enflurane. Donati & Bevan (1992) urged caution in interpreting the results of peripheral nerve stimulation and that although peripheral muscle appears to recover and ventilation is adequate, there still may be paralysis of muscles controlling the upper airway.

Vandenbrom et al (1991) described a method of measuring the effect of neuromuscular blocking agents on vocal cord movements and comparing the results with that of stimulation of the tibialis anterior muscle. Suxamethonium caused more pronounced blockade of the peripheral tibialis anterior muscle, as did tubocurarine and atracurium. Pancuronium and vecuronium appeared to cause an equal blockade of the intrinsic muscles of larynx and the tibialis anterior muscle.

The degree of magnitude of the blockade may vary using the train-of-four ratio ($T_4 : T_1$). Gwee & Cheah (1989) found that pancuronium was equipotent with tubocurarine but more potent than decamethonium and suxamethonium. What mustn't be forgotten is muscle fatigue and there are at least two processes involved in this, one of which is pH-dependent (Cady et al 1989). Adrenaline also influences muscle contraction by affecting extracellular calcium (Williams & Barns 1989).

The prior administration of suxamethonium leads to a reduction of the dose of atracurium to produce a similar degree of blockade when given by itself. Suxamethonium increases the volume of distribution of atracurium but decreases the atracurium concentration required to produce adequate blockade (Donati et al 1991). Inhalation anaesthetics such as enflurane can prolong the action of atracurium and vecuronium which were clinically irrelevant but care should be taken with the administration of pipecuronium and pancuronium (Swen et al 1989). During coronary artery surgery dopamine increased the elimination of pancuronium by increasing glomerular filtration rate but did not decrease tubular reabsorption. However, its elimination was increased during hypothermia (Mark et al 1990). These observations apply to animal experiments and Chang et al (1989) have drawn attention to species specificity in response to muscle relaxants. In mice, for example, suxamethonium causes sustained depolarization, by acting on the perijunctional receptor. Its response is different from the cat in that the neuromuscular blockade is due to attenuation of the endplate potential and not primarily due to depolarization.

Atracurium

Concern has been expressed about the metabolite of atracurium, laudanosine, which might accumulate during prolonged infusions of the muscle relaxant. Gwinnutt et al (1990) noted the increased levels in the cerebrospinal fluid (CSF) in patients with head injury, but failed to find any adverse effects. Nigrovic & Fox (1991) suggest that only two-thirds of atracurium administered is pharmacologically active, the remaining amount being responsible for the high initial concentrations of laudanosine.

Age may affect the potency of atracurium with prolonged recovery in the elderly (Kitts et al 1990). Obese patients require higher concentration of atracurium than those of normal weight to achieve comparable degree of neuromuscular blockade (Varin et al 1990), while respiratory alkalosis reduces the duration (Platt et al 1991). Renal failure has only a small influence on atracurium, although the terminal half-life of laudanosine is prolonged. If anything, there is resistance to the atracurium itself (Vandenbrom et al 1990). Resistance to atracurium has also been reported in a patient with carcinoma in whom the alpha$_1$ acid glycoprotein was raised (Tatman et al 1991). However, epidural analgesia with bupivacaine prolongs the neuromuscular blockage of atracurium (Toft et al 1990).

D-tubocurarine

Histamine release has been implicated in hypotension following the administration of d-tubocurarine, although ganglionic blockade is also said to be involved. Hatano et al (1990) demonstrated that the hypotension was due to the release of prostacyclin acting at H$_1$-receptors, and this effect can be attenuated by pretreatment with aspirin, DL-lysine or diphenhydramine.

Vecuronium

Pancuronium has been implicated in prolonged paralysis in patients being mechanically ventilated. It is believed that a short-acting relaxant such as vecuronium would be less hazardous but Margolis et al (1991) quoted 2 patients who developed prolonged reversible quadriplegia who were being ventilated for asthma and were receiving long-term infusion of vecuronium.

Doxacurium

Doxacurium is similar in action to pancuronium but has less effect on autonomic activity. There is also no histamine release. Although spontaneous recovery occurs following doxacurium, a non-depolarizing neuromuscular blocking agent, reversal with neostigmine is recommended (Faulds & Clissold 1991). Plasma clearance was significantly altered in patients with renal failure: this may result in prolonged blockade (Cook et al 1991).

Burns

Suxamethonium is not advocated in recent burns or disuse atrophy in which there appears to be increase efflux of potassium (Fung et al 1991). Tomera & Martyn (1989) found that the dose of tubocurarine required to inhibit twitch tension increased in proportion to the size of the burn. Cyclic adenosine monophosphate (AMP) levels were also increased, as well as prostaglandin (PGE$_2$). There was also resistance to atracurium in burns (Marathe et al 1989). There were significant reductions in twitch tension (in the mouse model) and this was related to the increased cyclic AMP levels. PGE$_2$ was also raised in burns; there was no relationship to twitch tension or the dose of d-tubocurarine. The response to tubocurarine is surprising as it would be expected that the weakened muscle would be sensitive to the muscle relaxant.

Interactions

Interactions between muscle relaxants and other drugs have been widely reported and recently Parr et al (1991) confirmed that betamethasone, a steroid, produced resistance to the neuromuscular blockade following vecuronium. Long-term therapy with dexamethasone or prednisone depresses plasma cholinesterase activity (Bradamante et al 1989). Metoclopramide also prolongs the effect of suxamethonium, presumably again by inhibiting plasma cholinesterase activity (Kao & Turner 1989). For genetic variation of human serum cholinesterase levels see Lockridge (1990).

Anticholinesterase

Concern has always been expressed about the ability of anticholinesterase to antagonize competitive neuromuscular blocking agents. Beemer et al (1991) emphasized that 'profound' neuromuscular blockade should be avoided towards the end of surgery, as otherwise the anticholinesterase may be ineffectual. Beemer et al (1991) advocated the use of neostigmine 0.08 mg/kg and commented that blockade from alcuronium was less likely to be reversed satisfactorily than atracurium. 'Air hunger' results from an increase in arterial Pco$_2$ and may occur even after complete reversal of neuromuscular blockade (Banzett et al 1990).

The place of anticholinesterases in organophosphate pesticide intoxication has been widely reported. Acute organophosphate intoxication can in fact result in prolonged effects involving memory, problem-solving and motor dexterity (Rosenstock et al 1991). Somani & Dube (1989) advised the use of pretreatment with physostigmine while Shockley (1989) reported favourably on the use of inhaled nebulized atropine. Besser et al (1990) reported favourably on the use of low-dose pancuronium while Caballero de Castro et al (1991) found that new bands of esterase activity appeared following prolonged exposure.

Increased levels of cholinesterase may appear in patients on valproic acid, carbamazepine and phenytoin, which are enzyme inducers (Puche et al 1989).

Physostigmine has been used in the management of alcohol withdrawal, acting by releasing beta-endorphin (Backon 1989), and also used to reverse respiratory depression caused by the use of intrathecal baclofen (Muller-Schwefe & Penn 1989).

Atropine is often administered to counterpart the side-effects of anti-cholinesterases, but Ziv et al (1992) have reported a novel use of pyridostigmine. Hyoscine used for the management of motion sickness has its side-effects and pyridostigmine (30 mg t.d.s.) is now being used to treat the side-effects of hyoscine.

Animal experiments indicate that even atropine may affect analgesia. Ghelardini et al (1990) have shown that atropine in low doses produced antinociception, had little effect in intermediate doses but produced hyperalgesia at high doses. Given that atropine crosses the blood–brain barrier, a decrease in cholinergic activity can reduce the level of surgical anaesthesia (Puil & El-Beheiry 1990).

Myasthenia gravis

Myasthenia gravis is an autoimmune disorder, of which three genetic groups are now recognized as well as ocular and neonatal groups. Remission is often achieved with steroids or with azathioprine in patients who do respond to thymectomy. Plasma exchange results in a temporary improvement in myasthenia. Most patients require treatment with anticholinesterase drugs (Havard & Fonseca 1990). Wirguin et al (1990) reported a patient in whom citrate increased the weakness by reducing the levels of ionized calcium.

In the Lambert–Eaton syndrome, a condition similar to myasthenia, 3,4-diaminopyridine was effective in reducing muscle weakness: it is extremely potent in release of acetylcholine at the neuromuscular junction and does not readily cross the blood–brain barrier (McEvoy et al 1989).

Snyder & Cardwell (1989) reported neuromuscular blockade in a patient with eclampsia being treated with nifedipine and magnesium sulphate. The mechanism for this has not yet been established, but it is possible that it had a place in that particular level. Resistance to atracurium has also been reported in a patient with carcinoma in whom alpha$_1$ acid glycoprotein was raised (Tatman et al 1991).

Malignant hyperthermia

Malignant hyperthermia still carries a high mortality and may be unrecognized despite a progressive rise in body temperature of 2°C per hour, increased muscle metabolism, metabolic acidosis and tachycardia. In animals with halothane-sensitive gene the rate of calcium release was markedly increased (Mickelson et al 1989). In cultured muscle cells, in addition to fast transient sodium currents and potassium outward current, there was a slow inward current associated with malignant hyperthermia (Wieland et al 1989). Following intense exercise, even of short duration the recovery of muscle pH was abnormal in patients with malignant hyperthermia (Allsop et al 1991). The gene for susceptibility for malignant hyperthermia can be detected by DNA markers (Healy et al 1991).

Some consider it advisable to have an anaesthetic machine which has never been contaminated by halothane available for all patients with malignant hyperthermia. McGraw & Keon (1989) recommend only removing the vaporizers, flushing the machine with oxygen at high flow for 15 min and using circuit tubing and carbon dioxide absorbers that have never been exposed to inhalational agents. In addition to avoiding agents which might trigger an attack of malignant hyperthermia prophylactic dantrolene has been recommended but Hackl et al (1990) found that this was unnecessary. Dantrolene can cause severe liver damage in patients who are on prolonged therapy for neurological disorders (Chan 1990).

There have been conflicting accounts of the possibility that malignant hyperthermia may occur in patients with Duchenne-type muscular dystrophy or the less severe form, the Becker type: many of the case reports are anecdotal but invariably halothane and suxamethonium have been administered. Bush & Dubowitz (1991) and McLeod & Creighton (1986) have described cases where suxamethonium was not used and anaesthesia consisted entirely of inhalational agents. One patient died during induction and the other had a cardiac arrest with high potassium and low calcium. Intense biochemical activity appears to occur in response to inhalational anaesthesia and special care should be taken with patients with a history of preoperative cramps and myoglobinuria. Severity of the disease does not seem to be critical as early cases appear to be more prone to develop severe biochemical changes. Hyperthermia may not necessarily be a feature of the response.

REFERENCES

Allsop P, Jorfeldt L, Rutberg H, Lennmarken C, Hall G M 1991 Delayed recovery of muscle pH after short duration, high intensity exercise in malignant hyperthermia susceptible subjects. Br J Anaesth 66: 541–545

Backon J 1989 Physostigmine induced beta-endorphin release as a mechanism for physostigmine management of early alcohol withdrawal. Med Hypotheses 29: 85–86

Banzett R B, Lansing R W, Brown R et al 1990 'Air hunger' from increased P_{CO_2} persists after complete neuromuscular block in humans. Respir Physiol 81: 1–18

Beemer G H, Bjorksten A R, Dawson P J et al 1991 Determinants of the reversal time of competitive neuromuscular block by anticholinesterases. Br J Anaesth 66: 469–475

Besser R, Vogt T, Gutmann L 1990 Pancuronium improves the neuromuscular transmission defect of human organophosphate intoxication. Neurology 40: 1275–1277

Bradamante V, Kunec-Vajic E, Lisic M et al 1989 Plasma cholinesterase activity in patients during therapy with dexamethasone or prednisone. Eur J Clin Pharmacol 36: 253–257

Bush A, Dubowitz V 1991 Fatal rhabdomyolysis complicating general anaesthesia in a child with Becker muscular dystrophy. Neuromuscular Disord 1: 201–204

Caballero de Castro A, Rosenbaum E A, Pechen De D'Angelo A 1991 Effect of malathion on bufo arenarum hensel development. Biochem Pharmacol 41: 491–495

Cady E B, Elshove H, Jones D A, Moll A 1989 The metabolic causes of slow relaxation in fatigued human skeletal muscle. J Physiol 418: 327–337

Chan C H 1990 Dantrolene sodium and hepatic injury. Neurology 40: 1427–1432

Chang C C, Chiou L C, Hwang L L 1989 Selective antagonism to succinylcholine-induced depolarization by alpha-bungarotoxin with respect to the mode of action of depolarizing agents. Br J Pharmacol 98: 1413–1419

Cook D R, Freeman J A, Lai A A et al 1991 Pharmacokinetics and pharmacodynamics of doxacurium in normal patients and in those with hepatic or renal failure. Anesth Analg 72: 145–150

Donati F, Bevan D R 1992 Editorial 1: Not all muscles are the same. Br J Anaesth 68: 235–236

Donati F, Gill S S, Bevan D R et al 1991 Pharmacokinetics and pharmacodynamics of atracurium with and without previous suxamethonium administration. Br J Anaesth 66: 557–561

Faulds D, Clissold S P 1991 Doxacurium. A review of its pharmacology and clinical potential in anaesthesia. Drugs 42: 673–689

Fung D L, White D A, Jones B R, Gronert G A 1991 The onset of disuse-related potassium efflux to succinylcholine. Anesthesiology 75: 650–653

Ghelardini C, Malmberg-Aiello P, Giotti A, Malcangio M, Bartolini A 1990 Investigation into atropine-induced antinociception. Br J Pharmcol 101: 49–54

Gwee M C E, Cheah L S 1989 In vitro time course studies on train-of-four fade induced by hexamethonium, pancuronium and decamethonium in the rat hemidiaphragm. Clin Exp Pharmacol Physiol 16: 897–903

Gwinnutt C L, Eddleston J M, Edwards D, Pollard B J 1990 Concentrations of atracurium and laudanosine in cerebrospinal fluid and plasma in three intensive care patients. Br J Anaesth 65: 829–832

Hackl W, Mauritz W, Winkler M et al 1990 Anaesthesia in malignant hyperthermia-susceptible patients without dantrolene prophylaxis; a report of 30 cases. Acta Anaesthesiol Scand 34: 534–537

Hatano Y, Arai T, Noda J et al 1990 Contribution of prostacyclin to d-tubocurarine-induced hypotension in humans. Anesthesiology 72: 28–32

Havard C W H, Fonseca V 1990 New treatment approaches to myasthenia gravis. Drugs 39: 66–73

Healy J M S, Heffron J A A, Lehan M et al 1991 Diagnosis of susceptibility to malignant hyperthermia with flanking DNA markers. Br Med J 303: 1225–1241

Isono S, Kochi T, Ide T et al 1992 Differential effects of vecuronium on diaphragm and geniohyoid muscle in anaesthetized dogs. Br J Anaesth 68: 239–243

Kao Y J, Turner D R 1989 Prolongation of succinylcholine block by metoclopramide. Anesthesiology 70: 905–908

Kitts J B, Fisher D M, Canfell C et al 1990 Pharmacokinetics and pharmacodynamics of atracurium in the elderly. Anesthesiology 72: 272–275

Lockridge O 1990 Genetic variants of human serum cholinesterase influence metabolism of the muscle relaxant succinylcholine. Pharmacol Ther 47: 35–60

McEvoy K, Windebank A J, Daube J R, Low P A 1989 3,4-diaminopyridine in the treatment of Lambert-Eaton myasthenic syndrome. N Engl J Med 321: 1567–1571

McGraw T T, Keon T P 1989 Malignant hyperthermia and the clean machine. Can J Anaesth 36: 530–532

McLeod M E, Creighton R E 1986 Anesthesia for pediatric neurological and neuromuscular diseases. J Child Neurol 1: 189–197

Marathe P H, Dwersteg J F, Pavlin E G et al 1989 Effect of thermal injury on the pharmacokinetics and pharmacodynamics of atracurium in humans. Anesthesiology 70: 752–755

Margolis B D, Khachikian D, Friedman Y, Gerrard C 1991 Prolonged reversible quadriparesis in mechanically ventilated patients who receive long-term infusions of vecuronium. Chest 100: 877–878

Mark J, Wierda K H, van der Starre P J A et al 1990 Pharmacokinetics of pancuronium in patients undergoing coronary artery surgery with and without low dose dopamine. Clin Pharmacokin 19: 491–498

Mickelson J R, Gallant E M, Rempel W E et al 1989 Effects of the halothane-sensitivity gene on sarcoplasmic reticulum function. Am J Physiol 287: C787–794

Muller-Schwefe G, Penn R D 1989 Physostigmine in the treatment of intrathecal baclofen overdose. J Neurosurg 71: 273–275

Nigrovic V, Fox J L 1991 Atracurium decay and the formation of laudanosine in humans. Anesthesiology 74: 446–454

Parr S M, Robinson B J, Rees D, Galletly D C 1991 Interaction between betamethasone and vecuronium. Br J Anaesth 67: 447–451

Platt M, Hayward A, Cooper A, Hirsch N 1991 Effect of arterial carbon dioxide tension on the duration of action of atracurium. Br J Anaesth 66: 45–47

Puche E, Garcia Morillas M, Garcia de la Serrana H, Mota C 1989 Probable pseudocholinesterase induction by valproic acid, carbamazepine and phenytoin leading to increased serum aspirin-esterase activity in epileptics. Int J Clin Pharmacol Res 9: 309–311

Puil E, El-Beheiry H 1990 Anaesthetic suppression of transmitter actions in neocortex. Br J Pharmacol 101: 61–66

Rosenstock L, Keifer M, Daniel W E et al 1991 Chronic central nervous system effects of acute organophosphate pesticide intoxication. Lancet 338: 223–227

Shockley L W 1989 The use of inhaled nebulized atropine for the treatment of malathion poisoning. Clin Toxicol 27: 183–192

Snyder S W, Cardwell M S 1989 Neuromuscular blockade with magnesium sulfate and nifedipine. Am J Obstet Gynecol 161: 35–36

Somani S M, Dube S N 1989 Physostigmine — an overview as pretreatment drug for organophosphate intoxication. Int J Clin Pharmacol Ther Toxicol 27: 367–387

Swen J, Rashkovsky O M, Ket J M et al 1989 Interaction between nondepolarizing neuromuscular blocking agents and inhalational anesthetics. Anesth Analg 69: 752–755

Tatman A J, Wrigley S R, Jones R M 1991 Resistance to atracurium in a patient with an increase in plasma alpha$_1$ globulins. Br J Anaesth 67: 623–625

Toft P, Nielsen H K, Severinsen I, Helbo-Hansen 1990 Effect of epidurally administered bupivacaine on atracurium-induced neuromuscular blockade. Acta Anaesthesiol Scand 34: 649–652

Tomera J F, Martyn J 1989 Mediators of burn-induced neuromuscular changes in mice. Br J Pharmacol 98: 921–929

Vandenbrom R H G, Mark J, Woerda K H, Agoston S 1990 Pharmacokinetics and neuromuscular blocking effects of atracurium besylate and two of its metabolites in patients with normal and impaired renal function. Clin Pharmacokin 19: 230–240

Vandenbrom R H G, Houwertjes M C, Agoston S 1991 A method for studying the pharmacodynamic profile of neuromuscular blocking agents on vocal cord movements in anaesthetized cats. Br J Pharmcol 102: 861–864

Varin F, Ducharme J, Theoret Y, Besner J-G, Bevan D R, Donati F 1990 Influence of extreme obesity on the body disposition and neuromuscular blocking effect of atracurium. Clin Pharmacol Therapeutics 48: 18–25

Wieland S J, Fletcher J E, Rosenberg H, Gong Q-H 1989 Malignant hyperthermia; slow sodium current in cultured human muscle cells. Am J Physiol 287: C759–765

Williams J H, Barns W S 1989 The positive inotropic effect of epinephrine on skeletal muscle: a brief review. Muscle Nerve 12: 968–975

Wirguin I, Brenner T, Shinar E, Argov Z 1990 Citrate-induced impairment of neuromuscular transmission in human and experimental autoimmune myasthenia gravis. Ann Neurol 27: 328–330

Ziv I, Versano D, Ruach M et al 1992 Prevention of peripheral side-effects of transdermal hyoscine by adjunctive therapy with low dosage of pyridostigmine. Br J Clin Pharmacol 33: 507–510

PHAEOCHROMOCYTOMA

Reference has been made in the previous volumes of the series to the usual presentation of phaeochromocytoma and recently Sardesai et al (1990) reported 6 cases who presented with sudden unexplained pulmonary oedema, and normal levels of catecholamine metabolites. Most of the patients died and at postmortem there was evidence of myocarditis, presumably due to the catecholamines. Techniques of anaesthesia for the removal of phaeochromocytoma depend on individual preference and experience: some employ a variety of alpha- and beta-adrenergic blocking agents as well as sodium nitroprusside. Zakowski et al (1989) reported on the use of esmolol, an ultra-short-acting beta-adrenergic blocking drug. Three cases are described in which nitroprusside was administered by infusion to control the blood pressure, and esmolol the heart rate. The recommended dose of esmolol was 500 mg/kg per min for 1 min followed by 100 mg/kg per min for 4 min, with the maintenance infusion rate of 25–300 µg/kg per min.

Propranolol, a non-specific beta-blocker used in the management of phaeochromocytoma, also inhibits the metabolism of paracetamol through oxidation and the glucuronide pathways (Baraka et al 1990).

REFERENCES

Baraka O Z, Truman C A, Ford J M, Roberts C J C 1990 The effect of propranolol on paracetamol metabolism in man. Br J Clin Pharmacol 29: 261–264
Sardesai S H, Mourant A J, Sivathandon Y et al 1990 Phaeochromocytoma and catecholamine induced cardiomyopathy presenting as heart failure. Br Heart J 63: 234–237
Zakowski M, Kaufman B, Berguson P et al 1989 Esmolol use during resection of pheochromocytoma: report of three cases. Anesthesiology 70: 875–877

RESUSCITATION

Cardiac arrest

Reports of the Scientific Meeting of the College of Anaesthetists in 1990 have recently been published (see Willatts 1991). Intravenous amiodarone has been recommended in the management of cardiac arrest when conventional resuscitation was of no avail (Williams et al 1989). This was in a highly selected series of patients whose cardiac arrest was initiated by tachyarrhythmia such as ventricular tachycardia or ventricular fibrillation.

REFERENCES

Willatts S M 1991 Fluids and electrolytes revisited. Br J Anaesth 67: 135–200
Williams M L, Woelfel A, Cascio W E et al 1989 Intravenous amiodarone during prolonged resuscitation from cardiac arrest. Ann Intern Med 110: 839–842

SPINAL AND EXTRADURAL ANALGESIA

Littrell (1991) has reviewed the anatomy and physiology of extradural analgesia, including the use of narcotic drugs.

Not only do spinal opioids produce satisfactory pain relief, but Hartell & Headley (1990) found that general anaesthetics such as methohexitone, althesin and ketamine caused a significant depression of spinal reflexes in response to noxious stimuli at doses well below those required for general anaesthesia. Clonidine given intrathecally potentiates the duration of sensory and motor blockade produced by hyperbaric bupivacaine. When clonidine was administered orally, it was without effect (Bonnet et al 1990). Other studies have confirmed that the addition of clonidine to extradural morphine enhances its effect although there may be a decrease in heart rate and blood pressure but no effect on the respiratory rate (Motsch et al 1990, Carabine et al 1992).

Hirabayashi et al (1990) have studied the effects of extradural compliance and resistance on the spread of local analgesic solutions administered extradurally and found that the number of segments blocked was inversely related to the extradural resistance. The dose required to block individual segments was also related to the extradural resistance. They commented that in the young, the extradural space has a low compliance and high resistance as the fat within this is tightly compressed. This results in less spread of the solution. In the elderly there is a degeneration of fatty tissue, with the result that the extradural space becomes less resistant and greater longitudinal spread of injected solution occurs.

The infusions of intravenous low-dose adrenaline resulted in a low level of plasma bupivacaine following extradural analgesia when compared with intravenous phenylephrine. This may be caused by the increased cardiac output following adrenaline and an increased volume of distribution (Sharrock et al 1991).

Nicol & Holdcroft (1992) have measured the density of many solutions which are now administered by the intrathecal route, commenting that the density of a drug in solution cannot accurately be predicted from a simple formula. They found that most drugs were isobaric at room temperature, but as they reached body temperature they became hypobaric. The effect of temperature had previously been reported by Williams (1984) who drew attention to the wide variation allowed by the British Pharmacopoeia assay limits ranging from 0.85% to 0.95% of sodium chloride. Callesen et al (1991) studied the influence of temperature and found that by adjusting it to 37°C in 0.5% bupivacaine produced a predictable and higher level of sensory blockade.

A variety of techniques have been used to identify the extradural space and the use of air or saline has been advocated. However Valentine et al (1991) found that the use of saline was less likely to produce unblocked segments when compared to air. The introduction of 32-gauge spinal catheters has been viewed with caution in view of the difficulty in threading the catheter, breakage or difficulty with removal. Kestin et al (1991) have reported the successful use of 32-gauge catheters for elective caesarean section with 0.5% bupivacaine, and found that the technique was easier and quicker than that for extradural anaesthesia. The incidence of post-spinal puncture headache was reduced with the use of 25-gauge pencil-point needle (Whitacre) (Lynch et al 1991).

The anatomy of the anterior spinal arteries is variable and Rodriguez-Baeza et al (1989) described three distinct types. This may account for transient neurological disorders with continuous extradural analgesia (Richardson & Bedder 1990). Rigler et al (1991) reported 4 cases of cauda equina syndrome which they suggessted were due to a relatively high dose of local anaesthetic solution. Ménière syndrome has been reported following extradural morphine but this was readily reversed by naloxone (Linder et al 1989). Pruritus is common following extradural morphine and this can be prevented by adding 50 mg of prednisone (Etchin et al 1990). Another problem is that of infection in patients receiving long-term extradural catheters for chronic pain relief. Infection of the tract leading to the extradural space can be treated by antibiotics and removal of the catheter which can be reinserted at a later date (Du Pen et al 1990).

A study on the effects of extradural analgesia on long-term sequelae in obstetric patients has shown that there was a high incidence of headache, backache and tingling in the hands and fingers as well as visual disturbances, fainting and paraesthesia in the legs (MacArthur et al 1992). However there was only an association between extradural analgesia and these symptoms and a randomized trial is required to verify this information.

Tipping et al (1990) have reported on the use of extradural meptazinol which rapidly crosses into the CSF, and in fact has a higher concentration in the CSF compared with plasma. The maximum concentration was reached at 17 min. There also appears to be an inversive relationship between potency and lipophilicity of drugs given intraspinally (McQuay et al 1989).

Intrathecal fentanyl appears to improve the efficiency of extradural analgesia with local anaesthetic solutions. Fassoulaki et al (1991) reported that 100 µg of fentanyl intravenously enhanced the spread of analgesia produced by spinal lignocaine, and this effect could be antagonized by naloxone. It is worthy of note that Lund et al (1985) found that 10 mg of intravenous morphine also enhanced the spread of analgesia of extradural bupivacaine.

Pethidine is known to have local anaesthetic properties as well as providing analgesia. Lewis et al (1992) found that intrathecal pethidine (1 mg/kg) produced adequate sensory blockade of short duration compared with bupivacaine for transurethral prostatectomy.

Whelan et al (1989) demonstrated that spinal anaesthesia has no effect on liver metabolism in drugs such as propranolol as there was no reduction in hepatic blood flow.

Spinal and extradural anaesthesia are contraindicated in patients with blood dyscrasias and in those receiving anticoagulants. It has generally been assumed that it is safe to administer anticoagulants after extradural technique has been performed, but Tekkok et al (1991) reported a case of extradural haematoma in a patient who was anticoagulated with heparin 5000 units intravenously after the catheter had been inserted. On the other hand anticoagulants are unnecessary as continuous extradural analgesia resulted in a decreased incidence of deep vein thrombosis (18%) when compared with general anaesthesia (59%) in patients undergoing knee arthroplasty (Jorgensen et al 1991). This is probably due to improvement in blood flow, reduction in blood viscosity and decrease in the ability of the blood to coagulate (Odoom 1989).

Rosenberg (1990) has reviewed the place of spinal analgesia in the treatment of severe pain, emphasizing the benefits of opioids compared with local analgesic solutions. Also discussed are the merits of the extradural route and the value of simultaneous infusion of opioids with local analgesic solutions in the extradural space for acute pain. Although 85% of patients suffering from carcinoma can still be managed with oral analgesics, the spinal opioids remain an alternative method of treatment.

Fedder (1990) has reported on the value of intrathecal morphine especially given continuously by a pump but complications such as respiratory depression still occur. However, it does improve the quality of life by eliminating or decreasing the use of systemic narcotics. Hogan et al (1991) reported that in 11 of their 16 cases treated with extradural morphine there were complications including dislodged or broken catheters, pain on injection, hyperaesthesia and bleeding or infection. Although the efficacy of the analgesia could be improved by adding bupivacaine, they were less enthusiastic about its use. There was cross-tolerance between systemic and extradural morphine especially regarding the respiratory-depressant action (Pfeifer et al 1989). Yoburn et al (1990) suggest that tolerance is due to changes in spinal delta and brain mu and delta mechanisms.

Stuart-Taylor et al (1992) have assessed the value of a nurse-administered service of extradural diamorphine to 800 patients and found it to be a safe and satisfactory method of providing postoperative analgesia. The incidence of respiratory depression was 0.9%. Following total knee arthroplasty effective analgesia was achieved with continuous infusion of extradural bupivacaine and an opioid resulting in more rapid rehabilitation (Mahoney et al 1990). Cholecystectomy is often followed by acute pain and Yamaguchi et al (1990) found that 0.06–0.12 mg intrathecal morphine produced adequate pain relief without respiratory depression and with a low incidence of vomiting and pruritus. Arendt-Nielsen et al (1991) have demonstrated a segmental effect of intrathecal morphine. Surprisingly, although it does produce excellent analgesia, there is little effect on the maximum allowable concentration of halothane (Licina et al 1991).

Postoperative pain control in the intensive care unit has been studied comparing the action of sufentanil 50 μg or morphine 5 mg given by continuous extradural infusion. With sufentanil there was a more rapid onset of analgesia and the forced vital capacity (FVC) was much better with sufentanil (Dyer et al 1990). In labour 0.2 mg intrathecal morphine and 0.125% bupivacaine provided better pain relief than either drug alone during labour (Abouleish et al 1991). However, Koren et al (1989) suggest that the analgesic and adverse effects of sufentanil are due to its central effects following systemic absorption.

The onset of action of spinal opioids is said to be related to lipid solubility and alfentanil was 3.7 times more permeable than morphine through all three meninges, but neither lipid-solubility nor molecular weight could explain the difference in permeability between morphine and alfentanil (Bernards & Hill 1990).

In a study of the afferent nervous feedback from working muscles to dynamic exercise, extradural analgesia was induced with bupivacaine. It was found that afferent neural activity was important for blood pressure regulation but does not necessarily have an influence on ventilation and heart rate (Fernandes et al 1990).

Following abdominal aortic surgery postoperative hypertension is not uncommon and it is associated with increased sympathetic activity. Extradural morphine attenuates this response (Breslow et al 1989). Papaverine appears to be effective in preventing ischaemic damage to the spinal cord during restriction of its blood supply (Svensson et al 1990).

Although extradural analgesia with bupivacaine may modulate the endocrine response to surgery, patient well-being was also thought to improve following operation. However, Zeiderman et al (1991) found that extradural analgesia had little effect on postoperative fatigue.

The addition of noradrenaline to local analgesic solutions prolongs the action of extradural analgesia and it is suggested that this may be due to a direct effect of the noradrenaline (Goto et al 1990). On the other hand infusion of extradural saline or Ringer's lactate can reverse and shorten the duration of bupivacaine-induced motor blockade without affecting sensation (Johnson et al 1990).

The rapid administration of 20 ml/kg over a 10-min period of crystalloid solution had little effect on hypotension following spinal analgesia for caesarean section (Rout et al 1992) and its place is under review, particularly with the possibility of the return of the use of vasopressors.

REFERENCES

Abouleish E, Rawal N, Shaw J et al 1991 Intrathecal morphine 0.2 mg versus epidural bupivacaine 0.125% or their combination: effects on parturients. Anesthesiology 74: 711–716
Arendt-Nielsen L, Anker-Moller E, Bjerring P, Spangsberg N 1991 Hypoalgesia following intrathecal morphine: a segmental dependent effect. Acta Anaesthesiol Scand 35: 402–406
Bernards C M, Hill H F 1990 Morphine and alfentanil permeability through the spinal dura, arachnoid and pia mater of dogs and monkeys. Anesthesiology 73: 1214–1219
Bonnet F, Buisson V B, Francois Y et al 1990 Effects of oral and subarachnoid clonidine on spinal anaesthesia with bupivacaine. Regional Anaesth 15: 211–214

Breslow M J, Jordan D A, Christopherson R et al 1989 Epidural morphine decreases postoperative hypertension by attenuating sympathetic nervous system hyperactivity. JAMA 261: 3577–3581

Callesen T, Jarnvig I, Thage B et al 1991 Influence of temperature of bupivacaine on spread of spinal analgesia. Anaesthesia 46: 17–19

Carabine U A, Milligan K R, Mulholldand D, Moore J 1992 Extradural clonidine infusions for analgesia after total hip replacement. Br J Anaesth 68: 338–343

Du Pen S L, Peterson D G, Williams A, Bogosian A J 1990 Infection during chronic epidural catheterization: diagnosis and treatment. Anesthesiology 73: 905–909

Dyer R A, Anderson B J, Michell W L, Hall J M 1990 Postoperative pain control with a continuous infusion of epidural sufentanil in the intensive care unit: a comparison with epidural morphine. Anaesth Analg 71: 130–136

Etchin A, Perl A, Bider D, Rafael Z B 1990 Prevention of a side effect of epidural morphine by epidural steroid administration in cesarean section. Gynecol Observ Invest 29: 305–306

Fassoulaki A, Sarantopoulos C, Chondreli S 1991 Systemic fentanyl enhances the spread of spinal analgesia produced by lignocaine. Br J Anaesth 67: 437–439

Fedder S L 1990 Intrathecal administration of morphine for pain of malignant origin. Surg Gynecol Obstet 170: 273–275

Fernandes A, Galbo H, Kjaer M et al 1990 Cardiovascular and ventilatory responses to dynamic exercise during epidural anaesthesia in man. J Physiol 420: 281–293

Goto F, Fujita N, Fujita T 1990 Cerebrospinal norepinephrine concentrations and the duration of epidural analgesia. Can J Anaesth 37: 839–843

Hartell N A, Headley P M 1990 Spinal effects of four injectable anaesthetics on nociceptive reflexes in rats: a comparison of electrophysiological and behavioral measurements. Br J Pharmacol 101: 563–568

Hirabayashi Y, Shimizu R, Matsuda I, Inoue S 1990 Effect of extradural compliance and resistance on spread of extradural analgesia. Br J Anaesth 65: 508–513

Hogan Q, Haddox J D, Abram S et al 1991 Epidural opiates and local anesthetics for the management of cancer pain. Pain 46: 271–279

Johnson M D, Burger G A, Mushlin P S et al 1990 Reversal of bupivacaine epidural anesthesia by intermittent epidual injections of crystalloid solutions. Anesth Analg 70: 395–399

Jorgensen L N, Rasmussen L S, Nielsen P T et al 1991 Antithrombotic efficacy of continuous extradural analgesia after knee replacement. Br J Anaesth 66: 8–12

Kestin I G, Madden A P, Mulvein J T, Goodman N W 1991 Comparison of incremental spinal anaesthesia using a 32-gauge catheter with extradural anaesthesia for elective caesarean section. Br J Anaesth 66: 232–236

Koren G, Sandler A N, Klein J et al 1989 Relationship between the pharmacokinetics and the analgesic and respiratory pharmacodynamics of epidural sufentanil. Clin Pharmacol Ther 46: 458–462

Lewis R P, Spiers S P W, McLaren I M et al 1992 Pethidine as a spinal anaesthetic agent — a comparison with plain bupivacaine in patients undergoing transurethral resection of the prostate. Euro J Anaesthesiol 9: 105–109

Licina M G, Schubert A, Tobin J E et al 1991 Intrathecal morphine does not reduce minimum alveolar concentration of halothane in humans: results of a double-blind study. Anesthesiology 74: 660–663

Linder S, Borgeat A, Biollaz M D J 1989 Ménière-like syndrome following epidural morphine analgesia. Anesthesiology 71: 782–783

Littrell R A 1991 Epidural analgesia. Am J Hosp Pharm 48: 2460–2474

Lund C, Hjortso N C, Mogensen T, Kehlet H 1985 Systemic morphine enhances spread of sensory analgesia during postoperative epidural bupivacaine infusion. Lancet 2: 1156–1157

Lynch J, Krings-Ernst I, Strick K et al 1991 Use of a 25-gauge Whitacre needle to reduce the incidence of postdural puncture headache. Br J Anaesth 67: 690–693

MacArthur C, Lewis M, Knox E G 1992 Investigation of long term problems after obstetric epidural anaesthesia. Br Med J 304: 1279–1282

McQuay H J, Sullivan A F, Smallman K, Dickenson A H 1989 Intrathecal opioids, potency and lipophilicity. Pain 36: 111–115

Mahoney O M, Noble P, Davidson J, Tullos H S 1990 The effect of continuous epidural analgesia on postoperative pain, rehabilitation and duration of hospitalization in total knee arthroplasty. Clin Orthop Rel Res 260: 30–37

Motsch J, Graber E, Ludwig K 1990 Addition of clonidine enhances postoperative analgesia from epidural morphine: a double-blind study. Anesthesiology 73: 1067–1073

Nicol M E, Holdcroft A 1992 Density of intrathecal agents. Br J Anaesth 68: 60–63

Odoom J A 1989 The influence of epidural and intrathecal anaesthesia with bupivacaine on haemostatic function. Pharm Weekbl [Sci] 12: 162–163

Pfeifer B L, Sernaker H L, Ter Horst U M, Porges S W 1989 Cross-tolerance between systemic and epidural morphine in cancer patients. Pain 39: 181–187

Richardson J, Bedder M 1990 Transient anterior spinal cord syndrome with continuous postoperative epidural analgesia. Anesthesiology 72: 764–766

Rigler M L, Drasner K, Krejcie T C et al 1991 Cauda equina syndrome after continuous spinal anesthesia. Anesth Analg 72: 275–281

Rodriguez-Baeza A, Muset-Lara A, Rodriguez-Pazos M, Domenech-Mateu J M 1989 Anterior spinal arteries. Origin and distribution in man. Acta Anatom 136: 217–221

Rosenberg P H 1990 Spinal analgesia — a modern approach to the treatment of severe pain. J Intern Med 227: 291–293

Rout C C, Akoojee S S, Rocke D A, Gouws E 1992 Rapid administration of crystalloid preload does not decrease the incidence of hypotension after spinal anaesthesia for elective caesarean section. Br J Anaesth 68: 394–397

Sharrock N E, Go G, Mineo R 1991 Effect of i.v low-dose adrenaline and phenylephrine infusions on plasma concentrations of bupivacaine after lumbar extradural anaesthesia in elderly patients. Br J Anaesth 67: 694–698

Stuart-Taylor M E, Billingham I S, Barrett R F, Church J J 1992 Extradural diamorphine for postoperative analgesia: first report of a nurse-administered service to 800 patients in a district general hospital. Br J Anaesth 68: 429–432

Svensson L G, Grum D F, Bednarski M et al 1990 Appraisal of cerebrospinal fluid alterations during aortic surgery with intrathecal papaverine administration and cerebrospinal fluid drainage. J Vasc Surg 11: 423–429

Tekkok I H, Cataltepe O, Tahta K, Bertan V 1991 Extradural haematoma after continuous extradural anaesthesia. Br J Anaesth 67: 112–115

Tipping T, Kay N H, Sear J W, McQuay H J 1990 Meptazinol disposition following extradural injection: plasma and CSF concentrations. Eur J Anaesthesiol 7: 381–388

Valentine S J, Jarvis A P, Shutt L E 1991 Comparative study of the effects of air or saline to identify the extradural space. Br J Anaesth 66: 224–227

Whelan E, Wood A, Shay S, Wood M 1989 Lack of effect of spinal anesthesia on drug metabolism. Anesth Analg 69: 307–312

Williams A R 1984 The pharmacist's approach to spinal analgesia. In: Kaufman L (ed) Anaesthesia review 2. Churchill Livingstone, London, pp 148–161

Yamaguchi H, Watanabe S, Motokawa K, Ishizawa Y 1990 Intrathecal morphine dose–response data for pain relief after cholecystectomy. Anesth Analg 70: 168–171

Yoburn B C, Lutfy K, Azimuddin S, Sierra V 1990 Differentiation of spinal and supraspinal opioid receptors by morphine tolerance. Life Sci 46: 343–350

Zeiderman M R, Welchew E A, Clark R G 1991 Influence of epidural analgesia upon postoperative fatigue. Br J Surg 78: 1457–1460

PAEDIATRICS

The major metabolites of morphine are morphine-3-glucuronide and morphine-6-glucuronide. In adults sulphation of morphine may also occur, but no children had detectable concentrations of morphine-6-sulphate and had only a small amount of morphine-3-sulphate. It seems that the analgesic effect of morphine in neonates and young children is likely to be due to morphine itself or to morphine-6-glucuronide (Choonara et al 1990). Cederholm et al (1990) reported on the use of high-dose morphine, ketamine and midazolam in a child with burns and, despite the high doses administered, there were no complications associated with the inadequate metabolism of the drugs.

The fate of codeine has been studied in adults in whom it is conjugated with glucuronic acid, but it may also be metabolized by N-O-demethylation, forming norcodeine and morphine. O-demethylation does not occur in the fetus but demethylation does. Quiding et al (1992) have shown that O-demethylation is present in infants of 6 months of age.

There is difficulty in agreeing the duration of starvation prior to induction of anaesthesia because of gastric contents, but on the other hand hypoglycaemia may develop, especially in young children. Splinter & Schaefer (1991) concluded that it is safe to administer clear fluid up to 3 hours prior to induction of anaesthesia.

There have been reports in the past of tragedies following dental anaesthesia especially in children, not only during the course of the procedures but also in the recovery period. Lanigan (1992) has drawn attention to oxygen desaturation occurring in the recovery period, and this was not reduced by the administration of oxygen. This undoubtedly was caused by obstruction of the airway which may be difficult to detect with the patient in the lateral position and restriction of the airway by oral packs.

REFERENCES

Cederholm I, Bengtsson M, Bjorkman S et al 1990 Long term high dose morphine, ketamine and midazolam infusion in a child with burns. Br J Clin Pharmacol 30: 901–905
Choonara I, Ekbom Y, Lindstrom B, Rane A 1990 Morphine sulphatin in children. Br J Clin Pharmacol 30: 897–900
Lanigan C J 1992 Oxygen desaturation after dental anaesthesia. Br J Anaesth 68: 142–145
Quiding H, Olsson G L, Boreus L O, Bondesson U 1992 Infants and young children metabolise codeine to morphine. A study after single and repeated rectal administration. Br J Clin Pharmacol 33: 45–49
Splinter W M, Schaefer J D 1991 Ingestion of clear fluids is safe for adolescents up to 3 H before anaesthesia. Br J Anaesth 66: 48–52

OBSTETRICS

The first confidential enquiry for the whole of the UK has recently been published (Report on confidential enquiries 1991), revealing that from 1985 to 1987 the maternal mortality rate was 7.6 per 100 000 total births. Although this is a decrease from the previous triennial report, there are still no grounds for complacency. While anaesthesia was a direct cause of 5 deaths, it was considered to be responsible for 16 other deaths due to poor postoperative management.

Hypertensive disorders of pregnancy, including pre-eclamptic toxaemia, were responisble for 25 deaths. Pre-eclamptic toxaemia is associated with increased vascular resistance and a reduced blood volume. The decrease in overall left ventricular output is due to the increased afterload rather than abnormalities of the ventricle and treatment is therefore directed towards the reduced preload and the increased afterload rather than the use of inotropes (Lang et al 1990). Calcium supplements after the 20th week reduced the risks of hypertension during pregnancy (Belizan et al 1991). Studies with nitro-prusside indicate that in severe pre-eclampsia there is decreased blood volume and increased venous tone and the use of nitroprusside results in hypovol-aemic hypotension. This is similar to that seen in severe haemorrhage and if there is reflex cardiac and vasomotor depression there is a fall in heart rate and a further fall in mean arterial pressure (Wasserstrum 1991). In hyperten-sion of pregnancy endothelin appears to have little place but it may contribute to fetal haemodynamic changes such as closure of the umbilical vessels at delivery (Nisell et al 1990).

Attempts to suppress the cardiovascular response to endotracheal intuba-tion, especially in patients with pregnancy-induced hypertension presenting for caesarean section, are not entirely successful. Rout & Rocke (1990) considered that alfentanil 10 μg/kg was just as effective as 2.5 μg/kg of fentanyl in suppressing the response, although in some patients it was ineffectual. Although it might be expected that alfentanil, being less fat-soluble than fentanyl, would be less likely to cross the placental barrier, the umbilical arterial Po_2 was lower in the fentanyl group.

It is generally considered that gastric emptying is delayed during pregnancy and is a causative factor of inhalation of gastric contents. MacFie et al (1991) adopted the rate of paracetamol absorption as a measure of gastric emptying and found that there was no significant delay during pregnancy. They also suggested that previous studies which found delay in gastric emptying were due to measurements made in patient in the supine position, which itself can cause delay in gastric emptying. Apparently gastric emptying is retarded in the left lateral position, but the right lateral position increases the rate of gastric emptying (Backon & Hoffman 1991). H_2-receptor blockers are often advocated but omeprazole, which inhibits H^+K^+ adenosine triphosphatase in a dose of 40 mg orally prior to elective caesarean section, markedly reduces intragastric volume and acidity (Gin et al 1990).

The introduction of epidural opioids in obstetrics has been controversial, but the addition of fentanyl potentiates the analgesic effects of bupivacaine, allowing less concentrated solution to be administered. However, Yau et al (1990) found that the combination of bupivacaine 0.125% with adrenaline 1.25 μg/ml and fentanyl 50 μg provided good pain relief for normal delivery. For elective caesarean section Howell et al (1990) recommended a mixture of bupivacaine and lignocaine in preference to 2% lignocaine with adrenaline. Kaufman (1988) reported on the successful use of intrathecal diamorphine in normal labour, although its duration of action appeared to be approximately 4 hours and during the second stage, nitrous oxide–oxygen supplementation was sometimes necessary. Keenan et al (1991) found that extradural diamorphine (5 mg in 8 ml saline) produced comparable analgesia to that of 8 ml of 0.375% bupivacaine; the duration of action was longer while the addition of 1 : 200 000 adrenaline augmented the quality and duration of analgesia. Unfortunately pruritus was a disturbing side-effect.

The addition of opioids to solution of bupivacaine given extradurally improved the quality of analgesia. Enever et al (1991) have in fact shown that diamorphine was more effective than fentanyl. Stevens et al (1991) confirmed that extradural diamorphine (3 mg) produced better analgesia than 10 mg of intramuscular morphine following caesarean section under extradural block-ade with bupivacaine. Unfortunately there was a higher incidence of vomiting and urinary retention. Noble et al (1991) noted that the addition of fentanyl to bupivacaine given extradurally in elective caesarean section produced superior analgesia compared with bupivacaine alone or bupivacaine with adrenaline.

Robson et al (1992) compared the effects of spinal and extradural analgesia during elective caesarean section and found that with extradural bupivacaine, there was an increase in cardiac output but if the drug is given by the spinal route, there was a decrease which would lead to a reduction in uteroplacental blood flow.

Preloading with crystalloids prior to caesarean section under epidural analgesia has become standard practice, but Wennberg et al (1990) have questioned the use of crystalloids in view of the possibility of producing pulmonary oedema and recommend the use of dextran 70. However Bhagwanjee et al (1990) found that compression of the legs with elasticated Esmarch bandages prevented hypotension following spinal anaesthesia ad-ministered for elective caesarean section.

Using Doppler techniques to assess maternal uterine and fetal blood flow showed that extradural analgesia using bupivacaine with adrenaline had little adverse effect on fetal circulation (Alahuhta et al 1991). A similar study (McLintic et al 1991) using lignocaine with or without adrenaline again found that extradural analgesia appeared to have little effect on the fetal circulation or the fetal outcome. In addition, episodes of hypotension and the effects of treatment with ephedrine also had little adverse effects. Dick et al (1992) also concluded that epidural analgesia was superior to general anaesthesia for caesarean section regarding fetal outcome, provided there were no adverse maternal or fetal factors.

Kestin (1991) has reviewed the place of spinal analgesia in obstetrics with techniques in current practice, especially in the USA. The advent of 32-gauge catheters has promoted the use of incremental doses of bupivacaine, but Kestin et al (1991) found that this offered no significant advantage over extradural bupivacaine as to the quality of blockade. There was little difference in the effects on the fetus provided hypotension was avoided. Kestin (1991) also compared the effects of combined spinal and extradural analgesia and also the use of opioids such as morphine and fentanyl. However there are very few controlled studies. Intrathecal opioids probably remain the method of choice for analgesia in labour in patients with severe cardiac or respiratory disorders.

Camann et al (1991) studied the maternal temperature during labour and found that systemic opioids had little effect, but following extradural analgesia there was a significant rise in temperature 5 hours later. The significance of this is not satisfactorily explained.

Macdonald (1991) had reviewed some of the potential hazards of aspirin and extradural analgesia in obstetrics. Low-dose aspirin inhibits platelet cyclo-oxygenase, which results in a reduction in thromboxane$_2$, leading to an increase in prostacyclin which inhibits platelet aggregation. It is suggested that aspirin should be discontinued 7–10 days before delivery and the bleeding time should be not longer than 10 min. Platelet count is also important. Concern is expressed regarding transfer of drugs across the placental barrier.

Atracurium and its metabolites do cross the placental barrier, but in such low doses that the drug is safe to use during caesarean section (Shearer et al 1991).

Matheson et al (1990) had drawn attention to the possible dangers of midazolam and nitrazepam reaching suckling infants from ingested breast milk. Although the milk concentrations of nitrazepam were found to increase significantly, Matheson et al (1990) concluded that both hypnotics may be used safely for a few days, but there may well be long-term effects of benzodiazepines on suckling infants.

Stevens & Wauchob (1991b) have successfully undertaken delivery of patients with dystrophia myotonica who presented in emergency and had to undergo caesarean section. The technique chosen was spinal analgesia with 2.5 ml of 0.5% heavy bupivacaine. They stressed the hazards of preoperative medication and also the danger of postoperative analgesia, emphasizing the need to nurse such patients in the intensive care unit postoperatively.

Liver function is altered during pregnancy and anabolic steroids may account for some of the physiological and biochemical changes. Acute fatty necrosis of the liver and hepatic function dysfunction association with pre-eclampsia are discussed by Anday & Cohen (1990). Pre-eclampsia, for example, leads to markedly elevated levels of alkaline phosphatase and gamma- glutamyl transferase near term. Serum bilirubin is also increased but significant rises suggest hepatic or haematological disorders.

Respiration function is altered in pregnancy with a fall in functional residual capacity and expiratory reserve volume. Respiratory muscle function remains normal but ventilatory drive and respiratory impedance increase. These effects in part may be due to an increase in progesterone levels (Contreras et al 1991).

REFERENCES

Alahuhta S, Rasanen J, Jouppila R et al 1991 Effects of extradural bupivacaine with adrenaline for Caesarean section on uteroplacental and fetal circulation. Br J Anaesth 67: 678–682
Anday E K, Cohen A 1990 Liver disease associated with pregnancy. Ann Clin Lab Sci 20: 233–238
Backon J, Hoffman A 1991 The lateral decubitus position may affect gastric emptying

through an autonomic mechanism: the skin pressure–vegetative reflex. Br J Clin Pharmacol 32: 138–139

Belizan J M, Villar J, Gonzalez L et al 1991 Calcium supplementation to prevent hypertensive disorders of pregnancy. N Engl J Med 325: 1399–1405

Bhagwanjee S, Rocke D A, Rout C C et al 1990 Prevention of hypotension following spinal anaesthesia for elective caesarean section by wrapping of the legs. Br J Anaesth 65: 819–822

Camann W R, Hortvet L A, Hughes N et al 1991 Maternal temperature regulation during extradural analgesia for labour. Br J Analg 67: 565–568

Contreras G, Gutierrez M, Beroiza T et al 1991 Ventilatory drive and respiratory muscle function in pregnancy. Am Rev Respir Dis 144: 837–841

Dick W, Traub E, Kraus H et al 1992 General anaesthesia versus epidural anaesthesia for primary Caesarean section — a comparative study. Eur J Anaesthesiol 9: 15–21

Enever G R, Noble H A, Kolditz D et al 1991 Epidural infusion of diamorphine with bupivacaine in labour. A comparison with fentanyl and bupivacaine. Anaesthesia 46: 169–173

Gin T, Ewart M C, Yau G, Oh T E 1990 Effect of oral omeprazole on intragastric pH and volume in women undergoing elective caesarean section. Br J Anaesth 65: 616–619

Howell P, Davies W, Wrigley M et al 1990 Comparison of four local extradural anaesthetic solutions for elective caesarean section. Br J Anaesth 65: 648–653

Kaufman L 1988 Intraspinal diamorphine: epidural and intrathecal. In: Scott D B (ed,) Diamorphine — its chemistry, pharmacology and clinical use. Woodhead-Faulkner, Cambridge p. 82–96

Keenan G M A, Munishankarappa S, Elphinstone M E, Milne M K 1991 Extradural diamorphine with adrenaline in labour: comparison with diamorphine and bupivacaine. Br J Anaesth 66: 242–246

Kestin I G 1991 Spinal anaesthesia in obstetrics. Br J Anaesth 66: 595–607

Kestin I G, Madden A P, Mulvein J T, Goodman N W 1991 Comparison of incremental spinal anaesthesia using a 32-gauge catheter with extradural anaesthesia for elective Caesarean section. Br J Anaesth 66: 232–236

Lang R M, Pridjian G, Feldman T et al 1990 Left ventricular mechanics in preeclampsia. Am Heart J 121: 1768–1775

Macdonald R 1991 Aspirin and extradural blocks. Br J Anaesth 66: 1–3

MacFie A G, Magides A D, Richmond M N, Reilly C S 1991 Gastric emptying in pregnancy. Br J Anaesth 67: 54–57

McLintic A J, Danskin F H, Reid J A, Thorburn J 1991 Effect of adrenaline on extradural anaesthesia, plasma lignocaine concentrations and the feto-placenta unit during elective caesarean section. Br J Anaesth 67: 683–689

Matheson I, Lunde P K M, Bredesen J E 1990 Midazolam and nitrazepam in the maternity ward: milk concentrations and clinical effects. Br J Clin Pharmacol 30: 787–793

Nisell H, Hemsen A, Lunell N-O et al 1990 Maternal and fetal levels of a novel polypeptide, endothelin: evidence for release during pregnancy and delivery. Gynecol Obstet Invest 30: 129–132

Noble D W, Morrison L M, Brockway M S, McClure J H 1991 Adrenaline, fentanyl or adrenaline and fentanyl as adjuncts to bupivacaine for extradural anaesthesia in elective caesarean section. Br J Anaesth 66: 645–650

Report on confidential enquiries into maternal deaths in the United Kingdom 1985–87: a summary of the main points 1991 Her Majesty's Stationery Office, London

Robson S C, Boys R J, Rodeck C, Morgan B 1992 Maternal and fetal haemodynamic effects of spinal and extradural anaesthesia for elective caesarean section, Br J Anaesth 68: 54–59

Rout C C, Rocke D A 1990 Effects of alfentanil and fentanyl on induction of anaesthesia in patients with severe pregnancy-induced hypertension. Br J Anaesth 65: 468–474

Shearer E S, Fahy L T, O'Sullivan E P, Hunter J M 1991 Transplacental distribution of atracurium, laudanosine and monoquaternary alcohol during elective caesarean section. Br J Anaesth 66: 551–556

Stevens J D, Wauchob T D 1991 Dystrophia myotonica — emergency caesarean section with spinal anaesthesia. Eur J Anaesthesiol 8: 305–308

Stevens J D, Braithwaite P, Corke C F et al 1991 Double-blind comparison of epidural diamorphine and intramuscular morphine after elective Caesarean section, with computerised analysis of continuous pulse oximetry. Anaesthesia 46: 256–259

Wasserstrum N 1991 Nitroprusside in preeclampsia. Circulatory distress and paradoxical bradycardia. Hypertension 18: 79–84

Wennberg E, Frid I, Haljamae H et al 1990 Comparison of Ringer's acetate with 3% dextran 70 for volume loading before extradural caesarean section. Br J Anaesth 65: 654–660

Yau G, Gregory M A, Gin T, Oh T E 1990 Obstetric epidural analgesia with mixtures of bupivacaine, adrenaline and fentanyl. Anaesthesia 45: 1020–1023

Index

Anaesthesia Review

Edited by Leon Kaufman

253

Contents of *Review 3*

ISBN 0443 03202 5
Published November 1985

Contents of *Review 4*

ISBN 0443 03450 8
Published May 1987

Contents of *Review* 5

ISBN 0443 03774 4
Published February 1988

Contents of *Review* 6

ISBN 0443 04024 9
Published July 1989

Contents of *Review 7*

ISBN 0443 04216 0
Published April 1990

Contents of *Review 8*

ISBN 0443 04384 1
Published April 1991

See p. ii for Contents of *Review 9*